W9-AVR-602

Spondyloarthritis

Guest Editors

JÜRGEN BRAUN, MD
JOACHIM SIEPER, MD

RHEUMATIC
DISEASE CLINICS
OF NORTH AMERICA

www.rheumatic.theclinics.com

August 2012 • Volume 38 • Number 3

SAUNDERS an imprint of ELSEVIER, Inc.

W.B. SAUNDERS COMPANY

A Division of Elsevier Inc.

1600 John F. Kennedy Blvd., Suite 1800 • Philadelphia, PA 19103-2899

http://www.theclinics.com

RHEUMATIC DISEASE CLINICS OF NORTH AMERICA Volume 38, Number 3

August 2012 ISSN 0889-857X, ISBN 13: 978-1-4557-5066-5

Editor: Pamela Hetherington

Rheumatic Disease Clinics of North America (ISSN 0889-857X) is published quarterly by Elsevier Inc., 360 Park Avenue South, New York, NY 10010-1710. Months of issue are February, May, August, and November. Business and editorial offices: 1600 John F. Kennedy Boulevard, Suite 1800, Philadelphia, PA 19103-2899. Periodicals postage paid at New York, NY and additional mailing offices. Subscription prices are USD 305.00 per year for US individuals, USD 534.00 per year for US institutions, USD 150.00 per year for US students and residents, USD 360.00 per year for Canadian individuals, USD 659.00 per year for Canadian institutions, USD 427.00 per year for international individuals, USD 659.00 per year for international institutions, and USD 210.00 per year for Canadian and foreign students/residents. To receive student/resident rate, orders must be accompanied by name of affiliated institution, date of term, and the *signature* of program/residency coordinator on institution letterhead. Orders will be billed at individual rate until proof of status received. Foreign air speed delivery is included in all *Clinics* subscription prices. All prices are subject to change without notice. **POSTMASTER:** Send address changes to *Rheumatic Disease Clinics of North America,* Elsevier Health Sciences Division, Subscription Customer Service, 3251 Riverport Lane, Maryland Heights, MO 63043. **Customer Service: 1-800-654-2452 (US and Canada). From outside of the US and Canada: 314-447-8871. Fax: 314-447-8029. For print support, e-mail: JournalsCustomerService-usa@elsevier.com. For online support, e-mail: JournalsOnline Support-usa@elsevier.com.**

Reprints. For copies of 100 or more of articles in this publication, please contact the Commercial Reprints Department, Elsevier Inc., 360 Park Avenue South, New York, New York, 10010-1710; Tel.: (+1) 212-633-3813, Fax: (+1) 212-462-1935, and E-mail: reprints@elsevier.com.

Rheumatic Disease Clinics of North America is covered in *MEDLINE/PubMed (Index Medicus), Current Contents/Clinical Medicine, Science Citation Index, ISI/BIOMED,* and *EMBASE/Excerpta Medica.*

Printed in the United States of America.

Contributors

CONSULTING EDITOR

MICHAEL H. WEISMAN, MD
Chief, Division of Rheumatology; Professor of Medicine, Cedars-Sinai Medical Center, Los Angeles, California

GUEST EDITORS

JÜRGEN BRAUN, MD
Head, Rheumazentrum Ruhrgebiet, and Ruhr Universität Bochum, Germany

JOACHIM SIEPER, MD
Head, Section of Rheumatology, Campus Benjamin Franklin, Charité University, Berlin, Germany

AUTHORS

XENOFON BARALIAKOS, MD
Rheumazentrum Ruhrgebiet, Herne, Germany

ANNELIES BOONEN, MD, PhD
Associate Professor of Rheumatology, Division of Rheumatology, Department of Medicine, Maastricht University Medical Center, Maastricht, The Netherlands

JÜRGEN BRAUN, MD
Head, Rheumazentrum Ruhrgebiet, and Ruhr Universität Bochum, Germany

MATTHEW A. BROWN, MBBS, MD, FRACP
Professor of Immunogenetics and Director, Princess Alexandra Hospital, University of Queensland Diamantina Institute, Brisbane, Woolloongabba, Queensland, Australia

RUBÉN BURGOS-VARGAS, MD
Professor, Department of Rheumatology, Hospital General de México; Faculty of Medicine, Universidad Nacional Autónoma de México, Mexico City, México

PHILIPPE CARRON, MD
Department of Rheumatology, Ghent University Hospital, Ghent, Belgium

DIRK ELEWAUT, MD, PhD
Department of Rheumatology, Ghent University Hospital, Ghent, Belgium

KAY-GEERT A. HERMANN, MD
Department of Radiology, Charité Medical School, Berlin, Germany

PEGGY JACQUES, MD, PhD
Department of Rheumatology, Ghent University Hospital, Ghent, Belgium

ROBERT B.M. LANDEWÉ, MD
Professor, Academic Medical Center, University of Amsterdam, Amsterdam, The Netherlands

RIK J.U. LORIES, MD, PhD
Laboratory for Skeletal Development and Joint Disorders, Department of Development and Regeneration, KU Leuven; Division of Rheumatology, University Hospitals Leuven, Leuven, Belgium

W.P. MAKSYMOWYCH, FRCP(C)
Department of Medicine, University of Alberta, Edmonton, Alberta, Canada

MICHAEL T. NURMOHAMED, MD, PhD
Departments of Rheumatology and Internal Medicine, VU University Medical Center; Department of Rheumatology, Jan van Breemen Research Institute, Reade, Amsterdam, The Netherlands

DENIS PODDUBNYY, MD
Research Associate, Rheumatology, Medical Department I, Campus Benjamin Franklin, Charité Universitätsmedizin Berlin, Berlin, Germany

JOHN D. REVEILLE, MD
Professor and Director, Division of Rheumatology and Clinical Immunogenetics, Department of Medicine, The University of Texas Health Science Center at Houston, Houston, Texas

PHILIP C. ROBINSON, MBChB, FRACP
Princess Alexandra Hospital, University of Queensland Diamantina Institute, Brisbane, Woolloongabba, Queensland, Australia

GEORG SCHETT, MD
Department of Internal Medicine 3, Institute for Clinical Immunology, University of Erlangen-Nuremberg, Erlangen, Germany

JOACHIM SIEPER, MD
Head, Section of Rheumatology, Campus Benjamin Franklin, Charité University, Berlin, Germany

I.H. SONG, MD, PhD
Department of Rheumatology, Charité Medical University, Campus Benjamin Franklin, Berlin, Germany

CARMEN STOLWIJK, MD
Division of Rheumatology, Department of Medicine, Maastricht University Medical Center, Maastricht, The Netherlands

FILIP VAN DEN BOSCH, MD, PhD
Department of Rheumatology, Ghent University Hospital, Belgium

DÉSIRÉE VAN DER HEIJDE, MD
Professor, Department of Rheumatology, Leiden University Medical Center, Leiden, The Netherlands

IRENE E. VAN DER HORST-BRUINSMA, MD, PhD
Associate Professor, Department of Rheumatology, VU University Medical Center; Jan van Breemen Research Institute, Reade, Amsterdam, The Netherlands

LIESBET VAN PRAET, MD
Department of Rheumatology, Ghent University Hospital, Ghent, Belgium

ASTRID VAN TUBERGEN, MD, PhD
Rheumatologist, Division of Rheumatology, Department of Medicine, Maastricht University Medical Center, Maastricht, The Netherlands

MICHAEL H. WEISMAN, MD
Chief, Division of Rheumatology; Professor of Medicine, Cedars-Sinai Medical Center, Los Angeles, California

Contents

Nonsteroidal anti-inflammatory drugs (NSAIDs) are considered a first-line therapy in patients with axial spondyloarthritis (axSpA), including ankylosing spondylitis. NSAIDs reduce pain and stiffness effectively in most patients, are able to reduce systemic and local inflammation, and can inhibit progression of structural damage in the spine. However, effective control of symptoms and retardation of radiographic progression often require continuous and long-term treatment, which raises safety concerns. This article discusses controversies related to the current role of NSAIDs in axSpA treatment, risks and benefits of this treatment, and current trends for individualized treatment.

Tumor necrosis factor α inhibitors (TNF blockers) have revolutionized the treatment of patients with ankylosing spondylitis. Despite clinical efficacy, there are questions and controversies treating rheumatologists face, which this review discusses: whether there are specific indications for specific TNF blockers; whether the dose of TNF blockers can be decreased; whether immunogenicity plays a role; what the role of residual active inflammation on MRI might be; and whether there is a window of opportunity to treat patients with ankylosing spondylitis and prevent radiographic progression. This article also summarizes evidence for switching between TNF blockers and addresses the question of malignancies.

There are 2 groups of drugs that have been shown effective in the treatment of patients with axial spondyloarthritis: nonsteroidal anti-inflammatory drugs and tumor necrosis factor α blockers. Conventional disease-modifying drugs and some other biologics have not been shown clinically efficacious in this disease. This overview discusses the available data on whether early treatment strategies in patients with axial spondyloarthritis have an effect on (1) the percentage of patients reaching clinical remission, (2) achieving drug-free remission, and (3) the progress of radiographic progression in the spine as a parameter for structural damage.

RHEUMATIC DISEASE CLINICS OF NORTH AMERICA

Foreword

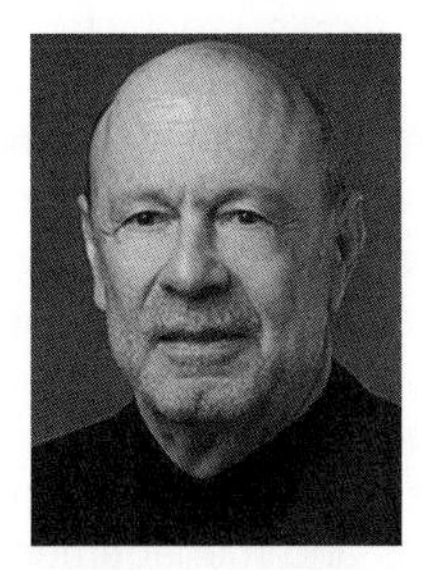

Michael H. Weisman, MD
Consulting Editor

This volume comprehensively reviews the state of the art of spondyloarthritis (SpA) diagnosis, prognosis, pathogenesis and genetic insights, and treatment. Sieper and Braun have done a spectacular job in putting the material together in readable and understandable format for rheumatologists at the early stages in their career or even for those seasoned rheumatologists who want to know more in depth and breadth. The worldwide burden of SpA now exceeds that of rheumatoid arthritis, and the time is right for this volume.

Boonen and Reveille discuss what is known about the epidemiology of ankylosing spondylitis (AS) worldwide and some of the difficulties we face to obtain accurate information—items such as the remarkable heterogeneity of the disease and the case definitions that vary from country to country. HLA-B27 prevalence is an excellent surrogate marker, but even this frequency will vary among different ethnic groups. Challenges remain and these authors address them.

Sieper and Braun address the now critical question facing all rheumatologists—what should we be telling our referring doctors about which case ascertainment strategy to use for referral of patients to the specialist. They address the important and complementary roles of B-27 testing and clinical evaluation of inflammatory back pain—yet these strategies may identify different phenotypes that are overlapping but may not all be the same.

Robinson and Brown describe the essential role of genetics in our understanding of AS. They point out the well-known anchor association with HLA-B27 in both European and Asian populations and the exciting new discovery of a gene-gene interaction with ERAP1 association restricted to HLA-B27-positive disease. In addition, multiple genes in the IL-23 and TNF pathways are now included in this polygenic disease with antigen

Rheum Dis Clin N Am 38 (2012) xiii–xv
http://dx.doi.org/10.1016/j.rdc.2012.09.005

presentation genes now taking the spotlight. They point out most importantly that some cohorts of axial SpA demonstrate a lower HLA-B27 carriage rate compared to cohorts of securely diagnosed AS. The meaning of these differences is currently being explored.

Baraliakos, Hermann, and Braun focus on imaging as a diagnostic tool for AS and SpA—pointing out the problems and pitfalls of using structural or inflammation changes as entry criteria into various classification schemes. However, the differential diagnosis of many of these laboratory, clinical, and imaging changes can be broad, and our efforts often have false positive and false negative challenges. They state imaging is but one tool in the toolkit, and it should be considered in that context.

Van der Horst-Bruinsma, Nurmohamed, and Landewe visit the extra-articular manifestations of SpA and validate our current approach to diagnosis and management. However, on the horizon there is accumulating evidence for the emergence of cardiovascular risk due to specific AS-related as well as atherosclerotic events—more investigations are needed, especially from large epidemiologic studies.

Lories and Schett are well aware of the controversies surrounding inflammation and new bone formation in AS; although some popular theories appear discordant, they point out that quite different mechanisms may trigger the bone phenotype seen in SpA. Further, they discuss what we do know as the key mechanisms of new bone formation in SpA, many of which these 2 investigators were pivotal into bringing forward in the first place. Bringing relevant animal models into discussions of human disease and reassessing proposed biomarker discoveries are their unique contributions and no one can do this better than Lories and Schett.

Burgos-Vargas and Weisman discuss separately, but essentially agree, that inflammatory back pain constitutes a real clinical entity but not a disease in the usual sense unless we accumulate more information about pathology and genetics of this specific group. In the meantime it serves a very useful purpose by providing the appropriate case definition for entry into a diagnostic algorithm involving imaging and genetics.

Elewaut and colleagues re-explore, based on new and emerging data, the clinical, genetic, and pathological relationship between AS and inflammatory bowel disease; they discuss these findings in terms of a therapeutic overlap. They suggest that it may be possible to broaden our therapeutic options based on what is being discovered anew about gut and joint inflammation.

It is not surprising that therapy is a big part of this volume because treatment advances and broad clinical experience have changed greatly over the past 5 years since this was last reviewed comprehensively in a single volume (Weisman MH, Reveille JD, van der Heijde D, editors. Ankylosing Spondylitis and the Spondyloarthropathies. Mosby Elsevier, 2008). Van den Bosch and colleagues provide a rational therapeutic approach, data driven, for the employment of different agents when the eye, skin, gut, and peripheral joints predominate. Poddubnyy and van der Heijde similarly discuss the evidence that supports the continuous use of NSAIDs to reduce structural damage progression in AS but they do warn about the risk of side effects. Song and Maksymowych review in depth the state of the art regarding TNF blockers addressing such issues as malignancy risk, the role of MRI assessing therapeutic response or lack therof, and whether there is a good time (or no time) for a treatment goal to specifically prevent radiographic progression. Sieper and Braun tackle the area of when to initiate treatment in axial SpA, noting the evidence that both radiographic and nonradiographic subsets do seem to respond more completely to TNF blocker therapy if started early. Questions still remain, however, in this disease as well as in RA or its subsets if treatment is started potentially too early; there may be some people who would have done well without the cost or the risk. As clearly warned by Sieper and

Braun, we are still defining and refining which groups are able to benefit in terms of retardation of radiographic progression.

Michael H. Weisman, MD
Chief
Division of Rheumatology
Cedars-Sinai Medical Center
8700 Beverly Boulevard, B-122
Los Angeles, CA 90048

E-mail address:
michael.weisman@cshs.org

Preface

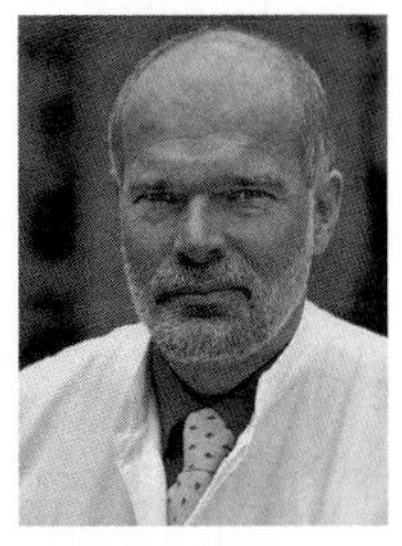
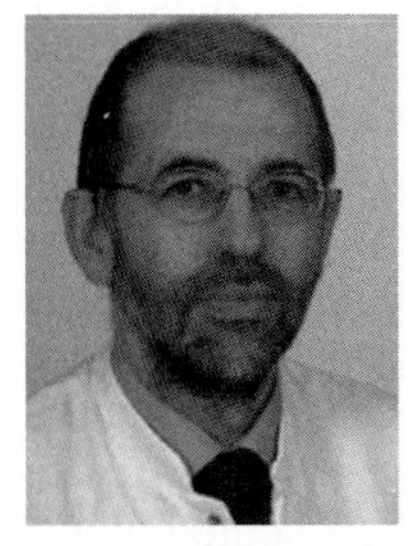

Jürgen Braun, MD Joachim Sieper, MD
Guest Editors

Ankylosing spondylitis (AS) is a chronic rheumatic disease with debilitating potential. AS mainly affects the spine, but the entheses, peripheral joints, and eye (anterior uveitis) are also commonly involved.[1] Since the diagnosis of AS has long been based on the 1984 modified New York criteria, it has been frequently delayed for several years. Therefore the "Assessments in Spondyloarthritis International Society" (ASAS) has developed new classification criteria to cover a wider spectrum of the disease that is now named as axial spondyloarthritis (axSpA).[2] These criteria also include earlier and more abortive stages of the disease as defined by the absence of structural damage in the sacroiliac joints (SIJ).[3] The role of structural changes in the spine such as syndesmophytes is less clear in this regard. However, on the described basis, the subsets AS and nonradiographic axial spondyloarthritis (nr-axSpA) may now be differentiated. Criteria for the definition of positive magnetic resonance imaging (MRI) findings for the SIJ[4] and the spine[5] in relation to and independent of the ASAS criteria have been proposed. Again, how the presence of active spinal inflammation in the absence of such changes in the SIJ is handled when classifying and diagnosing axSpA has not been clarified to date.

New classification criteria for peripheral SpA have also recently been developed.[6] In contrast to axSpA, in the absence of psoriasis, chronic inflammatory bowel disease, and a triggering infection suggestive of reactive arthritis, the term undifferentiated SpA is still sometimes used.

Since many patients with SpA are suffering from both axial and peripheral symptoms, it has been decided to take the predominant symptom as the one that determines between predominant axial and peripheral SpA. Inflammatory back pain is the most frequent and rather characteristic symptom of axSpA[7] but the (young) age of the patient and the degree of chronicity (>3 months) is even more relevant for classification and diagnosis. A data-based proposal to facilitate early referral has recently been made.[8] Young age at onset of back pain (<35 years) and improvement by movement and good response to nonsteroidal anti-inflammatory drugs (NSAIDs), but not morning stiffness, were identified as good predictors in

Rheum Dis Clin N Am 38 (2012) xvii–xxi
http://dx.doi.org/10.1016/j.rdc.2012.08.015 **rheumatic.theclinics.com**

combination with waking up the second half of the night and alternating buttock pain.

Our knowledge of risk factors for radiographic progression has also increased in the last years: next to gender and presence of syndesmophytes at baseline, C-reactive protein and the smoking status have recently been identified as being predictive of structural changes.[9]

More studies on the nature of the link between inflammation and new bone formation have been published. Clearly, there is more to the development of syndesmophytes and ankylosis than an initiating inflammation.[10] The development of fatty changes potentially preceding bone formation especially has recently attracted interest.[11,12]

The assessment of disease activity in AS has long relied on the BASDAI, but recent data have challenged the once arbitrarily proposed cutoff of 4.[13] In contrast, the AS-DAS that has been developed on a data-driven basis and that has now been evaluated in many studies[14] seems to perform superiorly in this regard. This includes the prediction of response to medical therapies.[15]

Anti-TNF therapy has changed the spectrum of treatment in AS and the whole group of AS and axSpA dramatically in the last decade.[16] The treatment effects may last several years,[17] and discontinuation of therapy has led to disease flares in the majority of patients. However, we still lack knowledge regarding the potential of dose-reducing strategies.

While the first studies on anti-TNF therapy were all performed with patients who had established AS for about 10 years, several more recent studies have concentrated on younger patients with a shorter disease duration.[18–21]

Although spinal inflammation as detected by MRI is largely reduced by anti-TNF therapy,[22] structural changes/progression (new bone formation) as detected by conventional radiography is not halted over 2 years.[23] However, function and mobility are still improving (mean), which may be more important for patients—within at least a few years.[24] Specific recommendations for anti-TNF therapy have recently been updated, and the whole group of axSpA has been included.[25] No other biologics can currently be recommended for the treatment of axSpA.[26]

In a recent update of the international recommendations on the management of AS, the role of NSAIDs as first-line therapy in AS has again been stressed.[27] This includes, on the 1 hand, a recommendation for continuous therapy in the maximally tolerated and approved dose in very and/or persistently active patients. On the other hand, there is a growing body of evidence that NSAIDs given continuously or in a high dose may reduce new bone formation[28,29]—thus they have DMARD function. Whether this also works in combination with TNF blockers is as yet unclear. The new standardized method proposed by ASAS to calculate the mean NSAID intake allows a comparison of the dosage between trials.[30]

In any case, the field of SpA is growing tremendously. It was not possible to mention all the important publications in the last years in this editorial. We would especially like to direct the attention of the readers to the various cohorts that have been initiated years ago, such as OASIS and GESPIC and the more recent DESIR, SPACE, and some others, which all greatly contribute to our knowledge about SpA. We are very thankful to the authors of this issue, who have helped so substantially to put the recent advances into perspective. The experiment of combining younger with more experienced authors has worked out very well.

Jürgen Braun, MD
Rheumazentrum Ruhrgebiet
Herne and Ruhr Universität Bochum
Germany

Joachim Sieper, MD
Section of Rheumatology
Campus Benjamin Franklin
Charité University
Berlin, Germany

E-mail addresses:
Juergen.Braun@vincenzgruppe.de (J. Braun)
joachim.sieper@charite.de (J. Sieper)

REFERENCES

1. Braun J, Sieper J. Ankylosing spondylitis. Lancet 2007;369(9570):1379–90.
2. Rudwaleit M, van der Heijde D, Landewé R, et al. The development of Assessment of SpondyloArthritis International Society (ASAS) classification criteria for axial spondyloarthritis (Part II): Validation and final selection. Ann Rheum Dis 2009 Mar 17. [Epub ahead of print].
3. Kiltz U, Baraliakos X, Karakostas P, et al. Patients with non-radiographic axial spondyloarthritis differ from patients with ankylosing spondylitis in several aspects. Arthritis Care Res (Hoboken) 2012 Apr 13. [Epub ahead of print].
4. Rudwaleit M, Jurik AG, Hermann KG, et al. Defining active sacroiliitis on magnetic resonance imaging (MRI) for classification of axial spondyloarthritis—a consensual approach by the ASAS/OMERACT MRI Group. Ann Rheum Dis 2009 May 18. [Epub ahead of print].
5. Hermann KG, Baraliakos X, van der Heijde DM, et al, on behalf of the Assessment in SpondyloArthritis international Society (ASAS). Descriptions of spinal MRI lesions and definition of a positive MRI of the spine in axial spondyloarthritis: a consensual approach by the ASAS/OMERACT MRI study group. Ann Rheum Dis 2012 May 14. [Epub ahead of print].
6. Rudwaleit M, van der Heijde D, Landewè R, et al. The development of Assessment of SpondyloArthritis International Society classification criteria for peripheral spondyloarthritis and spondyloarthritis in general. Ann Rheum Dis 2011;70: 25–31.
7. Braun J, Inman R. Clinical significance of inflammatory back pain for diagnosis and screening of patients with axial spondyloarthritis. Ann Rheum Dis 2010; 69(7):1264–8.
8. Braun A, Saracbasi E, Grifka J, et al. Identifying patients with axial spondyloarthritis in primary care: how useful are items indicative of inflammatory back pain? Ann Rheum Dis 2011;70(10):1782–7.
9. Poddubnyy D, Haibel H, Listing J, et al. Baseline radiographic damage, elevated acute phase reactants and cigarette smoking status predict radiographic progression in the spine in early axial spondyloarthritis. Arthritis Rheum 2012; 64(5):1388–98.
10. van der Heijde D, Machado P, Braun J, et al. MRI inflammation at the vertebral unit only marginally predicts new syndesmophyte formation: a multilevel analysis in patients with ankylosing spondylitis. Ann Rheum Dis 2012;71(3):369–73.
11. Chiowchanwisawakit P, Lambert RG, Conner-Spady B, et al. Focal fat lesions at vertebral corners on magnetic resonance imaging predict the development of new syndesmophytes in ankylosing spondylitis. Arthritis Rheum 2011;63(8): 2215–25.
12. Maksymowych WP, Morency N, Conner-Spady B, et al. Suppression of inflammation and effects on new bone formation in ankylosing spondylitis: evidence for

a window of opportunity in disease modification. Ann Rheum Dis 2012 May 5. [Epub ahead of print].
13. Kiltz U, Baraliakos X, Karakostas P, et al. The degree of spinal inflammation is similar in patients with axial spondyloarthritis who report high or low levels of disease activity: a cohort study. Ann Rheum Dis 2012 Apr 20. [Epub ahead of print].
14. van der Heijde D, Braun J, Dougados M, et al. Sensitivity and discriminatory ability of the ankylosing spondylitis disease activity score in patients treated with etanercept or sulphasalazine in the ASCEND trial. Rheumatology (Oxford); 2012 July 6. [Epub ahead of print].
15. Vastesaeger N, van der Heijde D, Inman RD, et al. Predicting the outcome of ankylosing spondylitis therapy. Ann Rheum Dis 2011 Mar 14. [Epub ahead of print].
16. Braun J, Brandt J, Listing J, et al. Treatment of active ankylosing spondylitis with infliximab—a double-blind placebo controlled multicenter trial. Lancet 2002;359: 1187–93.
17. Baraliakos X, Listing J, Fritz C, et al. Persistent clinical efficacy and safety of infliximab in ankylosing spondylitis after 8 years—early clinical response predicts long-term outcome. Rheumatology (Oxford); 2011 Jun 14. [Epub ahead of print].
18. Barkham N, Keen HI, Coates LC, et al. Clinical and imaging efficacy of infliximab in HLA-B27-positive patients with magnetic resonance imaging-determined early sacroiliitis. Arthritis Rheum 2009;60(4):946–54.
19. Song IH, Hermann K, Haibel H, et al. Effects of etanercept versus sulfasalazine in early axial spondyloarthritis on active inflammatory lesions as detected by whole-body MRI (ESTHER): a 48-week randomised controlled trial. Ann Rheum Dis 2011;70(4):590–6.
20. Song IH, Althoff CE, Haibel H, et al. Frequency and duration of drug-free remission after 1 year of treatment with etanercept versus sulfasalazine in early axial spondyloarthritis: 2 year data of the ESTHER trial. Ann Rheum Dis 2012 Mar 22. [Epub ahead of print].
21. Sieper J, Van der Heijde D, Dougados M, et al. Efficacy and safety of adalimumab in patients with non-radiographic axial spondyloarthritis: results of a randomised, placebo-controlled trial (ABILITY-1). Ann Rheum Dis 2012. [Epub ahead of print].
22. Braun J, Baraliakos X, Hermann KG, et al. Golimumab reduces spinal inflammation in ankylosing spondylitis: MRI results of the randomised, placebo-controlled GO-RAISE study. Ann Rheum Dis 2012;71(6):878–84.
23. Baraliakos X, Listing J, Brandt J, et al. Radiographic progression in patients with ankylosing spondylitis after 4 yrs of treatment with the anti-TNF-α antibody infliximab. Rheumatology (Oxford) 2007;46(9):1450–3.
24. Braun J, Sieper J. What is the most important outcome in ankylosing spondylitis? Rheumatology 2008;47(12):1738–40.
25. van der Heijde D, Sieper J, Maksymowych WP, et al, for the Assessment of SpondyloArthritis international Society. 2010 Update of the international ASAS recommendations for the use of anti-TNF agents in patients with axial spondyloarthritis. Ann Rheum Dis 2011;70(6):905–8.
26. Kiltz U, Heldmann F, Baraliakos X, et al. Treatment of ankylosing spondylitis in patients refractory to TNF-inhibition: are there alternatives? Curr Opin Rheumatol 2012;24(3):252–60.
27. Braun J, van den Berg R, Baraliakos X, et al. 2010 update of the ASAS/EULAR recommendations for the management of ankylosing spondylitis. Ann Rheum Dis 2011;70(6):896–904.

28. Poddubnyy D, Rudwaleit M, Haibel H, et al. Effect of non-steroidal anti-inflammatory drugs on radiographic spinal progression in patients with axial spondyloarthritis: results from the German Spondyloarthritis Inception Cohort. Ann Rheum Dis 2012 Mar 29. [Epub ahead of print].
29. Kroon F, Landewe R, Dougados M, et al. Continuous NSAID use reverts the effects of inflammation on radiographic progression in patients with ankylosing spondylitis. Ann Rheum Dis 2012. [Epub ahead of print].
30. Dougados M, Braun J, Szanto S, et al. NSAID-intake according to the ASAS score in clinical trials evaluating TNF blockers: The example of etanercept in advanced ankylosing spondylitis. Arthritis Care Res (Hoboken) 2012;64(2):290–4.

Epidemiology of Spondyloarthritis

Carmen Stolwijk, MD[a], Annelies Boonen, MD, PhD[a,*], Astrid van Tubergen, MD, PhD[a], John D. Reveille, MD[b]

KEYWORDS

• Spondyloarthritis • Ankylosing spondylitis • Psoriatic arthritis • Reactive arthritis • Epidemiology • Incidence • Prevalence

KEY POINTS

- Data on incidence and prevalence become increasingly important not only for clinicians when trying to understand disease patterns but also for policy makers for whom the prevalence of a disease has immediate impact on societal budgets and on population health. Hence, there is a need for accurate data on incidence and prevalence.
- The variation in incidence and prevalence of spondyloarthritis (SpA) as a disease and the SpA subtypes varies highly and this cannot only be attributed to geographic variation in the prevalence of HLA-B27. Because part of this variation likely is explained by variation in quality and bias of the methodologic approaches, the recent generic guidelines for performance of studies on incidence and prevalence could be adapted for use in the SpA.
- A particular challenge is to agree on a series of approaches with an acceptable (low) risk of bias that could operationalize the current classification criteria (which are developed for use in a [specialized] clinical setting) for use in large epidemiologic studies.
- Although a large part of the SpA subtypes in epidemiologic studies are classified as undifferentiated SpA (uSpA), this diagnosis will likely disappear with the acceptance of new concepts and classification of axial SpA and peripheral SpA. The application of these criteria in epidemiologic studies requires further consideration.
- Few data are available on the prevalence of inflammatory bowel disease (IBD)-related SpA and reactive arthritis (ReA). The new peripheral SpA criteria will likely encompass both entities, but the transient nature of ReA makes prevalence estimates challenging.

INTRODUCTION

SpA refers to a disease (ie, for which criteria have been developed) but also to a concept that represents a group of interrelated disorders. Classically, these disorders comprise ankylosing spondylitis (AS), psoriatic arthritis (PsA), ReA, SpA related

[a] Division of Rheumatology, Department of Medicine, Maastricht University Medical Center, PO Box: 5800, 6202 AZ Maastricht, The Netherlands; [b] Division of Rheumatology and Clinical Immunogenetics, Department of Medicine, The University of Texas Health Science Center at Houston, 6431 Fannin, MSB 5.270, Houston, TX 77030, USA
* Corresponding author.
E-mail address: a.boonen@mumc.nl

Rheum Dis Clin N Am 38 (2012) 441–476
http://dx.doi.org/10.1016/j.rdc.2012.09.003 **rheumatic.theclinics.com**
0889-857X/12/$ – see front matter

to IBD, and uSpA. More recently, a classification into axial and peripheral disease has been proposed. Phenotypically, these diseases have several features in common, including inflammatory back pain (IBP), peripheral arthritis (usually an oligoarthritis of the lower limbs), enthesitis, dactylitis, and extra-articular features, such as uveitis, psoriasis, and IBD. Genetically, the diseases are associated with the major histocompatibility complex class 1 antigen, HLA-B27.

Epidemiology is the study of the distribution and the determinants of diseases in human populations. The epidemiology of a disease is the most important determinant of the burden of a disease in a population. This article focuses on the epidemiology of SpA throughout the world by reviewing the literature on incidence and prevalence of the entire SpA group as well as the specific disorders belonging to SpA. Some challenges when determining the epidemiology of a disease are considered. First, the frequency of diseases reported in studies depends on criteria used for confirmation of the presence of a disease in the individual patients. For this purpose, classification criteria have been developed and, depending on the purpose and the methodologic approach, they can have different test characteristics. Second, numbers on prevalence and incidence may vary due to differences in study design, including the target population, sampling method, and approach to assess the disease criteria. These 2 aspects are discussed.

IMPORTANCE OF CLASSIFICATION CRITERIA AND DESIGN FOR EPIDEMIOLOGIC STUDIES

Classification Criteria and Their Use in Large Epidemiologic Studies

To reliably estimate the prevalence of a disease, criteria are needed to identify homogenous groups of patients. In the past 50 years, major advances have been made in the recognition and classification of SpA as an entity and the specific disorders belonging to SpA. Criteria developed for classification may not be useful, however, for conducting epidemiologic studies in the population but specifically designed for identification of patients attending specialized clinics and for inclusion in trials or observational studies. First, classification criteria, in contrast to diagnostic criteria, are designed for high specificity to avoid misclassification. As a result, they lack sensitivity at early or mild stages of disease, which may be a drawback in epidemiologic studies due to a possible underestimation of the incidence or prevalence of the disease, and, for diseases that are not frequent, large samples are needed to provide reliable estimates on incidence and prevalence. Second, classification criteria might include items, such as technical procedures (for instance, MRI), which might not be feasible for application in large population studies or items that require a specific physician diagnosis (for example, the presence of psoriasis).

Before classification criteria can be developed at all, disease has to be recognized as a morbus sui generis by physicians. It was mainly in the nineteenth and beginning of the twentieth centuries when physicians raised the idea of SpA as a distinct disease. In the mid-nineteenth century, several cases of psoriasis in association with arthritis were published by Rayner, Cazenave, Devergre, and Gilbert.[1] The name, *psoriasis arthritique*, was first introduced in 1860 by skin physician, Bazin. In the same century, the first cases of patients with IBP with limited mobility of the spine (or ankylosis in post-mortem studies) were reported by Travers (1824), Brody (1850), and later by Bechterev (1893), Strümpel (1897), and Marie (1898). Several names were proposed to distinguish this disease from rheumatoid arthritis, yet the term, *rheumatoid spondylitis*, was used for many years and only much later did the term AS become widely accepted. In 1916, Reiter contributed to the identification of the disease, ReA, for patients with arthritis, urethritis, and conjunctivitis, although even in 1507 a patient was reported with arthritis in association with urethritis. In the twentieth century, the association between ulcerative colitis and arthritis was first recognized (1930) and, in 1938, a patient with Crohn's disease was described who developed polyarthritis.[1] The ability to apply the rheumatoid factor (RF) test more widely in the 1950s (after its discovery by Waaler and Rose in 1940 and 1948, respectively) helped confirm that the entire group of disease (described previously) was distinct from rheumatoid arthritis because it lacked RF and, therefore, the term, *seronegative variants of rheumatoid arthritis*, was introduced. During the 1960s, Moll and Wright observed in family studies the striking association between sacroiliitis/AS and several other disorders, such as PsA, ulcerative colitis, and arthritis related to Crohn's disease. In 1974, Moll and Wright established the concept of these disorders and chose as a collective name, the term, *spondarthritides*.[2] Remarkably, their observation was done without consideration of the HLA-B27 associations (which had only been described the preceding year) but resulted from clinical and radiologic findings. The consideration of HLA-B27 in AS and other diseases in SpA, commencing during the 1970s, provided further confirmation of the concept.[3]

Once the diseases were well established in clinical rheumatology, the need for classification criteria was recognized to be able to create homogenous groups of patients for clinical or population studies. **Table 1** represents a chronologic overview of the main criteria proposed and used in either clinical or epidemiologic studies, with a brief description of the specific aim, methodologic approach, and description of items within the criteria that might hamper applicability in large epidemiologic studies. In 1961, criteria were proposed to identify patients with AS for population surveys (Rome criteria).[4] They required either the presence of 4 out of 5 clinical criteria or a sixth criterion (radiographic sacroiliitis) plus 1 of the clinical criteria. The Rome criteria were based on expert opinion but when evaluated later in a population study among American indigenous groups, the role of the radiographs was not found satisfactory.[5] This led to the revision of the Rome criteria as the New York (NY) criteria.[6] In New York City, an expert committee agreed that for epidemiologic purposes the diagnosis of AS should not be made without x-ray evidence of sacroiliitis, and, therefore, the presence of sacroiliitis was required for fulfillment of the criteria. Furthermore, the clinical items were revised in an attempt to make them more objective. In an evaluation of the NY criteria, Moll and Wright found that the clinical criteria failed in terms of sensitivity and specificity.[7] Therefore, a modification was proposed in 1984, the modified New York criteria (mNY), in which an item for IBP was added, but the radiographic criterion was kept.[8] Since then, the mNY criteria have been the most widely applied criteria in both clinical and epidemiologic studies in AS. The main restriction of these criteria for use in epidemiologic studies is that although they perform well in established disease, they lack sensitivity in the early disease stage, in which radiographic damage is not yet visible, which could cause a delay of up to 6 to 8 years in diagnosis.[9]

For PsA, the first classification criteria were proposed in 1973 by Moll and Wright[10] and required inflammatory arthritis, presence of psoriasis, and absence of RF. These criteria discriminated poorly between psoriatic and rheumatoid arthritis. More sensitive criteria for clinical studies were proposed by Vasey and Espinoza, McGonagle and colleagues, and Gladman, but none of them have been widely adopted nor validated at a satisfactory level.[11] Therefore, the Classification for Psoriatic Arthritis (CASPAR) criteria were developed in 2006.[12] The CASPAR criteria are easy to use and likely to perform well, although classifying early disease is the most important limitation of the criteria. Furthermore, the sensitivity of the CASPAR criteria for use in epidemiologic studies is not clear.

Table 1
Overview of the most commonly used classification criteria for SpA and specific diseases of the SpA concept showing some relevant characteristics when considering large epidemiologic studies

Classification Criteria, Year of Publication	Purpose	Method of Development	Entry or Required Criteria (Obliged)	Clinical Criteria	Radiographic or Laboratory Criteria
Rome criteria for AS,[4] 1963	Population studies	Clinical experience of rheumatologists	—	• Axial symptoms • Limitation in mobility • Extra-articular (uveitis)	• Sacroiliitis (radiographic)
NY criteria for AS,[6] 1966	Population studies	Clinical experience and results of a study of performance of Rome criteria	Radiographic sacroiliitis	• Axial symptoms • Limitation in mobility	• Sacroiliitis (radiographic)
mNY criteria for AS,[8] 1984	Diagnosis and clinical studies	Modification of NY criteria by experts based on results of study on Rome and NY criteria	Radiographic sacroiliitis	• Axial symptoms • Limitation in mobility	• Sacroiliitis (radiographic)
Amor criteria for SpA,[14] 1990	Clinical studies	Retrospective and prospective testing of candidate items (selected by experts)	—	• Axial symptoms • Peripheral symptoms • Extra-articular	• Sacroiliitis (radiographic) • HLA-B27
ESSG criteria for SpA,[15] 1991	Clinical studies	Statistical testing of candidate variables in patients with SpA (expert's opinion) and controls plus clinical reasoning	IBP or synovitis	• Axial symptoms • Peripheral symptoms • Extra-articular manifestations	• Sacroiliitis (radiographic)

ReA,[13] 2000	Clinical and epidemiologic studies	Expert opinion	Arthritis and preceding enteritis or urethritis	—	• Evidence of triggering infection or persistent synovial infection
CASPAR criteria for PsA,[12] 2006	Clinical studies	Statistical analysis of features in patients with PsA (based on expert's opinion) and control patients	Inflammatory articular disease	• Psoriasis • Dactylitis	• Radiographic new bone formation hands • Negative RF
ASAS axial SpA criteria,[19] 2009	Clinical studies	Candidate criteria (by experts based on clinical reasoning) tested prospectively (expert's opinion); final criteria based on statistical analysis and expert voting of candidate criteria	>3 mo Back pain and age at onset <45 y	• Axial symtpoms • Peripheral symptoms • Extra-articular manifestations	• Sacroiliitis (radiographic or MRI) • HLA-B27 • CRP
ASAS peripheral SpA criteria,[18] 2011	Clinical studies	Candidate criteria (by experts based on clinical reasoning) tested prospectively (expert's opinion); final criteria based on statistical analysis and expert voting of candidate criteria	Arthritis or enthesitis or dactylitis	• Axial symptoms • Peripheral symptoms • Extra-articular manifestations	• Sacroiliitis (radiographic or MRI) • HLA-B27

For ReA, despite several attempts, no universal validated classification or diagnostic criteria are available. Based on discussions at the 4th International Workshop on Reactive Arthritis in 1999, a consensus was achieved that the term ReA should be confined to patients who present with clinical features typical of ReA and in whom the preceding infection is caused by a microbe, which is commonly associated with ReA.[13] Furthermore, preliminary classification criteria for ReA were proposed but have never been validated. Along the same lines, no formal classification criteria for IBD-SpA or uSpA have been developed (to the authors' knowledge).

It was recognized that there also was a need for criteria to classify the whole spectrum of SpA, comprising the specified as well as unspecified forms of the disease. For this purpose, the European Spondyloarthropathy Study Group (ESSG) and Amor criteria were developed in the early 1990s.[14,15] They both cover the whole spectrum of SpA and include at the same time the axial and peripheral manifestations but also give weight to other features of the SpA concept not related to spinal or articular symptoms. The ESSG criteria are easy to apply and, therefore, often used in epidemiologic studies. It has been shown, however, that these criteria sets lack sensitivity and specificity.[16,17] Considering these drawbacks, efforts have been made in recent years to standardize and improve making an early diagnosis, and new classification criteria have been established by the Assessment of SpondyloArthritis International Society (ASAS).[18,19] According to these new ASAS classification criteria, SpA is divided into predominantly axial involvement and predominantly peripheral manifestations. According to the ASAS axial SpA criteria, suffering from chronic back pain for more than three months with age at onset before 45 years can be classified as having axial SpA if sacroiliitis on imaging (radiographs or MRI) is present plus at least 1 SpA feature or, in the absence of sacroiliitis on imaging, if HLA-B27 is positive plus at least 2 other SpA features. Patients can be classified as having peripheral SpA, if peripheral arthritis, enthesitis, or dactylitis is present, plus at least 1 or 2 other SpA features. The advantage of the ASAS axial SpA criteria is the inclusion of MRI, which is able to show inflammation of the sacroiliac joints in an early stage of disease. The ASAS axial SpA criteria have shown to perform well also in early stages of disease.[19] The inclusion of MRI and HLA-B27 testing, however, make them infeasible for use in large epidemiologic studies. Power requirements to determine the prevalence of an uncommon disease hamper the application in large studies when MRI is needed in a large proportion of patients. Not only are such examinations expensive but also classification of abnormalities on MRI should have sufficient specificity to avoid overdiagnosis. Including plain radiographs in large population studies is a challenge, however, not least because ethical committees would raise objections to radiographs in healthy subjects.

Having elaborated on classification criteria, the ASAS criteria cannot simply be applied in large epidemiologic (population) studies. Several alternative approaches can be seen in the literature. A 2-stage approach can be used, in which subjects are prescreened by questionnaires and are invited for further examinations in cases of suspicion based on the (sensitive) screening question. In addition, other criteria, such as *International Classification of Diseases (ICD)* codes, insurance claims, or patients' reported physician diagnoses have been used in epidemiologic studies. All these alternative choices make assumptions with regard to accuracy of the diagnosis but none of them is accurate against true evaluation by classification criteria.

Quality of Study Design for Prevalence and Incidence Studies

Decisions in policy and health care use are often influenced by prevalence and incidence of chronic diseases.[20] Therefore, studies on prevalence and incidence should be unbiased, high-quality studies. These studies are always observational, however, and this evidence is generally considered low. Two sets of guidelines can be recognized when considering quality of (observational) studies. First, guidelines can define how to conduct a study to the highest possible standards. For example, the initiative, Strengthening the Reporting of Observational Studies in Epidemiology (STROBE), developed a checklist of 22 items, with recommendations about what should be included in a more accurate and complete description of observational studies.[21] Second, guidelines may define how to assess the risk of bias of individual studies when aggregating them in a systematic review. This is important because a study may be performed to the highest possible standards yet still have a high risk of bias. In 2006, Mallen and colleagues reported that the assessment of the quality or risk of bias of reviews on observational studies was rarely done and often incomplete because of lack of instruments and guidance, in particular for studies on incidence and prevalence.[22] Since then, much effort has been done to improve this shortcoming. Sanderson and colleagues[23] identified in a review 86 approaches to assess risk of bias in observational studies and concluded there was a need for more reliable tools. Shamliyan and colleagues[24] reviewed tools to assess the quality and/or risk of bias of prevalence and incidence studies and reported the absence of agreement on type of items and way to score items, likely reflecting the need for extensive adaptations depending on the specific disease and population of interest. In the same article, they present a new checklist to assess the methodologic and reporting quality of observational studies of incidence and prevalence that was mainly based on the review of existing instruments and expert knowledge. Two aspects can be distinguished: (1) external validity, which is defined as the extent to which the results of a study can be generalized to the target population, and (2) internal validity, which is the extent to which the results of a study are correct for the subjects. When testing the tool, inter-rater agreement was poor and the investigators recommended further testing of checklists. Recently, Hoy and colleagues[25] developed another tool for risk of bias of prevalence studies. This tool makes a distinction between assessing whether the research was conducted to the highest possible standards (methodologic quality) and the extent to which results can be believed (risk of bias). The items in this risk of bias tool include the following questions (a *yes* answer implicates a low risk of bias and a *no* answer a high risk of bias):

External validity

1. Was the target population a close representation of the general population?
2. Was the sampling frame a close representation of the target population?
3. Was some form of random selection used to select the sample?
4. Was the likelihood of nonresponse bias minimal?

Internal validity

5. Were data collected directly from the subjects?
6. Was an acceptable case definition used?
7. Was the study instrument that measured the parameter of interest shown to have reliability and validity?
8. Was the same mode of data collection used for all subjects?
9. Was the length of the shortest prevalence period for the parameter of interest appropriate?
10. Were the numerator and denominator for the parameter of interest appropriate?

When interpreting studies on incidence and prevalence of SpA, these important questions were considered in the present review.

LITERATURE REVIEW ON PREVALENCE AND INCIDENCE SpA

Search Strategy and Appraisal

To be able to present a clear picture on the epidemiology of the SpA, an electronic search of PubMed was performed up to July 2012 using the following search terms: "spondyloarthritis," "spondyloarthropathy," "ankylosing spondylitis," "psoriatic arthritis," "reactive arthritis," undifferentiated spondyloarthritis," "incidence," "prevalence," and "epidemiology." The search was limited to original articles and reviews published in English. Furthermore, the reference lists of articles identified by the search strategy were searched. The search and selection of articles were done mostly by one person. Because this report did not have the intention to be a systematic review, no formal assessment or risk of bias was performed but during the data extraction the main items for external and internal validity were checked and included in the tables (**Tables 2–9**).

Distribution HLA-B27 Worldwide

The prevalence of SpA and SpA-related diseases shows considerable differences among ethnic groups and populations. This can be explained partly by differences in the prevalence of HLA-B27, to which the prevalence of SpA, in particular AS, is closely related. There are few studies on HLA-B27 prevalence, however, that are truly population based or nationally representative. The prevalence of HLA-B27 is highest in the Pawaia tribe in Papua New Guinea (53%),[26] the Haida indigenous peoples on the Queen Charlotte Islands in Western Canada (50%),[27] and Chukotka Eskimos in Eastern Russia (40%).[28] In Northern Scandinavian countries, HLA-B27 positivity is also reported as common (15%–25%).[29–31] In the Western European population, the prevalence of HLA-B27 is estimated at 4% to 13%, whereas HLA-B27 positivity is uncommon in the Arab countries (2%–5%)[32] and Japan (1%).[33] HLA-B27 is virtually absent among South American Indians, Australian Aborigines, and African blacks.[34]

Overall, most patients with AS possess HLA-B27. Approximately 90% of the patients with AS of Germanic and Northern European extraction are HLA-B27+. There are some racial differences, however. Among blacks, the B27− AS forms a much greater proportion of AS patients (<60%),[35] probably because of the increased significance of non-B27 alleles. Also, in the Middle East, the strength of the association is weak compared with Western countries (25%–75%),[36–38] and in sub-Saharan Africa the prevalence of HLA-B27 in patients with AS is reported as low. This was indirectly confirmed in a US multiracial/ethnic study. The National Health and Nutrition Examination Survey (NHANES) (2009) was the first nationally representative and population-based prevalence of HLA-B27 in the United States (6.1%) that was appropriately powered for whites (7.5%) and Mexican Americans (4.6%) but lacked power to guarantee the accuracy of the 1.1% frequency observed in African Americans.[39] The relation of HLA-B27 with other SpA subtypes is weaker compared with AS and is reported up to 70% in patients with ReA, 60% to 70% of patients with axial PsA, 25% of patients with peripheral PsA, and up to 70% in patients with IBD-SpA.[40,41] Different subtypes of HLA-B27 can be found throughout the world with different strengths of association with AS. HLA-B*2705 and B*2702 are the primary subtypes in whites, B*2704 and B*2705 in Eastern Asia, and B*2708 in Southern Asia.[40] Other subtypes (B*2706 and B*2709) were believed protective for the disease, although with both subtypes, AS cases have been reported.[41]

Incidence and Prevalence of Spondyloarthritis

Incidence

Only 4 studies reported the incidence of SpA as a disease entity that varied from 0.48/100,000 in Japan to 62.5/100,000 in Spain (see **Table 2**). The low prevalence in Japan

Table 2
Summary of studies on incidence of SpA

Author, Year	Target Population	Age	Sample	Method	Criteria	N Sample	Response (%)	Period	Incidence of SpA (/100,000)	Male:Female
Hukuda et al,[33] 2001	Japan	>15	All patients with SpA seen at institutes	Questionnaires to clinics for medical record review	Clinical and radiographic features	134 Institutes	70.9	1985–1996	0.48	4.5–3.0:1
Savolainen et al,[42] 2003	Kuopi, Finland	All	All referred patients	Examination by rheumatologist	Own study criteria	87,000	—	2000	52[a]	—
Kaipiainen and Aho,[43] 2000	5 Districts of Finland	—	All patients receiving drug reimbursement	Finish sickness insurance scheme and hospital records	Own study criteria	1,000,000	—	1995	18.6[a]	—
Munoz-Fernández et al,[44] 2010	Madrid, Spain	<45	All patients visiting GPs in Madrid	Referral of possible early SpA patients to specialized unit	ESSG criteria	111,941	—	2006	62.5	1:1

[a] Sum of prevalence of AS, PsA, ReA, and uSpA.

Table 3
Summary of studies on prevalence of SpA

Author, Year	Target Population	Age	Sample	Method	Criteria	N Sample	Response (%)	Men (%)	Mean Age	Prevalence of SpA (%, 95% CI)	Male:Female
Europe											
Bruges-Armas et al,[54] 2002	Terceira, Azores	>50	Random sample of osteoporosis survey	Interview + examination	ESSG	936	52	50	66.5	1.6 (0.8–2.7)	7:1
Saraux et al,[47] 2005	France	>18	Random sample of phone numbers	Phone screening question + phone rheumatologist interview (+ examination if needed)	Rheumatologist opinion	15,219	65	—	—	0.30 (0.17–0.46)	1:1
Trontzas,[124] 2005	9 Areas in Greece	>18	All residents in 7 areas + random sample 2 areas	Screening interview + examination	ESSG	10,647	81.2	48.8	47	0.49 (0.38–0.60)	5.5:1
De Angelis et al,[53] 2007	Marche, Central Italy	>18	Random sample of subjects of GPs	Screening questionnaire + examination	ESSG	3664	58.8	46.6	—	1.06 (0.78–1.38)	3.6:1
Adomaviciute et al,[49] 2008	2 Lithuanian cities	>18	Random sample of phone numbers	Phone interview	Rheumatologist ascertainment	6543	65.1	25.5	—	0.84 (0.53–1.21)	1.3:1
Haglund,[125] 2011	Southern Sweden	>15	Health care registery	*ICD-10* codes from health care register	*ICD-10* code	849,253	—	49	—	0.45 (0.44–0.47) (no ReA)	1:1
Onen et al,[52] 2008	Izmir, Turkey	>20	Random selection of persons from 2 urban areas	Screening interview + examination	ESSG	2887	98 78 83	45.3	43.7	1.05 (0.70–1.50)	0.72:1

Braun et al,[50] 1998	Berlin, Germany	—	HLA-B27+ and HLA-B27−blood donors	Screening questionnaires + examination	ESSG	348	85.3 71.4	67	38.5	1.9	3:1
North America											
Reveille et al,[56] 2012	United States	20–69	Representative sample of US adults	Interview + examination	Amor + ESSG (incomplete)	5013	—	48.4	—	Amor: 0.9 (0.7–1.1), ESSG: 1.4 (1.0–1.9)	0.5:1
Alexeeva,[126] 1994	Chukotka, Russia	>12	All residents of 2 settlements	Questionnaire + examination	ESSG/Amor	355	71.3%	44.2	—	2.5	—
Asia											
Hukuda et al,[33] 2001	Japan	>15	All patients with SpA seen at institutes	Questionnaires for medical record review	Clinical and roentgenographic features	134 Institutes	70.9	—	—	0.0095	4.5–3:1
Farooqi,[127] 1998	North Pakistan	>15	Sample of 3 localities	Screening COPCORD questionnaire + examination	Unclear	2090	95	—	—	0.10	—
Minh Hoa et al,[59] 2003	Urban Vietnam	>15	Total population of Trung Liet	Screening COPCORD questionnaire + examination	Unclear	2119	86–94	—	—	0.28	2:1
Davatchi et al,[73] 2008	Tehran, Iran	>15	Sample of zip codes + adjacent houses	Screening COPCORD questionnaire + examination	Unclear	10,291	74.9	47.4	—	0.23	
Liao,[128] 2009	Dalang Town, China	>16	All residents of Dalang Town	Screening questionnaire + examination	ESSG	10,921	88.8	52.1	—	0.78 (0.62–0.95) (axial SpA)	1.4:1
Boyer et al,[46] 1994	Alaskan Eskimos	>20	2 Populations enrolled in Alaska Area Native Health Service	Review of records + further evaluation of possible SpA	ESSG/Amor	6749	89	—	—	2.5	0.9:1

Table 4
Summary of studies on incidence of AS

Author, Year	Target Population	Age	Sample	Method	Criteria	N Sample	Period	Incidence of as (/100,000)	Male:Female
Hanova et al,[65] 2010	Czechoslovakia	>16	2 Regions, all referred patients	Examination by rheumatologist	mNY	15,374	2002–2003	6.4 (4.5–14.4)	3.3:1
Savolainen et al,[42] 2003	Kuopio, Finland	All	All referred patients	Examination by rheumatologist	Study[a]	87,000	2000	5.8 (1.6–14.8)	4:0
Kaipiainen et al,[63] 1997	Finland	>16	5 Regions	Patients under nationwide sickness insurance to receive medication for AS	Specially reimbursed medication for AS	1,000,000	1980–1990	6.9 (6.0–7.8)	2.3:1
Alamanos,[66] 2004	Northwest Greece	>16	Patients referred to rheumatology clinics	Medical records review	mNY	488,435	1983–2002	1.5 (0.4–2.5)	4.7:1
Geirsson,[129] 2010	Iceland	>18	AS patients seen by rheumatologists	Review of medical records + database genetic study, confirmation examination	mNY	220,441	1947–2005	0.44 to 5.48	1.9:1
Bakland et al,[64] 2005	Northern Norway	>16	Patients registered with AS at hospital	Medical records review	mNY	217,000	1960–1993	7.3 (5.3–9.2)	3.1:1
Carbone et al,[62] 1992	Rochester, MN	—	AS patients registered in record system	Diagnosis from record system	mNY	18,000–69,000	1935–1989	7.3 (6.1–8.4)	4:1
Hukuda et al,[33] 2001	Japan	>15	All AS patients seen at institutes	Questionnaires for medical record review	Clinical and roentgenographic features	134 Institutes	70.9	0.48	—

[a] Back pain > 3 months and bilateral sacroiliitis grade 2 or more or syndesmophytes or squared vertebrae in radiographs.

coincides with a low prevalence of HLA-B27 (<0.5%). The study was based on a nationwide questionnaire survey in which physicians of institutes with possible SpA patients were asked to review the medical records.[33] SpA was classified based on clinical and radiographic features. The incidence was determined with the assumption that at least one-tenth of the SpA population was recruited by the survey and was estimated not to exceed 0.48/100,000 person-years. The 2 most prevalent SpA subtypes were AS (68.3% of SpA) and PsA (12.7% of SpA). In a study from Finland, based on referrals to rheumatology outpatient clinics, the annual incidence of SpA was 52/100,000 person years,[42] with PsA the most prevalent subtype (44.4%), followed by uSpA (25%). Another study from Finland, which used records of a nationwide insurance program, estimated an overall incidence of SpA of 19/100,000. This study only included patients who needed medical treatment for their condition.[43] Also in this study, PsA was the most frequent subtype (37%), followed by AS (32%).

In past years, the importance of an early diagnosis of SpA became clear and efforts were made to diagnose patients in an early stage. In a study from Spain, general practitioners in Madrid were asked and trained to refer all patients under age 45 years with either IBP or asymmetric arthritis of lower limbs with 3 to 24 months' symptom duration to a specialized early arthritis clinic during 6 consecutive months.[44] Case definition was based on the ESSG criteria. The annual estimated incidence of SpA was 62.5/100,000, suggesting a high incidence of early SpA. ESSG criteria, however, were used as gold standard, although it has been described that only 50% of the patients who fulfill the ESSG criteria are still classified as SpA 5 years later.[16]

Prevalence

Sixteen studies reported data on the prevalence of SpA, which varied from 0.01% in Japan to 2.5% in Alaska (see **Table 3**). The highest prevalence of 2.5% in Alaskan Eskimos was based on combined ESSG and Amor criteria.[45,46] Most studies on prevalence of SpA, however, are conducted in Europe. In a study from France, prevalence of SpA was estimated to be 0.30%.[47] The study was based on a telephone survey in which a random sample of telephone numbers was selected and patients were asked if a diagnosis of SpA was ever made. Only patients with suspected SpA were called by a rheumatologist. This method probably underestimated the prevalence of SpA because only patients with a diagnosis were captured. Another telephone survey population study from France revealed a prevalence of 0.47%, which was nearly similar to the prevalence of rheumatoid arthritis in the same survey.[48] A study from Lithuania, using the same methodology as the study from France, estimated a SpA prevalence of 0.84%.[49] As discussed previously, not only the sensitivity of the initial screening question but also possible bias in persons having or having not a telephone (possibly disfavoring persons of lower socioeconomic status) should be taken into account when interpreting the results. In a German study, 348 blood donors, of whom half were HLA-B27+, were screened for SpA using the ESSG criteria and included the use of MRI for diagnosing early AS.[50] The estimated prevalence of SpA among the adult population was estimated at 1.9%, although this number was later adjusted to 1.73% (to adjust for selection bias when generalizing blood donors to the general populaton).[51] It is doubtful, however, if blood donors are a representative sample of the general population. In a Turkish population study, 145 out of 2887 subjects who responded positively on a questionnaire were evaluated by a rheumatologist and showed a prevalence of 1.05% according to the ESSG criteria.[52] A comparable prevalence of SpA was reported in a study in Central Italy (1.1%), despite the low HLA-B27 prevalence in Italy.[53] In this study, the most common form of SpA was PsA (38%) followed by AS (34%). A population study in persons older than 50 years of age from the

Table 5
Summary of studies on prevalence of AS

Author, Year	Target Population	Age	Sample	Method	Criteria	N Sample	Response (%)	Men (%)	Mean Age	Prevalence of AS (%, 95% CI)	Male:Female
Europe											
Hanova,[65] 2010	Czechoslovakia	>16	2 Regions, all referred patients	Examination by rheumatologist	mNY	15,374	—	—	—	0.09 (0.08–0.11)	4.6:1
Saraux,[47] 2005	France	>18	Random sample of phone numbers	Phone screening question + phone rheumatologist interview (+examination if needed)	Physician confirmation by phone or examination	15,219	65	—	—	0.08 (0.03–0.15)	—
Kaipiainen,[63] 1997	Finland	>30	Representative population sample	Examination	Specially reimbursed medication for AS	8000	90	—	—	0.15 (0.08–0.27)	2.7:1
Trontzas,[124] 2005	Greece	>18	9 Areas	Visiting households + interview	mNY	10,647	81.2	48.8	47	0.24 (0.16–0.32)	6.1:1
Alamanos,[66] 2004	Northwest Greece	>16	Patients referred to rheumatology clinics	Medical records review	mNY	488,435	—	—	—	0.03 (0.03–0.03)	4.7:1
Geirsson,[129] 2010	Iceland	>18	AS patients seen by rheumatologists	Review of medical records + confirmation examination	mNY	220,441	91.4	—	—	0.13 (0.11–0.14)	1.9:1
De Angelis,[53] 2007	Marche, Central Italy	>18	Random sample of subjects of GPs	Screening questionnaire, + examination	mNY	3664	58.8	46.6	—	0.37 (0.23–0.49)	—
Van Der Linden,[68] 1983	Zoetermeer, the Netherlands	>44	2 Districts of the town	X-ray followed by examination	mNY	2957	NA	—	—	0.24	—

Johnsen et al,[31] 1992	Norwegian Samis (Lapps)	20–64	Inhabitants 2 cities	Questionnaire + examination	NY	1723	78.2	53.7	—	1.8 (0.9–3.2)	2.7:1
Bakland et al,[64] 2005	Northern Norway	>16	A hospital-based AS patient registry	Medical records review	mNY	217,000	—	51	—	0.26	3.1:1
Gran et al,[29] 1985	Northern Norway	20–54	All inhibitants of Tromsø invited	Questionnaire + examination of random sample of positive responders	NY	21,329	77.9 and 56	54.5	—	1.1–1.4	3.9–6.1:1
Haglund,[125] 2011	Southern Sweden	>15	AS patients registered	*ICD-10* codes from health care register	*ICD-10* code	849,253	—	49	—	0.12 (0.11–0.12)	2.1:1
Onen et al,[52] 2008	Izmir, Turkey	>20	Random selection of persons from 2 urban areas	Screening interview + examination	mNY	2887	98 78 83	45.3	43.7	0.49 (0.26–0.85)	1.2:1
Braun et al,[50] 1998	Berlin	—	HLA-B27+ and HLA-B27– blood donors	Screening questionnaires + examination	mNY	348	85.3 71.4	67	38.5	0.86	—
North America											
Carter et al,[69] 1979	Rochester, MN		AS patients registered	Medical record review	NY	33,000–52,000	—	—	—	0.13	3:1
Maurer,[70] 1979	United States	25–74	Complex multistage probability design	Questionnaire + radiograph (in women only ih >50 y)	X-ray sacroiliitis	6913	4903 (X rays available)			0.73 (men); 0.30 (women)	
Boyer et al,[46] 1994	Alaskan Eskimos	>20	2 populations enrolled in Alaska Area Native Health service	Review of records + further evaluation of possible SpA	NY	6749	89	—	—	0.4	
Latin America											
Alverez-Nemegyei et al,[75] 2011	Southeast Mexico	>18	Random sample of residents of Yucatán	Screening COPCORD questionnaire + examination	mNY	3195		38.2	42.7	0.02	

(*continued on next page*)

Table 5 (*continued*)

Author, Year	Target Population	Age	Sample	Method	Criteria	N Sample	Response (%)	Men (%)	Mean Age	Prevalence of AS (%, 95% CI)	Male:Female
Asia											
Hukuda et al,[33] 2001	Japan population	>15	All patients seen at medical institutes	Questionnaires for medical record review	Either Rome or NY	134 Institutes	70.9	—	—	0.0065	—
Chou et al,[71] 1994	Taiwan	>20	Random subjects from 3 areas	Screening questionnaire + examination	NY	8998	49	50.7		0.19–0.54	0.7–4.6:1
Liao et al,[128] 2009	Dalang Town, China	>16	All residents of Dalang Town	Screening questionnaire + examination	mNY	10,921	88.8	52.1	—	0.25 (0.16–0.35)	
Alexeeva et al,[126] 1994	Chukotka, Russia		All residents of 2 settlements	Questionnaire + examination	NY	355	71.3%	44.2	—	1.1	—
Davatchi et al,[73] 2008	Tehran, Iran	>15	Sample of zip codes + adjacent houses	Screening COPCORD questionnaire + examination	Unclear	10,291	74.9	47.4	—	0.12	

Table 6
Summary of studies on incidence of PsA

Author, Year	Target Population	Age	Sample	Method	Criteria	N Sample	Period	Incidence of PsA (/100,000)	Male:Female
Hukuda et al,[33] 2001	Japan	>15	All AS patients seen at institutes	Questionnaires for medical record review	ESSG/Amor (clinical and radiographic)	134 Institutes	70.9	0.1	—
Hanova et al,[65] 2010	Czechoslovakia	>16	2 Regions, all referred patients	Examination by rheumatologist	Vasey and Espinoza	15,374	2002–2003	3.6 (1.4–7.6)	1.3:1
Savolainen et al,[42] 2003	Kuopio, Finland	All	All referred patients	Examination by rheumatologist	Study specific[a]	87,000	2000	23.1 (13.2–37.5)	1.6:1
Söderlin et al,[90] 2002	South Sweden	>16	All referred patients in Kronoberg County	Examination by rheumatologist	Psoriasis + arthritis, RF−	140,000	1999–2000	8 (4–15)	0.4:1
Shbeeb et al,[89] 1999	Minnesota	—	All medical records	Medical records review	Inflammatory arthritis + psoriasis	—	1982–1991	6.6 (5.0–8.2)	0.9:1
Wilson,[93] 2009	Minnesota	—	All Medical records	Medical record review	CASPAR	124,277	1970–1999	7.2 (6.0–8.4)	1.7:1
Soriano et al,[92] 2011	Buenos Aires, Argentina	>18	Members of a private health system insurance	Medical records review	CASPAR	138,288	2000–2006	6.3 (4.2–8.3)	1.9:1
Kaipiainen et al,[88] 1996	5 districts in Finland	>16	all patients recieving drug reimbursment	Finish sickness insurance scheme and hospital records	psoriasis + arthritis or spinal involvement	1.000.000	1990	6	1.3:1
Alamanos et al,[91] 2003	north-west Greece	>16	patients attending 2 hospitals and private rheumatology clinics	medical records review	ESSG	488,435	1982-2001	3.02 (1.55-4.49)	1:1

[a] Peripheral arthritis with psoriasis, excluding RF-positive polyarthritis or spondylitis with psoriasis.

Table 7
Summary of studies on prevalence of PsA

Author, Year	Target Population	Age	Sample	Method	Criteria	N Sample	Response	Men (%)	Mean Age	Prevalence of PsA (%, 95% CI)	Male:Female
Europe											
Hanova et al,[65] 2010	Czechoslovakia	>16	2 Regions, all referred patients	Examination by rheumatologist	Vasey and Espinoza	15,374	—	—	—	0.05 (0.04–0.06)	0.85:1
Saraux et al,[47] 2005	France	>18	Random sample of phone numbers	Phone screening question + phone rheumatologist interview (+ examination if needed)	Physician diagnosis by phone or examination	15,219	65	—	—	0.19 (0.09–0.35)	—
Trontzas,[124] 2005	Greece	>18	9 Areas	Visiting households for interview	ESSG + psoriasis	10,647	81.2	48.8	47	0.17 (0.10–0.24)	4.8:1
De Angelis et al,[53] 2007	Marche, Central Italy	>18	Random sample of subjects of GPs	Screening questionnaire + examination)	mNY	3664	58.8	46.6	—	0.42 (0.31–0.61)	—
Haglund,[125] 2011	Southern Sweden	>15	All PsA patients registered	*ICD-10* codes from health care register	*ICD-10* code	849,253	—	49	—	0.25 (0.24–0.26)	0.81:1
Braun et al,[50] 1998	Berlin, Germany	—	HLA-B27+ and HLA-B27− blood donors	Screening questionnaires + examination	ESSG	348	85.3 71.4	67	38.5	0.29	
Love et al,[95] 2007	Reykjavik, Iceland	>18	Psoriasis database + hospital records for diagnosis of PsA	Confirming interview + examination	SwePsA	134,253	—	—	—	0.14 (0.11–0.17)	0.57:1

Madland et al,[94] 2005	Western Norway	>20	All PsA patients at rheumatology centers	*ICD* codes, 4 rheumatology centers	Psoriasis + arthritis or axial SpA	321,454	—	—	—	0.20 (1.8–2.1)	1.7:1
North America											
Shbeeb et al,[89] 1999	Minnesota	—	All PsA patients registered	Medical record review	Inflammatory arthritis + psoriasis	—	—	—	—	0.10 (0.08–0.12)	—
Wilson et al,[93] 2009	Minnesota	—	All PsA patients registered	Medical record review	CASPAR	124,277	—	—	—	0.16 (0.13–0.19)	1.5:1
Boyer et al,[46] 1994	Alaskan Eskimos	>20	2 populations enrolled in Alaska Area Native Health Service	Review of records + further evaluation of possible SpA	ESSG/Amor	6749	89	—	—	<0.1	
Latin-America											
Soriano et al,[92] 2011	Buenos Aires, Argentina	>18	Members of a private health system insurance	Medical records review	CASPAR	138,288	—	—	—	0.07 (0.06–0.09)	1.7:1
Alverez-Nemegyei,[75] 2011	Southeast Mexico	>18	Random sample	Screening COPCORD questionnaire + examination	mNY	3195	—	38.2	42.7	0.02	—
Asia											
Hukuda et al,[33] 2001	Japan population	>15	All patients seen at medical institutes	Questionnaires for medical record review	ESSG/Amor (clinical and radiographic features)	134 Institutes	70.9	—	—	0.001	—
Liao,[128] 2009	Dalang Town, China	>16	All residents of Dalang Town	Questionnaire + examination	ESSG	10921	88.8	52.1	—	0.02	—
Alexeeva,[126] 1994	Chukotka, Russia		All residents of 2 settlements	Questionnaire + examination	Unclear	355	71.3%	44.2	—	0.3	

Table 8
Summary of studies on prevalence of IBD-related SpA

Author, Year	Target Population	Age	Sample	Method	Criteria	N Sample	Response	Men (%)	Mean Age	Prevalence of IBD-SpA (%, 95% CI)
De Angelis et al,[53] 2007	Marche, Central Italy	>18	Random sample of subjects of GPs	Screening questionnaire, + examination	ESSG+ IBD	3664	58.8	46.6	—	0.09 (0.04–0.16)
Haglund,[125] 2011	Southern Sweden	>15	All registered patients	*ICD-10* codes from health care register	*ICD-10* code	849,253	—	49	—	0.02 (0.01–0.02)

Table 9
Summary of studies on incidence of ReA

Author, Year	Target Population	Age	Sample	Method	Criteria	N Sample	Period	Incidence of ReA (/100,000)	Male:Female
Söderlin et al,[90] 2002	South Sweden	>16	All referred patients in Kronoberg County	Examination by rheumatologist	Inflammatory joint disease preceded by infection	140,000	1999–2000	28 (20–39)	0.6:1
Hanova et al,[65] 2010	Czechoslovakia	>16	2 Regions, all referred patients	Examination by rheumatologist	Vasey and Espinoza	15,374	2002–2003	9.3 (5.5–14.8)	0.7:1
Townes,[117] 2008	Minnesota and Oregon	>1	Patients with culture infection reported to Foodnet	Screening telephone interview + examination	Inflammatory joint disease preceded by infection	6379	2002–2004	0.6–3.1	0.66:1
Savolainen et al,[42] 2003	Kuopio, Finland	All	All referred patients	Examination by rheumatologist	Study specific[a]	87,000	2000	10 (4.1–20.8)	—
Isomäki,[118] 1987	Finland	>16	Referred patients in 29 counties surrounding Heinola	Examination	Peripheral synovitis preceded by gastrointestinal or urogenial infection	260,000	1974–1975	27	0.75:1
Kvien,[119] 1993	Oslo, Norway	18–60	All referred patients with suspected ReA	Examination by rheumatologist + follow-up	Arthritis with positive stool, culture or antibody titer	271,726	1988–1990	9.6	1:0.86

[a] Previous gastrointestinal or urogenital tract infection associated with peripheral synovitis or with inflammatory signs in sacroiliac, glenohumeral, or hip joints and positive stool culture or positive LCR test for *C. trachomatis* or elevated levels of antibodies against enteric bacteria associated with ReA.

Azores, Portugal, estimated the overall prevalence of SpA according to the ESSG criteria at 1.6%, and remarkably only 1 in 7 patients had a previous diagnosis of SpA.[54] In a population-based epidemiologic study in Greece, the estimated prevalence of SpA was 0.49%.[55]

Recently, a prevalence study of SpA has been conducted in the United States. Both ESSG (using 4 of 7 items) and Amor criteria (using 6 of 11 items) were assessed in a representative sample of 5013 US adults ages 20 to 69 years in the 2009–2010 NHANES study. The overall age adjusted prevalence of SpA using the Amor criteria was 0.9% and when using the ESSG criteria 1.4%.[56] Not all items required for the ESSG and Amor criteria could be assessed because the study concerned a self-report questionnaire excluding items based on spinal mobility, laboratory assessment, or radiography.

In most parts of Asia, the prevalence of SpA tends to be lower than in other countries in the world. A recent review from China estimated the prevalence between 0.49% and 0.93%.[57] A remarkably lower prevalence of SpA of 0.0095%, however, was reported in the study from Japan.[33] In Thailand and Vietnam, prevalence rates were estimated at 0.12% and 0.28%, respectively.[58,59] In the Middle East, the prevalence of SpA is low. A study from Iran estimated a prevalence of 0.23% and in Pakistan of 0.1%. The studies from China, Thailand, Vietnam, Iran, and Pakistan were Community Oriented Programme for the Control of Rheumatic Disease (COPCORD) studies, which is a program to estimate the burden of pain, arthritis, and disability in the community with the aim of improving musculoskeletal health. Providing accurate prevalence information is not the main focus of the program.

The few studies that performed further subtyping suggested invariably that within patients with SpA a large proportion have uSpA, a disease entity that cannot be classified further into AS, PsA, or ReA.[46,48,50]

Phenotypic variations within SpA

Table 3 shows that data on gender diversity in the occurrence of SpA are conflicting. A recent English study in patients with SpA showed that female disease was at least as severe as male disease.[60] In the same study, a slightly different phenotype was found between genders. Women predominantly suffered from upper axial disease, together with stiffness, fatigue, and enthesitis. In contrast, men predominantly suffered from peripheral joint disease, whereas back pain was equally frequent in both genders. A study from Brazil found that female gender was more frequently associated with peripheral SpA, upper limb arthritis, dactylitis, psoriasis, nail involvement, and family history of SpA, and male gender with pure axial involvement, radiographic sacroiliitis, and HLA-B27+. The number of painful and swollen joints was significantly higher in women.[61]

Epidemiology of Ankylosing Spondylitis

Incidence

Eight studies addressed the incidence of AS, which varied from 0.44/100,000 persons in Iceland to 7.3/100,000 in the United States and Northern Norway (see **Table 4**). Using data from the population-based Rochester Epidemiology Project, collected between 1935 and 1989, the overall age-adjusted and sex-adjusted incidence rate in Minnesota was 7.3/100,000 person-years.[62] This incidence rate tended to decline between 1935 and 1989, but there was little change in the age at symptom onset or at diagnosis over the 55-year study period. A Finnish study using the nationwide sickness insurance scheme estimated the incidence of AS requiring antirheumatic medications at 6.9/100,000 with no change over time.[63] Studies from Norway and

Czechoslovakia showed comparable incidences of AS of 7.3/100,000 and 6.4/100,000, respectively.[64,65] The incidence in a study from Greece was found lower (1.5/100,000).[66] The incidence in Japan was estimated at 0.48/100,000.[33]

Prevalence

Thirty-one studies reported on the prevalence of AS, which varied from less than 0.01% in Japan to 1.8% in Norwegian Samis (Lapps) (see **Table 5**). Most studies were conducted in Europe and prevalence of AS followed the geographic distribution of HLA-B27, with the highest prevalence of AS in Northern Norway. A study of Samis (Lapps), in whom the prevalence of HLA-B27 is 24%, reported a prevalence of 1.8% whereas an epidemiologic survey among men and women in the young middle-aged population in Tromsø showed a prevalence of 1.1% to 1.4%.[29,31] In contrast, a third study from Northern Norway showed a prevalence of only 0.31%.[64] This study was hospital based using medical record data, however, and, therefore, only included patients with AS under care of a rheumatologist, likely representing the severe spectrum of the disease. In Central and Western Europe, population-based studies from Czechoslovakia and Germany reported a high prevalence of AS (0.9% and 0.86%, respectively).[50,65] The prevalence of AS in the German blood donor study was later adjusted (for representativeness of blood donors for the general population) to 0.55% to account for sampling among blood donors.[51] According to a population-based study in Turkey, the prevalence of AS in urban areas is 0.49%.[52] Lower prevalence rates of AS in Europe have been reported in population-based studies from Greece (0.24%),[66] a sample study of the Finish population greater than or equal to 30 years of age (0.15%),[63] and in studies from Hungary (0.23%)[67] and the Netherlands (0.24%).[68] In an older study in the United States, the overall prevalence of AS in a mainly white population was reported to be 0.13%.[69] This study included only patients who sought medical care for their condition, and, therefore, the reported number is probably an underestimation. Alternatively, NHANES I (1971–1975) examined 6913 participants between the ages of 25 and 74, obtaining pelvic radiographs in all but 2010 of these individuals (the latter being women under the age of 50 years).[70] The prevalence of severe or moderate radiographic sacroiliitis in men was 7.3 per 1000 in men (0.73%) and in women over age 50 3.0 per 1000 (0.3%). How many had AS by mNY criteria was not ascertained, because questions regarding IBP or measurements of spinal mobility were not done. The prevalence of AS in black Americans might be approximately one-third of that in whites, although there is only indirect evidence for this.[35] Only a few studies reported on the prevalence of AS in Asia. The lowest prevalence of AS was found in Japan (0.0065%).[33] The prevalence in Taiwan was somewhat higher: 0.19% to 0.54%.[71] In China, a recent review reported prevalence rates of AS ranging from 0.11% to 0.41% in different studies.[57] For the Middle East, few available data showed that AS is uncommon in this part of the world. In Iraq, a prevalence was reported of 0.07%[72] and in Iran of 0.14%.[73] For Australia, there is no evidence to support the occurrence of AS in the indigenous Australian Aborigines with pure ancestry, probably related to the low frequency of HLA-B27 in this population.[74] Studies from Latin America and Africa are scarce. A community-based COPCORD door-to-door study in 4059 subjects, aged older than 18 years, in Mexico estimated a prevalence of AS of 0.02%.[75] AS is virtually absent in African blacks. In a study from Togo, there were only 9 Togolese AS patients seen among all 2030 patients attending the rheumatology unit of a teaching hospital over a period of 27 months.[76] Also other studies from South Africa and Zimbabwe showed that AS was extremely rare among African blacks.[77] This can be expected due to the low prevalence of HLA-B27 in these populations. In addition, a study from Gambia found that the risk of developing AS was also small in HLA-B27+ Gambians, compared with those of HLA-B27− whites, suggesting a non-B27 protective factor reducing the prevalence of AS in this population.[77]

HLA-B27 as risk for occurrence and phenotypic heterogeneity of AS

The prevalence of AS among persons carrying HLA-B27 varies substantially in epidemiologic reports throughout the world. In the Netherlands, 2% of HLA-B27+ subjects suffer from AS,[68] but in northern Norway, 6.7% of HLA-B27+ may develop AS,[29] and according to the blood donor study from Germany 6.4%.[50] Furthermore, it has been shown that the risk of developing AS is much higher for HLA-B27+ first-degree relatives of HLA-B27+ AS patients (10%–30%).[68]

The phenotype of the disease also differs among HLA-B27+ and HLA-B27− patients. In a large study of 1080 patient with AS, HLA-B27− patients were significantly older at disease onset.[78] The distribution in age and disease onset was significantly wider in HLA-B27− AS than in HLA-B27+ AS. The percentages with childhood disease did not differ significantly, whereas the percentage of late onset was significantly greater among HLA-B27− patients with AS. With respect to clinical manifestations, HLA-B27+ patients more frequently suffered from acute anterior uveitis than HLA-B27− patients.[76] Observations were conformed in some smaller studies.[79,80]

Differences between male and female patients with AS

AS is traditionally considered as a predominantly male disease, with a commonly reported male:female ratio of approximately 3:1. A study of 3000 members of the German Ankylosing Spondylitis Society, however, found a continuous increase in the percentage of women among patients diagnosed with AS in recent decades.[81] In 1960, only 10% of diagnosed AS patients were women, increasing to 46% of the patients diagnosed since 1990. This suggests that the male predominance in AS may be, at least in part, an artifact induced by deficits in the diagnosis of AS among women many decades ago. In the same study, it was shown that the age of disease onset was not significantly different between men and women, but there was a significantly longer delay in diagnosis among women. Moreover, a slower progression rate for spinal ankylosis was found in female patients, although they reported significantly more pain and need for drug therapy.

In a study from Mexico, it has been suggested that women have less severe disease, resulting in less disability.[82] A study with 769 patients with AS from the United States (556 men and 213 women) showed no gender differences in cervical or lumbar radiographic severity.[83]

Prevalence of extra-articular SpA features in AS

Although the Rome and mNY criteria focused only on axial features to classify AS, extra-articular manifestations, including uveitis, psoriasis, and IBD, are also inherently part of the SpA concept because they occur more frequently in patients with SpA/AS than expected in the general population. In the new ASAS axial SpA classification criteria, these features are part of the classification. When summarizing the literature, the prevalence of uveitis was reported as 33.2% (SD 0.8) in patients with a mean disease duration of 17.0 (SD 1.0) years.[84] The prevalence increased with longer disease duration. There are no exact data on the prevalence of psoriasis and IBD in AS; estimates vary for psoriasis from 10% to 25% and for IBD from 5% to 10% of patients.[85] In 236 AS patients included in the German Spondyloarthritis Inception Cohort (GESPIC), psoriasis was present in 10.2% of AS patients and IBD in 2.6%

patients.[86] Another cohort from France (Devenir des Spondylarthropathies Indifferenciées Récentes [DESIR]) included 181 patients fulfilling the mNY criteria. IBD was present in 7.2% and psoriasis in 14.4% of patients.[87]

Epidemiology of Psoriatic Arthritis

Incidence

The incidence of PsA reported in 7 studies varies from 0.1/100,000 in the Japan to 23.1/100,0000 in Finland (see **Table 6**). The lowest incidence was reported in a study from Japan and was based on a questionnaire sent to all medical institutions of the country potentially attended by patients with SpA.[33] Physicians at the institutes were asked to review the medical records. The incidence rates reported in several studies from Finland, Sweden, Czechoslovakia, Greece, Argentina, and the United States were fairly uniform, ranging from 3.0/100,000 to 8/100,000.[65,88–92] Data from 2 Finnish studies, however, were conflicting. In one study that examined all patients who were entitled under the nationwide sickness insurance scheme to receive medication for PsA, the annual incidence was 6/100,000 between 1990 and 1995.[88] In a second study, the incidence was higher (23/100,000).[42] In this study, information about the study was given through a local newspaper, and subjects attended 1 health center and 2 local hospitals for study. Classification was based on the presence of psoriasis and arthritis, excluding RF+ polyarthritis or spondylitis with psoriasis.

A study in the United States used the population-based data resources of the Rochester Epidemiology Project to identify all cased of inflammatory arthritis with a definite diagnosis of psoriasis between 1982 and 1991. The age-adjusted and sex-adjusted annual incidence rate was 6.6/100,000.[89] A recent study in the same population identified a population-based incidence cohort of subjects aged 18 years or over, who fulfilled the CASPAR criteria, between 1970 and 1999 and studied time trends of PsA incidence.[93] The overall age-adjusted and sex-adjusted incidence of PsA per 100,000 significantly increased from 3.6 between 1970 and 1979 to 9.8 between 1990 and 2000.

Prevalence

The prevalence of PsA is reported for 16 studies and ranged between 0.001% in Japan to 0.42% in Italy (see **Table 7**). The majority of studies were performed in Europe and the United States.[47,66,89,94,95] Cross-sectional population surveys that collect data directly from subjects reported a higher prevalence than retrospective studies, which were based on medical record review. Most studies used the coexistence of psoriasis and arthritis, others the ESSG criteria. In a study from South America (Argentina) based on the CASPAR criteria, the prevalence was 0.07%.[88] In a North American study that used the CASPAR criteria (the Rochester Epidemiology Project), the point prevalence was 0.16% in 2000.[93] In a study from Japan, the prevalence was low: 0.001%.[33] Studies from Africa, large parts of Asia, and South America are lacking.

Prevalence in patients with psoriasis

Among patients with psoriasis, the prevalence of PsA ranges between 6% and 42% in studies from Europe, the United States, and South Africa, but rates are lower in Asian countries (1%–9%).[96] Some recent studies base the classification on the CASPAR criteria: in a study from the United Kingdom, the prevalence was 13.8% among psoriasis patients,[97] and a Chinese study found a prevalence of 5.8%.[98] Furthermore, it is recognized that the underdiagnosis of PsA is probably high. In a study of 100 consecutive psoriasis patients without known PsA, the disease was diagnosed in 29%.[99]

Epidemiology of IBD-SpA

Prevalence

Epidemiologic studies of IBD-related SpA are scarce and present only data on prevalence. A prevalence of 0.09% was estimated in an Italian population study and of 0.02% in a Swedish study (**Table 10**). In patients with different forms of SpA, approximately 60% to 70% have gut inflammation, which is mainly chronic inflammation discovered by endoscopy.[100–102] In 7% of SpA patients, this develops to overt IBD.[103]

Prevalence of SpA in patients with IBD

IBD has an estimated prevalence in the general population ranging from 0.01% to 0.5%, with highest numbers reported in studies from Western Europe and the United States.[104] Any spinal or articular SpA manifestation was found in 17% to 62% of patients. Peripheral arthritis has been reported in 5% to 28% of patients, predominantly in Crohn disease[105–111]; 12% to 46% of patients with IBD fulfilled classification of SpA when applying the ESSG criteria and 2% to 10% of patients fulfilled the mNY criteria.[105–110,112–114] Radiologic evidence of sacroiliitis has been reported more frequently: in 2% to 18% on plain radiographs and in 29% of patients on CT, of whom only 3% were symptomatic.[106,107,109,112,114,115] The frequency of HLA-B27 is generally not increased in the IBD population. The prevalence of HLA-B27 in a study in 406 patients with IBD from Norway was 13%, comparable with the general population in that area (10%), whereas in patients with AS, the prevalence of HLA-B27 was 73%.[112]

Epidemiology of Reactive Arthritis

Incidence

In 6 studies on the incidence of ReA, reports varied from 0.6/100,000 in Minnesota and Oregon to 28/100,000 in South Sweden (see **Table 9**). Most epidemiologic data of ReA are based on outbreak studies in which patients with joint symptoms during and after the infection are traced with questionnaire or other investigations. The large difference in criteria used, but more importantly in the population sampled, resulted in a wide variation in the estimate of the incidence of ReA, which varies between 0.6/100,000 and 28/100,000 subjects in population studies.[116] In a study from the United States, telephone interviews were performed with individuals who had a confirmed infection of Campylobacter, *Escherichia coli*, Salmonella, Shigella, or Yersinia, and patients were asked for new-onset rheumatologic symptoms.[117] Possible ReA patients were invited for physical examination. The estimated incidence of ReA was 0.6/100,000 subjects in the area of the outbreak when assuming that none of the nonresponders had SpA, and up to 3.1/100,000 when assuming that the nonresponders were equally likely as the responders to have had ReA. In this study, no association between ReA and HLA-B27 was found. In a study from Czechoslovakia, patients with suspected symptoms of ReA were referred by their general physician to a rheumatologist. An age-standardized incidence of 9.3/100,000 subjects was found.[65] Because the course of ReA may be self-limiting, not everyone with ReA might have sought help. Higher incidence rates (10/100,000–28/100,000) were found in studies from Scandinavian countries, where the prevalence of HLA-B27 is high.[42,90,118,119] The highest incidence of 28/100,000 was found in a study from Sweden, in which all suspected patients were referred from primary health care centers to a rheumatologist.[90] A recent review showed that, in outbreak studies, the occurrence of ReA after an infection of Campylobacter have been reported in 0.7% to 1.8% of patients; after a Shigella infection in 0% to 6.9% of patients; after a Yersinia infection in 0% to 21% of patients; and after a Salmonella infection in 0% to 29% of patients.[116]

Table 10
Summary of studies on prevalence of ReA

Author, Year	Target Population	Age	Sample	Method	Criteria	N Sample	Response %	Men (%)	Mean Age	Prevalence of ReA (%, 95% CI)	Male:Female
Hanova et al,[65] 2010	Czechoslavakia	>16	2 Regions, all referred patients	Examination by rheumatologist	Third international workshop on ReA	15,374	—	—	—	0.09 (0.07–0.11)	1.2:1
Saraux et al,[47] 2005	France	>18	Random sample of phone numbers	Phone screening question + phone rheumatologist interview (+ examination if needed)	Physician confirmation by phone or examination	15,219	65	—	—	0.04 (0.01–0.07)	
De Angelis et al,[53] 2007	Marche, Central Italy	>18	Random sample of subjects of GPs	Screening questionnaire + examination	ESSG + prior urogenital or gastrointestinal infection	3664	58.8	46.6	—	0.09 (0.04–0.16)	
Braun et al,[50] 1998	Berlin	—	HLA-B27+ and HLA-B27– blood donors	Screening questionnaires + examination	ESSG	348	85.3 71.4	67	38.5	0.1	—
Alexeeva,[126] 1994	Chukotka, Russia	—	All residents of 2 settlements	Questionnaire + examination	Unclear	355	71.3	44.2	—	0.6	—
Boyer et al,[46] 1994	Alaskan Eskimos	>20	2 Populations enrolled in Alaska Area Native Health service	Review of records + further evaluation of possible SpA	ESSG and Amor (clinical and radiographic features)	6749	89	—	—	1.0	

Prevalence

The prevalence of acute ReA arthritis has been estimated between 0.09% and 1.0%, depending on criteria used for diagnosis, racial/ethnic differences, and the setting in which the study was undertaken (hospital series vs single-source outbreaks vs community-based series) (see **Table 9**).[120] No data are available from Scandinavian countries.

HLA-B27 in ReA

In contrast to the population-based study from the United States, the risk of ReA in HLA-B27+ patients has been reported in another study to be up to 50 times higher after the exposure of a triggering infection compared with HLA-B27− patients in hospital-based studies.[121] This number, however, is possibly (partly) biased due to inclusion of the most severe cases in hospital-based studies.

EPIDEMIOLOGY OF USPA

No formal definition or classification criteria for uSpA exist. Case definitions used comprise either incomplete forms of distinctly defined entities (preradiographic phase of mNY AS or SpA not fulfilling all required ESSG or Amor criteria) or disease descriptions that fulfill ESSG or Amor criteria but cannot be specified further into a specific SpA disease. There are few data on prevalence and incidence of uSpA. Few data from Europe[48,50] and Alaska[46] suggest that approximately 40% of patients with SpA have uSpA. Some longitudinal studies are available in which patients with uSpA are followed prospectively. In a study from Brazil, 111 patients with uSpA fulfilling the ESSG and Amor criteria were followed-up for 10 years. During the follow-up, 27 patients progressed to AS (24.3%) and 3 to PsA (2.7%), whereas 25 patients (22.5%) went into remission. HLA-B27 and buttock pain were independently associated with progression to AS.[122]

EPIDEMIOLOGY OF AXIAL SpA ACCORDING TO THE NEW CLASSIFICATION CRITERIA

Axial SpA comprises AS and nonradiographic axial SpA. Epidemiologic studies applying these criteria are not yet available and, as discussed previously, these criteria were not developed for use in large population studies. There is a report, however, that applied the criteria in a general practitioner setting. In a study in Rotterdam, the Netherlands, 364 patients with chronic low back pain were identified from general practitioner (GP) records. They underwent a complete history and physical examination by a rheumatologist, HLA-B27 was assessed, and sacroiliac joints were imaged by conventional radiography and MRI. The overall point prevalence of axial SpA was 21.5% using the ASAS criteria, of which 67.5% were diagnosed by MRI and 15.5% were diagnosed by a positive HLA-B27 and 2 other SpA features. Of all patients, 6.6% fulfilled the mNY criteria for AS. In this study, 3 times as many patients were diagnosed compared with the mNY criteria using conventional radiographs alone. Adding HLA-B27 increased the likelihood of diagnosis of SpA by 68%, and using radiographs increased the likelihood by 75%.[123]

SUMMARY

Data on prevalence and incidence of the SpA have become particularly important in recent years since more treatments have become available, making it necessary to gain insight into whether or not patients have sought medical attention and to know what the impact on society is in terms of health and costs when all patients require a specific treatment approach.

Large variations in the population incidence and prevalence rates of SpA (as a disease entity) and its subtypes, however, were seen when reviewing the literature. These variations could in part be attributed to geographic distribution of HLA-B27, a main risk factor for SpA, and explaining high rates in the Northern countries and low rates in Japan and Middle Africa. When concentrating on data from Western European countries and the United States, however, large differences remained, not only differences in the way the target population was sampled but also large differences in the approach to operationalize criteria to identify cases contributing to such differences. Overall, SpA as a disease is prevalent with rates in Western European countries between 0.3% and 2.5%. When subtyping SpA, uSpA seems to make up approximately 40% of these cases. Prevalence rates of AS and PsA seem approximately similar in Western countries, up to 0.53%. Although the prevalence rates for of ReA and IBD-SpA seem somewhat lower, it should also be realized there were fewer studies available and likely the case findings in epidemiologic studies are even more challenging. Recently it was proposed to facilitate classification and distinguish within SpA the axial and peripheral subtype. Moreover, the axial Spa criteria aim to encompass not only patients having bilateral grade 2 sacroiliitis but also patients with nonradiographic axial SpA. It should be emphasized both new criteria sets have been used for application in a clinical seting. It would be particular challenging to operationalise these concepts/criteria for application in epidemiological studies.

REFERENCES

1. Wright V, Moll JM. Seronegative polyarthritis. Amsterdam: Publishing Co; 1976.
2. Moll JM, Haslock I, Macrae IF, et al. Associations between ankylosing spondylitis, psoriatic arthritis, Reiter's disease, the intestinal arthropathies, and Behcet's syndrome. Baltimore: Medicine; 1974. p. 343–64.
3. Brewerton DA, Hart FD, Nicholls A, et al. Ankylosing spondylitis and HL-A 27. Lancet 1973;1(7809):904–7.
4. Kellgren JH. Diagnostic criteria for population studies. Bull Rheum Dis 1962;13: 291–2.
5. Gofton JP, Lawrence JS, Bennett PH, et al. Sacro-ilitis in eight populations. Ann Rheum Dis 1966;25(6):528–33.
6. Bennett PH. Population studies of the rheumatic diseases. Amsterdam: Excerpta Medica Foundation; 1968.
7. Moll JM, Wright V. New York clinical criteria for ankylosing spondylitis. A statistical evaluation. Ann Rheum Dis 1973;32(4):354–63.
8. van der Linden S, Valkenburg HA, Cats A. Evaluation of diagnostic criteria for ankylosing spondylitis. A proposal for modification of the New York criteria. Arthritis Rheum 1984;27(4):361–8.
9. Mau W, Zeidler H, Mau R, et al. Clinical features and prognosis of patients with possible ankylosing spondylitis. Results of a 10-year followup. J Rheumatol 1988;15(7):1109–14.
10. Moll JM, Wright V. Psoriatic arthritis. Semin Arthritis Rheum 1973;3(1):55–78.
11. Helliwell PS, Taylor WJ. Classification and diagnostic criteria for psoriatic arthritis. Ann Rheum Dis 2005;64(2):ii3–8.
12. Taylor W, Gladman D, Helliwell P, et al. Classification criteria for psoriatic arthritis: development of new criteria from a large international study. Arthritis Rheum 2006;54(8):2665–73.

13. Braun J, Kingsley G, van der Heijde D, et al. On the difficulties of establishing a consensus on the definition of and diagnostic investigations for reactive arthritis. Results and discussion of a questionnaire prepared for the 4th International Workshop on Reactive Arthritis, Berlin, Germany, July 3-6, 1999. J Rheumatol 2000;27(9):2185–92.
14. Amor B, Dougados M, Mijiyawa M. Criteria of the classification of spondylarthropathies. Rev Rhum Mal Osteoartic 1990;57(2):85–9 [in French].
15. Dougados M, van der Linden S, Juhlin R, et al. The European Spondylarthropathy Study Group preliminary criteria for the classification of spondylarthropathy. Arthritis Rheum 1991;34(10):1218–27.
16. Collantes E, Veroz R, Escudero A, et al. Can some cases of 'possible' spondyloarthropathy be classified as 'definite' or 'undifferentiated' spondyloarthropathy? Value of criteria for spondyloarthropathies. Spanish Spondyloarthropathy Study Group. Joint Bone Spine 2000;67(6):516–20.
17. Collantes-Estevez E, Cisnal del Mazo A, Munoz-Gomariz E. Assessment of 2 systems of spondyloarthropathy diagnostic and classification criteria (Amor and ESSG) by a Spanish multicenter study. European Spondyloarthropathy Study Group. J Rheumatol 1995;22(2):246–51.
18. Rudwaleit M, van der Heijde D, Landewe R, et al. The Assessment of SpondyloArthritis International Society classification criteria for peripheral spondyloarthritis and for spondyloarthritis in general. Ann Rheum Dis 2011;70(1):25–31.
19. Rudwaleit M, van der Heijde D, Landewe R, et al. The development of Assessment of SpondyloArthritis international Society classification criteria for axial spondyloarthritis (part II): validation and final selection. Ann Rheum Dis 2009; 68(6):777–83.
20. Fox DM. Evidence of evidence-based health policy: the politics of systematic reviews in coverage decisions. Health Aff 2005;24(1):114–22.
21. Malta M, Cardoso LO, Bastos FI, et al. STROBE initiative: guidelines on reporting observational studies. Rev Saude Publica 2010;44(3):559–65.
22. Mallen C, Peat G, Croft P. Quality assessment of observational studies is not commonplace in systematic reviews. J Clin Epidemiol 2006;59(8):765–9.
23. Sanderson S, Tatt ID, Higgins JP. Tools for assessing quality and susceptibility to bias in observational studies in epidemiology: a systematic review and annotated bibliography. Int J Epidemiol 2007;36(3):666–76.
24. Shamliyan TA, Kane RL, Ansari MT, et al. Development quality criteria to evaluate nontherapeutic studies of incidence, prevalence, or risk factors of chronic diseases: pilot study of new checklists. J Clin Epidemiol 2011;64(6): 637–57.
25. Hoy D, Brooks P, Woolf A, et al. Assessing risk of bias in prevalence studies: modification of an existing tool and evidence of interrater agreement. J Clin Epidemiol 2012;65(9):934–9.
26. Bhatia K, Prasad ML, Barnish G, et al. Antigen and haplotype frequencies at three human leucocyte antigen loci (HLA-A, -B, -C) in the Pawaia of Papua New Guinea. Am J Phys Anthropol 1988;75(3):329–40.
27. Gofton JP, Chalmers A, Price GE, et al. HL-A 27 and ankylosing spondylitis in B.C. Indians. J Rheumatol 1984;11(5):572–3.
28. Benevolenskaia LI, Erdes S, Krylov M, et al. The epidemiology of spondyloarthropathies among the native inhabitants of Chukotka. 2. The prevalence of HLA-B27 in the population and among spondyloarthropathy patients. Ter Arkh 1994;66(5):41–4 [in Russian].

29. Gran JT, Husby G, Hordvik M. Prevalence of ankylosing spondylitis in males and females in a young middle-aged population of Tromso, northern Norway. Ann Rheum Dis 1985;44(6):359–67.
30. Gran JT, Mellby AS, Husby G. The prevalence of HLA-B27 in Northern Norway. Scand J Rheumatol 1984;13(2):173–6.
31. Johnsen K, Gran JT, Dale K, et al. The prevalence of ankylosing spondylitis among Norwegian Samis (Lapps). J Rheumatol 1992;19(10):1591–4.
32. Mustafa KN, Hammoudeh M, Khan MA. HLA-B27 prevalence in Arab populations and among patients with ankylosing spondylitis. J Rheumatol 2012; 39(8):1675–7.
33. Hukuda S, Minami M, Saito T, et al. Spondyloarthropathies in Japan: nationwide questionnaire survey performed by the Japan Ankylosing Spondylitis Society. J Rheumatol 2001;28(3):554–9.
34. Khan MA. HLA-B27 and its subtypes in world populations. Curr Opin Rheumatol 1995;7(4):263–9.
35. Khan MA. Race-related differences in HLA association with ankylosing spondylitis and Reiter's disease in American blacks and whites. J Natl Med Assoc 1978; 70(1):41–2.
36. al-Arfaj A. Profile of ankylosing spondylitis in Saudi Arabia. Clin Rheumatol 1996; 15(3):287–9.
37. Alharbi SA, Mahmoud FF, Al Awadi A, et al. Association of MHC class I with spondyloarthropathies in Kuwait. Eur J Immunogenet 1996;23(1):67–70.
38. Uppal SS, Abraham M, Chowdhury RI, et al. Ankylosing spondylitis and undifferentiated spondyloarthritis in Kuwait: a comparison between Arabs and South Asians. Clin Rheumatol 2006;25(2):219–24.
39. Reveille JD, Hirsch R, Dillon CF, et al. The prevalence of HLA-B27 in the United States: data from the U.S. National Health and Nutrition Examination Survey, 2009. Arthritis Rheum 2012;64(5):1407–11.
40. Reveille JD. Major histocompatibility genes and ankylosing spondylitis. Best Pract Res Clin Rheumatol 2006;20(3):601–9.
41. Thomas GP, Brown MA. Genetics and genomics of ankylosing spondylitis. Immunol Rev 2010;233(1):162–80.
42. Savolainen E, Kaipiainen-Seppanen O, Kroger L, et al. Total incidence and distribution of inflammatory joint diseases in a defined population: results from the Kuopio 2000 arthritis survey. J Rheumatol 2003;30(11):2460–8.
43. Kaipiainen-Seppanen O, Aho K. Incidence of chronic inflammatory joint diseases in Finland in 1995. J Rheumatol 2000;27(1):94–100.
44. Munoz-Fernandez S, de Miguel E, Cobo-Ibanez T, et al. Early spondyloarthritis: results from the pilot registry ESPIDEP. Clin Exp Rheumatol 2010;28(4): 498–503.
45. Boyer GS, Lanier AP, Templin DW. Prevalence rates of spondyloarthropathies, rheumatoid arthritis, and other rheumatic disorders in an Alaskan Inupiat Eskimo population. J Rheumatol 1988;15(4):678–83.
46. Boyer GS, Templin DW, Cornoni-Huntley JC, et al. Prevalence of spondyloarthropathies in Alaskan Eskimos. J Rheumatol 1994;21(12):2292–7.
47. Saraux A, Guillemin F, Guggenbuhl P, et al. Prevalence of spondyloarthropathies in France: 2001. Ann Rheum Dis 2005;64(10):1431–5.
48. Saraux A, Guedes C, Allain J, et al. Prevalence of rheumatoid arthritis and spondyloarthropathy in Brittany, France. Societe de Rhumatologie de l'Ouest. J Rheumatol 1999;26(12):2622–7.

49. Adomaviciute D, Pileckyte M, Baranauskaite A, et al. Prevalence survey of rheumatoid arthritis and spondyloarthropathy in Lithuania. Scand J Rheumatol 2008; 37(2):113–9.
50. Braun J, Bollow M, Remlinger G, et al. Prevalence of spondylarthropathies in HLA-B27 positive and negative blood donors. Arthritis Rheum 1998;41(1):58–67.
51. Akkoc N, Khan MA. Overestimation of the prevalence of ankylosing spondylitis in the Berlin study: comment on the article by Braun et al. Arthritis Rheum 2005; 52(12):4048–9 [author reply: 9–50].
52. Onen F, Akar S, Birlik M, et al. Prevalence of ankylosing spondylitis and related spondyloarthritides in an urban area of Izmir, Turkey. J Rheumatol 2008;35(2): 305–9.
53. De Angelis R, Salaffi F, Grassi W. Prevalence of spondyloarthropathies in an Italian population sample: a regional community-based study. Scand J Rheumatol 2007;36(1):14–21.
54. Bruges-Armas J, Lima C, Peixoto MJ, et al. Prevalence of spondyloarthritis in Terceira, Azores: a population based study. Ann Rheum Dis 2002;61(6): 551–3.
55. Andrianakos A, Trontzas P, Christoyannis F, et al. Prevalence of rheumatic diseases in Greece: a cross-sectional population based epidemiological study. The ESORDIG Study. J Rheumatol 2003;30(7):1589–601.
56. Reveille JD, Witter JP, Weisman MH. Prevalence of axial spondylarthritis in the United States: estimates from a cross-sectional survey. Arthritis Care Res (Hoboken) 2012;64(6):905–10.
57. Ng SC, Liao Z, Yu DT, et al. Epidemiology of spondyloarthritis in the People's Republic of China: review of the literature and commentary. Semin Arthritis Rheum 2007;37(1):39–47.
58. Chaiamnuay P, Darmawan J, Muirden KD, et al. Epidemiology of rheumatic disease in rural Thailand: a WHO-ILAR COPCORD study. Community Oriented Programme for the Control of Rheumatic Disease. J Rheumatol 1998;25(7): 1382–7.
59. Minh Hoa TT, Darmawan J, Chen SL, et al. Prevalence of the rheumatic diseases in urban Vietnam: a WHO-ILAR COPCORD study. J Rheumatol 2003;30(10): 2252–6.
60. Roussou E, Sultana S. Spondyloarthritis in women: differences in disease onset, clinical presentation, and Bath Ankylosing Spondylitis Disease Activity and Functional indices (BASDAI and BASFI) between men and women with spondyloarthritides. Clin Rheumatol 2011;30(1):121–7.
61. de Carvalho HM, Bortoluzzo AB, Goncalves CR, et al. Gender characterization in a large series of Brazilian patients with spondyloarthritis. Clin Rheumatol 2012;31(4):687–95.
62. Carbone LD, Cooper C, Michet CJ, et al. Ankylosing spondylitis in Rochester, Minnesota, 1935-1989: is the epidemiology changing? Arthritis Rheum 1992; 35(12):1476–82.
63. Kaipiainen-Seppanen O, Aho K, Heliovaara M. Incidence and prevalence of ankylosing spondylitis in Finland. J Rheumatol 1997;24(3):496–9.
64. Bakland G, Nossent HC, Gran JT. Incidence and prevalence of ankylosing spondylitis in Northern Norway. Arthritis Rheum 2005;53(6):850–5.
65. Hanova P, Pavelka K, Holcatova I, et al. Incidence and prevalence of psoriatic arthritis, ankylosing spondylitis, and reactive arthritis in the first descriptive population-based study in the Czech Republic. Scand J Rheumatol 2010; 39(4):310–7.

66. Alamanos Y, Papadopoulos NG, Voulgari PV, et al. Epidemiology of ankylosing spondylitis in Northwest Greece, 1983-2002. Rheumatology (Oxford) 2004; 43(5):615–8.
67. Gomor B, Gyodi E, Bakos L. Distribution of HLA B27 and ankylosing spondylitis in the Hungarian population. J Rheumatol Suppl 1977;3:33–5.
68. van der Linden S, Valkenburg H, Cats A. The risk of developing ankylosing spondylitis in HLA-B27 positive individuals: a family and population study. Br J Rheumatol 1983;22(4 Suppl 2):18–9.
69. Carter ET, McKenna CH, Brian DD, et al. Epidemiology of Ankylosing spondylitis in Rochester, Minnesota, 1935-1973. Arthritis Rheum 1979;22(4):365–70.
70. Maurer K. Basic data on arthritis: knee, hip, and sacroiliac joints in adults ages 25–74 years, united states, 1971–1975. Vital Health Stat 1979;11(213): 1–31.
71. Chou CT, Pei L, Chang DM, et al. Prevalence of rheumatic diseases in Taiwan: a population study of urban, suburban, rural differences. J Rheumatol 1994; 21(2):302–6.
72. Al-Rawi ZS, Al-Shakarchi HA, Hasan F, et al. Ankylosing spondylitis and its association with the histocompatibility antigen HL-A B27: an epidemiological and clinical study. Rheumatol Rehabil 1978;17(2):72–5.
73. Davatchi F, Jamshidi AR, Banihashemi AT, et al. WHO-ILAR COPCORD Study (Stage 1, Urban Study) in Iran. J Rheumatol 2008;35(7):1384.
74. Roberts-Thomson RA, Roberts-Thomson PJ. Rheumatic disease and the Australian aborigine. Ann Rheum Dis 1999;58(5):266–70.
75. Alvarez-Nemegyei J, Pelaez-Ballestas I, Sanin LH, et al. Prevalence of musculoskeletal pain and rheumatic diseases in the southeastern region of Mexico. A COPCORD-based community survey. J Rheumatol Suppl 2011;86:21–5.
76. Mijiyawa M. Spondyloarthropathies in patients attending the rheumatology unit of Lome Hospital. J Rheumatol 1993;20(7):1167–9.
77. Stein M, Davis P, Emmanuel J, et al. The spondyloarthropathies in Zimbabwe: a clinical and immunogenetic profile. J Rheumatol 1990;17(10):1337–9.
78. Feldtkeller E, Khan MA, van der Heijde D, et al. Age at disease onset and diagnosis delay in HLA-B27 negative vs. positive patients with ankylosing spondylitis. Rheumatol Int 2003;23(2):61–6.
79. Linssen A. B27+ disease versus B27- disease. Scand J Rheumatol Suppl 1990; 87:111–8 [discussion: 8–9].
80. Awada H, Abi-Karam G, Baddoura R, et al. Clinical, radiological, and laboratory findings in Lebanese spondylarthropathy patients according to HLA-B27 status. Joint Bone Spine 2000;67(3):194–8.
81. Feldtkeller E, Bruckel J, Khan MA. Scientific contributions of ankylosing spondylitis patient advocacy groups. Curr Opin Rheumatol 2000;12(4):239–47.
82. Jimenez-Balderas FJ, Mintz G. Ankylosing spondylitis: clinical course in women and men. J Rheumatol 1993;20(12):2069–72.
83. Jang JH, Ward MM, Rucker AN, et al. Ankylosing spondylitis: patterns of radiographic involvement–a re-examination of accepted principles in a cohort of 769 patients. Radiology 2011;258(1):192–8, T80.
84. Zeboulon N, Dougados M, Gossec L. Prevalence and characteristics of uveitis in the spondyloarthropathies: a systematic literature review. Ann Rheum Dis 2008;67(7):955–9.
85. El Maghraoui A. Extra-articular manifestations of ankylosing spondylitis: prevalence, characteristics and therapeutic implications. Eur J Intern Med 2011; 22(6):554–60.

86. Rudwaleit M, Haibel H, Baraliakos X, et al. The early disease stage in axial spondylarthritis: results from the German Spondyloarthritis Inception Cohort. Arthritis Rheum 2009;60(3):717–27.
87. Dougados M, d'Agostino MA, Benessiano J, et al. The DESIR cohort: a 10-year follow-up of early inflammatory back pain in France: study design and baseline characteristics of the 708 recruited patients. Joint Bone Spine 2011;78(6):598–603.
88. Kaipiainen-Seppanen O. Incidence of psoriatic arthritis in Finland. Br J Rheumatol 1996;35(12):1289–91.
89. Shbeeb M, Uramoto KM, Gibson LE, et al. The epidemiology of psoriatic arthritis in Olmsted County, Minnesota, USA, 1982-1991. J Rheumatol 2000;27(5):1247–50.
90. Soderlin MK, Borjesson O, Kautiainen H, et al. Annual incidence of inflammatory joint diseases in a population based study in southern Sweden. Ann Rheum Dis 2002;61(10):911–5.
91. Alamanos Y, Papadopoulos NG, Voulgari PV, et al. Epidemiology of psoriatic arthritis in northwest Greece, 1982-2001. J Rheumatol 2003;30(12):2641–4.
92. Soriano ER, Rosa J, Velozo E, et al. Incidence and prevalence of psoriatic arthritis in Buenos Aires, Argentina: a 6-year health management organization-based study. Rheumatology (Oxford) 2011;50(4):729–34.
93. Wilson FC, Icen M, Crowson CS, et al. Time trends in epidemiology and characteristics of psoriatic arthritis over 3 decades: a population-based study. J Rheumatol 2009;36(2):361–7.
94. Madland TM, Apalset EM, Johannessen AE, et al. Prevalence, disease manifestations, and treatment of psoriatic arthritis in Western Norway. J Rheumatol 2005;32(10):1918–22.
95. Love TJ, Gudbjornsson B, Gudjonsson JE, et al. Psoriatic arthritis in Reykjavik, Iceland: prevalence, demographics, and disease course. J Rheumatol 2007; 34(10):2082–8.
96. Tam LS, Leung YY, Li EK. Psoriatic arthritis in Asia. Rheumatology (Oxford) 2009;48(12):1473–7.
97. Ibrahim G, Waxman R, Helliwell PS. The prevalence of psoriatic arthritis in people with psoriasis. Arthritis Rheum 2009;61(10):1373–8.
98. Yang Q, Qu L, Tian H, et al. Prevalence and characteristics of psoriatic arthritis in Chinese patients with psoriasis. J Eur Acad Dermatol Venereol 2011;25(12): 1409–14.
99. Haroon M, Kirby B, Fitzgerald O. High prevalence of psoriatic arthritis in patients with severe psoriasis with suboptimal performance of screening questionnaires. Ann Rheum Dis 2012. [Epub ahead of print].
100. De Vos M, Cuvelier C, Mielants H, et al. Ileocolonoscopy in seronegative spondylarthropathy. Gastroenterology 1989;96(2 Pt 1):339–44.
101. Mielants H, Veys EM, Goemaere S, et al. Gut inflammation in the spondyloarthropathies: clinical, radiologic, biologic and genetic features in relation to the type of histology. A prospective study. J Rheumatol 1991;18(10):1542–51.
102. Simenon G, Van Gossum A, Adler M, et al. Macroscopic and microscopic gut lesions in seronegative spondyloarthropathies. J Rheumatol 1990;17(11):1491–4.
103. De Vos M, Mielants H, Cuvelier C, et al. Long-term evolution of gut inflammation in patients with spondyloarthropathy. Gastroenterology 1996;110(6):1696–703.
104. Molodecky NA, Soon IS, Rabi DM, et al. Increasing incidence and prevalence of the inflammatory bowel diseases with time, based on systematic review. Gastroenterology 2012;142(1):46–54.e42 [quiz: e30].
105. Beslek A, Onen F, Birlik M, et al. Prevalence of spondyloarthritis in Turkish patients with inflammatory bowel disease. Rheumatol Int 2009;29(8):955–7.

106. de Vlam K, Mielants H, Cuvelier C, et al. Spondyloarthropathy is underestimated in inflammatory bowel disease: prevalence and HLA association. J Rheumatol 2000;27(12):2860–5.
107. Lanna CC, Ferrari Mde L, Rocha SL, et al. A cross-sectional study of 130 Brazilian patients with Crohn's disease and ulcerative colitis: analysis of articular and ophthalmologic manifestations. Clin Rheumatol 2008;27(4):503–9.
108. Protzer U, Duchmann R, Hohler T, et al. Enteropathic spondylarthritis in chronic inflammatory bowel diseases: prevalence, manifestation pattern and HLA association. Med Klin (Munich) 1996;91(6):330–5 [in German].
109. Rodriguez VE, Costas PJ, Vazquez M, et al. Prevalence of spondyloarthropathy in Puerto Rican patients with inflammatory bowel disease. Ethn Dis 2008;18(2 Suppl 2): S2-225–S2-229.
110. Salvarani C, Vlachonikolis IG, van der Heijde DM, et al. Musculoskeletal manifestations in a population-based cohort of inflammatory bowel disease patients. Scand J Gastroenterol 2001;36(12):1307–13.
111. Palm O, Moum B, Jahnsen J, et al. The prevalence and incidence of peripheral arthritis in patients with inflammatory bowel disease, a prospective population-based study (the IBSEN study). Rheumatology (Oxford) 2001;40(11):1256–61.
112. Palm O, Moum B, Ongre A, et al. Prevalence of ankylosing spondylitis and other spondyloarthropathies among patients with inflammatory bowel disease: a population study (the IBSEN study). J Rheumatol 2002;29(3):511–5.
113. Scarpa R, del Puente A, D'Arienzo A, et al. The arthritis of ulcerative colitis: clinical and genetic aspects. J Rheumatol 1992;19(3):373–7.
114. Turkcapar N, Toruner M, Soykan I, et al. The prevalence of extraintestinal manifestations and HLA association in patients with inflammatory bowel disease. Rheumatol Int 2006;26(7):663–8.
115. Scott WW Jr, Fishman EK, Kuhlman JE, et al. Computed tomography evaluation of the sacroiliac joints in Crohn disease. Radiologic/clinical correlation. Skeletal Radiol 1990;19(3):207–10.
116. Hannu T. Reactive arthritis. Best Pract Res Clin Rheumatol 2011;25(3):347–57.
117. Townes JM, Deodhar AA, Laine ES, et al. Reactive arthritis following culture-confirmed infections with bacterial enteric pathogens in Minnesota and Oregon: a population-based study. Ann Rheum Dis 2008;67(12):1689–96.
118. Isomaki H, Raunio J, von Essen R, et al. Incidence of inflammatory rheumatic diseases in Finland. Scand J Rheumatol 1978;7(3):188–92.
119. Kvien TK, Glennas A, Melby K, et al. Reactive arthritis: incidence, triggering agents and clinical presentation. J Rheumatol 1994;21(1):115–22.
120. Pope JE, Krizova A, Garg AX, et al. Campylobacter reactive arthritis: a systematic review. Semin Arthritis Rheum 2007;37(1):48–55.
121. Aho K, Ahvonen P, Lassus A, et al. HL-A antigen 27 and reactive arthritis. Lancet 1973;2(7821):157.
122. Sampaio-Barros PD, Bortoluzzo AB, Conde RA, et al. Undifferentiated spondyloarthritis: a longterm followup. J Rheumatol 2010;37(6):1195–9.
123. Hoeven van L, Luime J, Han H, et al. Striking prevalence of axial spondyloarthritis in primary care patients with chronic low back pain; a cross-sectional study. Arthritis and Rheumatism 2010;62:2180.
124. Trontzas P, Andrianakos A, Miyakis S, et al. Seronegative spondyloarthropathies in Greece: a population-based study of prevalence, clinical pattern, and management. The ESORDIG study. Clin Rheumatol 2005;24(6):583–9.
125. Haglund E, Bremander AB, Petersson IF, et al. Prevalence of spondyloarthritis and its subtypes in southern Sweden. Ann Rheum Dis 2011;70(6):943–8.

126. Alexeeva L, Krylov M, Vturin V, et al. Prevalence of spondyloarthropathies and HLA-B27 in the native population of Chukotka, Russia. J Rheumatol 1994; 21(12):2298–300.
127. Farooqi A, Gibson T. Prevalence of the major rheumatic disorders in the adult population of north Pakistan. Br J Rheumatol 1998;37(5):491–5.
128. Liao ZT, Pan YF, Huang JL, et al. An epidemiological survey of low back pain and axial spondyloarthritis in a Chinese Han population. Scand J Rheumatol 2009;38(6):455–9.
129. Geirsson AJ, Eyjolfsdottir H, Bjornsdottir G, et al. Prevalence and clinical characteristics of ankylosing spondylitis in Iceland—a nationwide study. Clin Exp Rheumatol 2010;28(3):333–40.

Classification, Diagnosis, and Referral of Patients with Axial Spondyloarthritis

Jürgen Braun, MD[a], Joachim Sieper, MD[b,*]

KEYWORDS

- Axial spondyloarthritis • Classification • Diagnosis • Referral

KEY POINTS

- The concepts for classification, diagnosis and referral of patients with axial spondyloarthitis differ, although they of course basically relate to the same disease. While classification criteria and referral strategies concentrate largely on patients with chronic back pain with an age at onset before 45 years, the rheumatologist can make a diagnosis of axial SpA in patients with late onset or in patients with back pain for only some weeks if other items are fulfilled.
- Early recognition of patients with axial SpA is important to establish the diagnosis, potentially start therapeutic interventions and avoid unnecessary health care procedures.

axSpA, including ankylosing spondylitis (AS) and nonradiographic axSpA (nr-axSpA), is a chronic inflammatory rheumatic disease that predominantly affects the axial skeleton. It typically starts in young adulthood, at between 20 and 30 years of age, and more than 90% of patients are younger than 45 years when the first symptoms appear. Men are slightly more affected than women.[1] Several recent clinical trials have shown that anti-inflammatory therapy with anti–TNF-directed biologics is effective, especially in patients with axSpA who had a short disease duration, which may reach Assessment of SpondyloArthritis International Society (ASAS) partial remission in approximately 50% of patients treated.[2–4] In line with that, young age is predictive of response to therapy.[5–7] Although it is unclear whether (early) treatment is able to prevent structural changes (early) at all, consequent inhibition of sacroiliac and spinal inflammation seems, at present, the only intervention that may have this effect. In addition, NSAIDs seem to have an influence on new bone formation[8,9] in established disease but recent data have suggested that this may be different in early disease.[10]

Early recognition of axSpA is not an easy challenge. There is a well-reported delay between the first onset of symptoms—usually IBP (discussed later)[11,12]—and the

[a] Rheumazentrum Ruhrgebiet, Herne and Ruhr Universität Bochum, Germany; [b] Section of Rheumatology, Campus Benjamin Franklin, Charité University, Hindenburgdamm 30, Berlin 12200, Germany

* Corresponding author.

E-mail address: Joachim.sieper@charite.de

Rheum Dis Clin N Am 38 (2012) 477–485
http://dx.doi.org/10.1016/j.rdc.2012.08.002 rheumatic.theclinics.com

diagnosis of AS, which is frequently reported to be between 5 and 10 years.[13] The main reasons for this are (1) the high prevalence of back pain in the population, (2) the lack of knowledge in a substantial proportion of general practitioners and orthopedic surgeons, and (3) the requirement of structural changes in the sacroiliac joints, which may last several years to become visible on conventional radiographs.[14]

The process of development of structural changes may take many years in some patients but this may be different in others: in one study, approximately 20% of patients with IBP for less than 2 years already had structural changes.[15,16] To clarify one issue of terminology: due to the known limitations of conventional radiography the term *radiographic sacroiliitis* reflects structural damage as the consequence of inflammation rather than active ongoing inflammation. Patients who do not (yet) fulfill this criterion have recently been named as having, *non-radiographic axSpA* (*nr-axSpA*)[17,18]—this is included in the ASAS classification criteria of axSpA (**Box 1**),[19] which addresses both patients with radiographic axSpA (AS) and those with nr-axSpA and in combination with peripheral SpA (perSpA) (**Box 2**),[20] which includes both patients with radiographic axSpA (AS) and those with nr-axSpA. These criteria for the first time allow patients with early and also with abortive forms of the disease to be classified.

Since the first definition of the leading clinical symptom in AS, IBP, in 1977,[21] it has been regarded as the most important clinical sign for the identification of patients with axSpA. Different sets of criteria have been proposed that have comparable sensitivity and specificity of approximately 80%.[11,12,22] They include morning stiffness, wakening up in the second half of the night because of back pain, and improvement by exercise but not by rest. Differences between the items may be relevant for referral because items behave differently when used in primary versus tertiary care.[17]

Box 1
ASAS classification criteria for axial spondyloarthritis (SpA, [19])

1. Patients must have had ≥3 months of back pain (with/without peripheral manifestations) and age at onset should have been <45 years.
2. In addition, there should be either sacroiliitis[a] on imaging plus ≥1 SpA feature or HLA-B27 needs to be positive plus ≥2 other SpA features

SpA features

- Iflammatory back pain (IBP)
- Arthritis
- Enthesitis (heel)
- Uveitis
- Dactylitis
- Psoriasis
- Crohn disease/ulcerative colitis
- Good response to non-steroidal anti-inflammatory drugs (NSAIDs)
- Family history for SpA
- HLA-B27
- Elevated C-reactive protein (CRP)

[a] Either by conventional radiographs according to the New York criteria[34] or by MRI according to the ASAS definition.[24]

Box 2
ASAS classification criteria for peripheral spondyloarthritis (SpA, [20])

1. Patients with peripheral manifestations only who have
2. Arthritis,[a] and/or enthesitis and/or dactylitis and in addition either
   a. ≥1 of these SpA features
      i. (Anterior) uveitis
      ii. Psoriasis
      iii. Crohn disease/ulcerative colitis
      iv. Preceding infection
      v. HLA-B27
      vi. Sacroiliitis on imaging

or

   b. ≥2 of these SpA features
      i. Arthritis
      ii. Enthesitis
      iii. Dactylitis
      iv. Inflammatory back pain (IBP) ever
      v. Family history of SpA

[a] Usually lower limb and/or asymmetric arthritis.

DIAGNOSIS AND CLASSIFICATION

The concept of SpA has been discussed since the publication by Moll and colleagues in 1974,[32] which appeared a year after the discovery of the association of AS with HLA-B27.[33] Thereafter, more proposals for classification have widened the spectrum of SpA.[34–36] The performance of the new classification criteria for SpA has recently been intensively discussed.[37] This article focuses on the consequences for the nomenclature and the diagnosis of SpA. Terminology and placement of the main groups and the subgroups are as follows:

(Predominant) axSpA
- nr-axSpA
- AS = radiographic axSpA
- Both can be associated with psoriasis and/or inflammatory bowel disease (IBD)

(Predominant) perSpA
- Psoriatic arthritis (PsA) and/or perSpA associated with psoriasis
- perSpA associated with IBD: type I and type II
- Reactive arthritis
- Undifferentiated perSpA

This proposal is further defined by the following statements and definitions:

The term, axSpA, covers both AS as defined by the 1984 New York criteria[34] and nr-axSpA as defined by the ASAS criteria.[19]

axSpA can be subdivided into 3 stages: nonradiographic stage I, stage II as defined by structural changes in the sacroiliac joints but no structural changes in the spine, and stage III as defined by structural changes in the spine. There is, however, no international agreement on this. The role of inflammatory changes in the spine requires further study. Late onset of SpA has been reported.[38]

The term, *undifferentiated*,[39] is no longer used for SpA patients with predominant axial involvement who have no structural changes in the axial skeleton. This subgroup is now named nr-axSpA. The authors believe this should also mean that there are no definite structural changes in the spine (syndesmophytes). There is currently no agreement, however, on this and patients with syndesmophytes are allowed to be included in trials with nr-axSpA patients (if they have no definite changes in the sacroiliac joints).

No further differentiation is made between primary axSpA and secondary axSpA, including AS. Cases of axSpA with concomitant psoriasis and/or chronic IBD are described as "in association with."

All patients with peripheral arthritis who have present or past psoriasis are named as having PsA, according to the Classification Criteria for Psoriatic Arthritis (CASPAR)[40]—unless their clinical presentation is typical for SpA.[41] Formally, the 2 definitions of PsA and/or perSpA associated with psoriasis could be differentiated by the ASAS explanation of arthritis, usually lower limb and/or asymmetric arthritis[20], versus the CASPAR definition[40], that a patient must have inflammatory articular disease (joint, spine, or entheseal). This should be handled liberally, however, because a precise definition of a cutoff does not seem to work practically. Therefore, the authors propose leaving the decision of terminology to rheumatologists, knowing that PsA is the most frequently used term. This term could be preferentially used for the patients with a clinical picture that is more reminiscent of rheumatoid arthritis. If arthritis of the lower limbs and/or enthesitis is the predominant feature, the term, *perSpA associated with psoriasis*, may be preferred. In patients with peripheral symptoms suggestive of SpA who have a history of psoriasis, the term, *perSpA associated with psoriasis*, may be preferred. In cases of definite erosive or osteoproliferative changes, the old term, *PsA sine psoriase*, also seems ok. The authors also would not change the terminology for the synovitis, acne, pustolosis, hyperostosis, and osteitis (SAPHO) syndrome.[42]

Osteodestructive changes in peripheral joints occur mainly in PsA and AS but also may rarely occur in other subtypes.

Peripheral arthritis associated with IBD can be subdivided into types I and II, as proposed several years ago.[43]

Reactive arthritis is diagnosed mainly in patients with a clinically convincing preceding infection in the urogenital tract, enteral tract, or respiratory tract—unless a significant change in antibody titers or a positive polymerase chain reaction result for *Chlamydia* is available either from synovial fluid or a smear from the urogenital tract.[44] IBP may occur after reactive arthritis but is a rare event.[45]

In cases of joint pain and/or entheseal pain in patients with a suspicion of SpA based on clinical symptoms laboratory assessments, CRP and HLA-B27 should be performed, and imaging results, obtained by MRI, ultrasound, or, in special cases, scintigraphy, may be needed to make a diagnosis. In case of positive findings these patients can be classified as (undifferentiated) perSpA.

Which patients could potentially be diagnosed as axSpA who do not fulfill the ASAS classification criteria for axSpA?

Patients with predominant axial symptoms

- With <3 months back pain
- With an age at onset >45 years
- With evidence of sacroiliitis on imaging but without ≥1 SpA feature
- Without evidence of sacroiliitis on imaging but with ≥1 SpA feature
- With HLA-B27+ but with <2 other SpA features
- Without HLA-B27+ but with ≥2 other SpA features
- Without
  - IBP
  - Arthritis
  - Heel enthesitis
  - (Anterior) uveitis
  - Dactylitis
  - Psoriasis
  - Crohn disease/colitis
  - Good response to NSAIDs
  - Family history of SpA
  - HLA-B27
  - Elevated CRP

With evidence of spondylitis (MRI)
With evidence of structural changes in the spine (syndesmophytes or ankylosis)
With a preceding infection

Which patients could potentially be diagnosed as perSpA who do not fulfill the ASAS classification criteria for perSpA?

Patients with peripheral manifestations only

- With arthritis and/or enthesitis and/or dactylitis but not ≥1 SpA features (uveitis, psoriasis, Crohn disease/colitis, preceding infection, HLA-B27)
- With arthritis, enthesitis, or dactylitis but not ≥2 SpA features (arthritis, enthesitis, dactylitis, family history for SpA, sacroiliitis on imaging)
- Without arthritis, enthesitis, or dactylitis but ≥1 SpA features (uveitis, psoriasis, Crohn disease/colitis, preceding infection, HLA-B27)
- Without arthritis but enthesitis or dactylitis plus ≥1 SpA features (uveitis, psoriasis, Crohn disease/colitis, preceding infection, HLA-B27)
- Without enthesitis arthritis or dactylitis plus ≥1 SpA features (uveitis, psoriasis, Crohn disease/colitis, preceding infection, HLA-B27)
- Without dactylitis but arthritis or enthesitis plus ≥2 SpA features (arthritis, enthesitis, dactylitis, family history for SpA, sacroiliitis on imaging)
- With pain at/around joints and/or entheses plus any signs of SpA
- With spondylitis on imaging (MRI) only
- With definite structural changes in peripheral joints
- With definite structural changes in the spine

These lists may be incomplete but presumably they cover the spectrum of SpA. They mark the difference between classification and diagnostic criteria in SpA. Because the classification criteria have been extensively tested, approximately 20% of the patients who have undergone the process of classification for SpA have either false-positive or false-negative results. Thus, the best strategy in daily clinical practice is to work on the basis of classification criteria but to give a reason when a diagnosis of SpA is made when the classification criteria are not fulfilled.

REFERRAL

Based on the classification criteria, several proposals have been made as to how to diagnose axSpA patients early in the course of the disease.[23] Inflammatory changes in the subchondral bone marrow (osteitis) of the sacroiliac joints are important in this regard,[24] whereas the role of spinal inflammation[25] is less clear in this early stage of the disease. The interpretation of conventional radiographs and MRI can be difficult. Often, an experienced rheumatologist or radiologist is needed for proper interpretation. Therefore, many experts discourage the extensive use of imaging in primary care.[26]

An early referral from primary care to a rheumatologist is important for several reasons but it is not clear how this is best managed. Based on early data from the United Kingdom, the authors believe that axSpA can be identified as a cause of chronic back pain in only approximately 5% of patients presenting with chronic back pain to general practitioners.[27] Thus, Which parameters should be taught to physicians in primary care that are easy to use and result in an acceptable rate of patients referred to the rheumatologist who end up diagnosed as axSpA?

More than 2000 patients have been included in referral studies in past years.[17,28–31] The most important conclusions are

1. A consistent percentage of 30% to 40% of patients received a final diagnosis of axSpA using different referral strategies in many countries in several parts of the world. Thus, referral strategies for an earlier diagnosis of axSpA seem effective.
2. Using IBP as a single referral parameter seems to work and many referring physicians seem to have chosen this as their main signaling tool, but there was large disagreement between referring physicians and rheumatologists about the true rate of IBP.
3. In comparison, HLA-B27 positivity performs better than IBP as a referral parameter, but in comparison to IBP it is less often used as a referral parameter.
4. A higher number of referral parameters may perform better than just one but this was only tested against IBP alone.
5. A simple set of referral parameters was at least as good as a more complicated set and should, therefore, be preferred.
6. nr-axSpA is an important subgroup among newly diagnosed axSpA patients, with a proportion close to 50% of patients, depending on the setting of the study.

REFERENCES

1. Braun J, Sieper J. Ankylosing spondylitis. Lancet 2007;369:1379–90.
2. Haibel H, Rudwaleit M, Listing J, et al. Efficacy of adalimumab in the treatment of axial spondyloarthritis without radiographically defined sacroiliitis: results of a 12-week, randomized controlled trial followed by an open-label extension up to week fifty-two. Arthritis Rheum 2008;58:1981–91.
3. Barkham N, Keen HI, Coates LC, et al. Clinical and imaging efficacy of infliximab in HLA-B27-positive patients with magnetic resonance imaging determined early sacroiliitis. Arthritis Rheum 2009;60:946–54.
4. Song IH, Hermann K, Haibel H, et al. Effects of etanercept versus sulfasalazine in early axial spondyloarthritis on active inflammatory lesions as detected by whole-body MRI (ESTHER): a 48-week randomised controlled trial. Ann Rheum Dis 2011;70:590–6.
5. Rudwaleit M, Schwarzlose S, Hilgert ES, et al. Magnetic Resonance Imaging (MRI) in predicting a major clinical response to anti-TNF-treatment in ankylosing spondylitis. Ann Rheum Dis 2008;67(9):1276–81.

6. Baraliakos X, Listing J, Fritz C, et al. Persistent clinical efficacy and safety of infliximab in ankylosing spondylitis after 8 years—early clinical response predicts long-term outcome. Rheumatology (Oxford) 2011;50(9):1690–9.
7. Vastesaeger N, van der Heijde D, Inman RD, et al. Predicting the outcome of ankylosing spondylitis therapy. Ann Rheum Dis 2011;70(6):973–81.
8. Wanders A, Heijde D, Landewé R, et al. Nonsteroidal antiinflammatory drugs reduce radiographic progression in patients with ankylosing spondylitis: a randomized clinical trial. Arthritis Rheum 2005;52(6):1756–65.
9. Kroon F, Landewé R, Dougados M, et al. Continuous NSAID use reverts the effects of inflammation on radiographic progression in patients with ankylosing spondylitis. Ann Rheum Dis 2012. [Epub ahead of print].
10. Poddubnyy D, Rudwaleit M, Haibel H, et al. Effect of non-steroidal anti-inflammatory drugs on radiographic spinal progression in patients with axial spondyloarthritis: results from the German Spondyloarthritis Inception Cohort. Ann Rheum Dis 2012. [Epub ahead of print].
11. Rudwaleit M, Metter A, Listing J, et al. Inflammatory back pain in ankylosing spondylitis: a reassessment of the clinical history for application as classification and diagnostic criteria. Arthritis Rheum 2006;54:569–78.
12. Braun J, Inman R. Clinical significance of inflammatory back pain for diagnosis and screening of patients with axial spondyloarthritis. Ann Rheum Dis 2010; 69(7):1264–8.
13. Feldtkeller E, Khan MA, van der Heijde D, et al. Age at disease onset and diagnosis delay in HLA-B27 negative vs positive patients with ankylosing spondylitis. Rheumatol Int 2003;23:61–6.
14. Mau W, Zeidler H, Mau R, et al. Evaluation of early diagnostic criteria for ankylosing spondylitis in a 10 year follow-up. Z Rheumatol 1990;49:82–7.
15. Heuft-Dorenbosch L, Landewé R, Weijers R, et al. Combining information obtained from magnetic resonance imaging and conventional radiographs to detect sacroiliitis in patients with recent onset inflammatory back pain. Ann Rheum Dis 2006;65(6):804–8.
16. van Onna M, Jurik AG, van der Heijde D, et al. HLA-B27 and gender independently determine the likelihood of a positive MRI of the sacroiliac joints in patients with early inflammatory back pain: a 2-year MRI follow-up study. Ann Rheum Dis 2011;70(11):1981–5.
17. Braun A, Saracbasi E, Grifka J, et al. Identifying patients with axial spondyloarthritis in primary care: how useful are items indicative of inflammatory back pain? Ann Rheum Dis 2011;70:1782–7.
18. Kiltz U, Baraliakos X, Karakostas P, et al. Patients with non-radiographic axial spondyloarthritis differ from patients with ankylosing spondylitis in several aspects. Arthritis Care Res (Hoboken) 2012. http://dx.doi.org/10.1002/acr.21688.
19. Rudwaleit M, van der Heijde D, Landewe R, et al. The development of Assessment of SpondyloArthritis international Society classification criteria for axial spondyloarthritis (part II): validation and final selection. Ann Rheum Dis 2009; 68:777–83.
20. Rudwaleit M, van der Heijde D, Landewe R, et al. The Assessment of SpondyloArthritis international Society classification criteria for peripheral spondyloarthritis and for spondyloarthritis in general. Ann Rheum Dis 2011;70:25–31.
21. Calin A, Porta J, Fries JF, et al. Clinical history as a screening test for ankylosing spondylitis. JAMA 1977;237:2613–4.
22. Sieper J, van der Heijde D, Landewe R, et al. New criteria for inflammatory back pain in patients with chronic back pain: a real patient exercise by experts from the

Assessment of SpondyloArthritis international Society (ASAS). Ann Rheum Dis 2009;68:784–8.

23. Rudwaleit M, van der Heijde D, Khan MA, et al. How to diagnose axial spondyloarthritis early. Ann Rheum Dis 2004;63:535–43.
24. Rudwaleit M, Jurik AG, Hermann KG, et al. Defining active sacroiliitis on magnetic resonance imaging (MRI) for classification of axial spondyloarthritis: a consensual approach by the ASAS/OMERACT MRI group. Ann Rheum Dis 2009;68:1520–7.
25. Hermann KG, Baraliakos X, van der Heijde DM, et al, On behalf of the assessment in SpondyloArthritis international Society (ASAS). Descriptions of spinal MRI lesions and definition of a positive MRI of the spine in axial spondyloarthritis: a consensual approach by the ASAS/OMERACT MRI study group. Ann Rheum Dis 2012;71(8):1278–88.
26. Sieper J, Rudwaleit M. Early referral recommendations for ankylosing spondylitis (including preradiographic and radiographic forms) in primary care. Ann Rheum Dis 2005;64:659–63.
27. Underwood MR, Dawes P. Inflammatory back pain in primary care. Br J Rheumatol 1995;34:1074–7.
28. Brandt HC, Spiller I, Song IH, et al. Performance of referral recommendations in patients with chronic back pain and suspected axial spondyloarthritis. Ann Rheum Dis 2007;66:1479–84.
29. Poddubnyy D, Vahldiek J, Spiller I, et al. Evaluation of 2 screening strategies for early identification of patients with axial spondyloarthritis in primary care. J Rheumatol 2011;38:2452–60.
30. Hermann J, Giessauf H, Schaffler G, et al. Early spondyloarthritis: usefulness of clinical screening. Rheumatology (Oxford) 2009;48:812–6.
31. Sieper J, Srinivasan S, Zamani O, et al. Comparing 2 referral strategies to diagnose axial spondyloarthritis: RADAR study. Ann Rheum Dis 2011;70(Suppl 3):81.
32. Moll JM, Haslock I, Macrae IF, et al. Associations between ankylosing spondylitis, psoriatic arthritis, Reiter's disease, the intestinal arthropathies, and Behcet's syndrome. Medicine (Baltimore) 1974;53:343–64.
33. Brewerton DA, Hart FD, Nicholls A, et al. Ankylosing spondylitis and HL-A 27. Lancet 1973;1(7809):904–7.
34. van der Linden S, Valkenburg HA, Cats A. Evaluation of diagnostic criteria for ankylosing spondylitis. A proposal for modification of the New York criteria. Arthritis Rheum 1984;27:361–8.
35. Amor B, Dougados M, Mijiyawa M. Criteria of the classification of spondylarthropathies. Rev Rhum Mal Osteoartic 1990;57:85–9.
36. Dougados M, van der Linden S, Juhlin R, et al. The European Spondylarthropathy Study Group preliminary criteria for the classification of spondylarthropathy. Arthritis Rheum 1991;34:1218–27.
37. van Tubergen A, Weber U. Diagnosis and classification in spondyloarthritis: identifying a chameleon. Nat Rev Rheumatol 2012;8(5):253–61.
38. Olivieri I, Padula A, Pierro A, et al. Late onset undifferentiated seronegative spondyloarthropathy. J Rheumatol 1995;22:899–903.
39. Zochling J, Brandt J, Braun J. The current concept of spondyloarthritis with special emphasis on undifferentiated spondyloarthritis. Rheumatology (Oxford) 2005;44(12):1483–91.
40. Taylor W, Gladman D, Helliwell P, et al, CASPAR Study Group. Classification criteria for psoriatic arthritis: development of new criteria from a large international study. Arthritis Rheum 2006;54(8):2665–73.

41. van den Berg R, van Gaalen F, van der Helm-van Mil A, et al. Performance of classification criteria for peripheral spondyloarthritis and psoriatic arthritis in the Leiden early arthritis cohort. Ann Rheum Dis 2012;71(8):1366–9.
42. Magrey M, Khan MA. New insights into synovitis, acne, pustulosis, hyperostosis, and osteitis (SAPHO) syndrome. Curr Rheumatol Rep 2009;11(5):329–33.
43. Orchard TR, Wordsworth BP, Jewell DP. Peripheral arthropathies in inflammatory bowel disease: their articular distribution and natural history. Gut 1998;42(3):387–91.
44. Braun J, Kingsley G, van der Heijde D, et al. On the difficulties of establishing a consensus on the definition of and diagnostic investigations for reactive arthritis. Results and discussion of a questionnaire prepared for the 4th International Workshop on Reactive Arthritis, Berlin, Germany, July 3–6, 1999. J Rheumatol 2000;27(9):2185–92.
45. Laasila K, Laasonen L, Leirisalo-Repo M. Antibiotic treatment and long prognosis of reactive arthritis. Ann Rheum Dis 2003;62(7):655–8.

Inflammatory Back Pain

Rubén Burgos-Vargas, MD[a,b,*], Jürgen Braun, MD[c]

KEYWORDS

- Inflammatory back pain • Back pain • Spondyloarthritis • Ankylosing spondylitis

KEY POINTS

- The characteristics of back pain in patients with AS and axSpA include nocturnal pain and improvement with exercise, but not with rest in most cases.
- Several sets of criteria for the identification of IBP have been developed.
- Several characteristics of IBP have been essential in the classification of AS and axSpA.
- In some cases, the differentiation of IBP and non-inflammatory back pain is sometimes difficult.

INTRODUCTION

Low back pain (LBP), a subcategory of back pain (BP), refers to the lumbar segment of the spinal column and is one of the most common musculoskeletal complaints of human beings. It is also a common reason for medical visits in the United States.[1,2] Approximately 80% of the population has at least 1 episode of acute LBP at some time in a lifetime[3,4] that sometimes leads to medical consultation. Many patients, however, do not seem to seek medical care[5] and the majority of those attending primary care do not receive a specific diagnosis,[6–8] which has given rise to the term, *nonspecific LBP*.

LBP is classified as chronic when symptoms last for more than 3 months. The prevalence of chronic LBP in the population is lower than that of acute LBP and often depends on age; gender; mechanical factors, such as heavy or unusual load activities; pathologic conditions, such as musculoligamentous sprains and strains; herniated disks and spondylolistesis; and even psychosocial factors. Primary care physicians, orthopedic surgeons, and chiropractors take care of most patients with acute and chronic LBP. Regardless of treatment, greater than 90% have complete relief of their BP within 6 weeks.[2,9]

[a] Department of Rheumatology, Hospital General de México Eduardo Liceaga, Dr Balmis 148, México DF 06720, Mexico; [b] Faculty of Medicine, Universidad Nacional Autónoma de México, Mexico DF, México; [c] Rheumazentrum Ruhrgebiet, Landgrafenstrasse 15, D-44652, Herne and Ruhr-University, Bochum, Germany
* Corresponding author.
E-mail address: burgosv@prodigy.net.mx

Rheum Dis Clin N Am 38 (2012) 487–499
http://dx.doi.org/10.1016/j.rdc.2012.08.014 **rheumatic.theclinics.com**
0889-857X/12/$ – see front matter

The interest of rheumatologists in LBP is primarily from the identification of patients with rheumatic diseases, in particular those related to inflammatory arthritides affecting the spine and sacroiliac joints, such as ankylosing spondylitis (AS). AS is now part of a larger spectrum of spondyloarthritides (SpAs), and the whole subset is named, *axial SpAs (axSpAs)*. The term covers AS and the nonradiographic form that is defined by the absence of structural changes. This article concentrates largely on AS, because most of the published studies have used AS criteria. Knowledge of the signs and symptoms that distinguish the inflammatory involvement of the spine from that of noninflammatory—mainly mechanical—conditions is fundamental for the identification of patients with AS and other SpAs in clinics. BP is also seen in rheumatic diseases, such as osteoarthritis, osteoporosis, and rheumatoid arthritis.

Regarding localization, the involvement of the spine in patients with AS and other SpAs is usually not limited to the lumbar region; rather, it extends from the sacroiliac joints up to the thoracic, lumbar, and cervical segments. Instead of LBP—the term most commonly used for the group of mechanical, noninflammatory conditions—the involvement of the spine in patients with AS is usually referred as *inflammatory back pain (IBP)*.

CONCEPT DEVELOPMENT

Conceptually, IBP consists of a group of symptoms either present or absent, representing the most important characteristic clinical features of spinal and sacroiliac involvement in patients with AS and axSpAs. IBP is neither a complaint nor a symptom but a group of positive and negative variables. The most relevant characteristics of IBP were described approximately in the 1950s by several investigators.[10–12] Hart and colleagues[10] and Wilkinson and Bywaters[12] recognized the role of physical rest and physical activity on BP in patients with AS. For example, in their study of 202 patients with AS, Wilkinson and Bywaters[12] described, "most patients with a spinal onset noticed definite aggravation of the pain after resting, pain and stiffness being most marked on rising from bed and again after reclining in an armchair in the evening. Many found relief after activity, and a few found it necessary to get out of bed during the night to 'limber up' before completing their night's rest." They also noticed, "many, including some with quiescent disease, found that their pain was aggravated by heavy exertion or by jolting the spine." Hart and colleagues[10] had previously described something similar: "A frequent feature of the pain and stiffness was the aggravation caused by immobility. Waking in the morning stiff and in pain, the patient gradually became more supple during the day, feeling at his best from the afternoon until bedtime."

Such clinical features were acknowledged and, therefore, included in the 1961 Rome criteria for the diagnosis of AS.[13] Two of 5 clinical criteria referred to "Low back pain and stiffness for more than 3 months which is not relieved by rest" and "Pain and stiffness in the thoracic region." The 1966 New York[14] revision of Rome's criteria[13] which resulted in the New York criteria for AS[14] changed those two parameters to one: "History or the presence of pain at the dorso-lumbar junction or in the lumbar spine." This simplification process eliminated the 2 most important features of IBP and reduced the specificity of the New York criteria. van der Linden and colleagues[15] analyzed the diagnostic value of the Rome criteria[13] and the New York criteria[14] in patients with AS, first-degree relatives (with and without sacroiliitis and with and without HLA-B27), and healthy controls (with and without HLA-B27) and proposed modifying the latter by reincorporating "Low back pain and stiffness for more than 3 months which improves with exercise, but is not relieved by rest."

IBP was also important for the recognition of the SpAs as a group. The involvement of the axial skeleton in Amor and colleagues' article[16] refers to "lumbar or dorsal pain during the night, or morning stiffness of lumbar or dorsal spine"—which does not mention other features of IBP—and "buttock pain if affecting alternately the right or the left buttock." The European Spondyloarthropathy Study Group (ESSG) criteria[17] refer to "inflammatory spinal pain" affecting the back, dorsal, or cervical region, as defined by the presence of 4 out of 5 criteria proposed by Calin and colleagues[18] in 1977—these were the first data based study on IBP.

Today, IBP is 1 of the clinical parameters for the classification of axSpA[19] and peripheral SpA[20] proposed by the Assessment of SpondyloArthritis International Society (ASAS). The definition of IBP for axSpA corresponds to the ASAS definition of IBP[21] whereas that for peripheral SpA refers to IBP in the past "according to the rheumatologist's judgment." axSpA also includes "buttock pain alternating between right and left gluteal areas" in reference to axial involvement.

THE RECOGNITION OF PATIENTS WITH IBP

One of the initial steps in the identification of patients with AS or SpAs who complain of BP is the identification of IBP features. For that reason, clinicians have developed some sets of criteria and tools for the classification and diagnosis of IBP.[18,21–23] Their diagnostic value—sensitivity as well as specificity and likelihood ratio (LR)—has been determined in various clinical settings in patients with AS, SpAs, or other diseases and in healthy individuals.

Calin and colleagues[18] developed 17 questions addressing the characteristics of BP as well as 1 each on familial aggregation, age at onset, physician consultation, and past radiographic studies for screening patients with nonspecific causes of BP and to identify those with possible AS. These questions were tested in HLA-B27–positive AS as well as in HLA-B27–negative patients with normal sacroiliac joints from an orthopedic clinic and in healthy controls. A positive response to 4 of 5 specific questions allowed the differentiation of AS BP and nonspecific BP with 95% sensitivity and 85% specificity (**Box 1**). Yet, in other studies, sensitivity was as low as 23% and 38% and specificity 75%.[15,24–26] Despite these later findings, Calin and colleagues' criteria had been widely used in clinical and epidemiologic studies.

Rudwaleit and colleagues[22] developed a set of criteria for IBP, which included some changes to Calin and colleagues'[18] criteria, specifically patient's maximum age, the addition of 2 parameters (morning stiffness and improvement with exercise), and the removal of 2 other parameters (duration of symptoms and insidious onset) (**Box 2**). Another major difference is that the criteria set tested required that patients

Box 1
Screening test for ankylosing spondylitis[a]

Age of onset less than 40 years

Insidious onset

Duration of at least 3 months

Association with morning stiffness

Improvement with exercise

[a] Calin and colleagues' criteria for inflammatory BP.[18]

Box 2
Proposed new criteria for inflammatory back pain in young to middle-aged adults (50 years old) with chronic back pain and application as classification and diagnostic criteria[a]

1. Morning stiffness of ≤30 minutes' duration
2. Improvement in BP with exercise but not with rest
3. Awakening because of BP during the second half of the night only
4. Alternating buttock pain

[a] Berlin criteria for inflammatory BP.[22]

must have chronic BP and be less than 45 years old at onset. When intended for IBP classification, the presence of at least 2 parameters raises the sensitivity to 70.3%, the specificity to 81.2%, and the positive LR to 3.7. For IBP diagnosis, the presence of at least 3 parameters yields low sensitivity (33.6%) but high specificity (97.3%) and positive LR (12.4). If none of the parameters is present, sensitivity lowers to 10.9%, specificity to 57.1%, and positive LR to 0.25.

The diagnostic value of IBP as a unique manifestation of SpA (using 75% sensitivity, 76% specificity, 3.1 positive LR, and 0.33 negative LR) is markedly increased when HLA-B27 and MRI of the sacroiliac joints are positive (90% sensitivity and specificity, 9 positive LR, and 0.11 negative LR). The combination of IBP with other SpA features, specifically those listed in Amor and colleagues'[16] or ESSG[17] criteria, yields variations in the diagnostic properties of the Berlin criteria.

The ASAS set of criteria for IBP resulted from an exercise with real cases in which 13 experts determined whether 20 patients with BP of diverse causes had IBP or not.[21] Thus, 8 items related to IBP were assessed and considered positive or negative by each expert. According to the experts' opinion, 61 of 109 (56%) judgments on the nature of BP corresponded to IBP. The concordance rate of global judgment on the presence or absence of IBP was 0.83. Except for BP duration greater than 3 months, the frequency of age at onset greater than 40 years, insidious onset, morning stiffness of the back, improvement with exercise, no improvement with rest, alternating buttock pain, and pain at night with improvement on getting out of bed were significantly higher in the group of patients judged with IBP versus those with non-IBP. The final set of IBP parameters in ASAS proposal included those that in the logistic regression analysis were independently contributory to IBP (**Box 3**).

Weisman and colleagues[23] developed an ascertainment tool for the identification of patients with AS based on the presence of IBP among patients with chronic BP. The

Box 3
Inflammatory back pain parameters, according to experts[a]

1. Age at onset, 40 years
2. Insidious onset
3. Improvement with exercise
4. No improvement with rest
5. Pain at night (with improvement on getting up)

[a] ASAS expert criteria for IBP.[21]

first phase of the study included a literature review in search of potential items as well as their selection of by board members and finally the item generation by focus groups of patients with AS according to disease duration. The next phases included a feasibility study of the tool in AS and chronic BP patients, item reduction, and tool validation in 145 patients with AS and 308 patients with chronic BP. The final version of the tool included 12 items with which investigators expect to identify patients with AS in early stages of the disease (**Box 4**). Two of these items refer to symptoms on non-IBP, mechanical complaints that might exclude the diagnosis of IBP.

In addition, Braun and colleagues[27] identified which clinical parameters were predictive for a diagnosis of axSpA in patients with chronic BP presenting in primary care. For a diagnosis of axSpA, the items, age at onset less than or equal to 35 years, improvement by exercise, improvement with nonsteroidal anti-inflammatory drugs, waking up in the second half of the night, and alternating buttock pain, had 47.8% sensitivity, 86.1% specificity (area under the curve [AUC] 71.3%), positive LR of 3.4, and negative LR of 0.6. For the diagnosis of AS, greater than or equal to 3 criteria had a sensitivity of 57.4%, specificity of 85.6% (AUC 75.7%), positive LR of 4.0, and negative LR of 0.5. Finally, for a diagnosis of nonradiographic SpA, the presence of greater than or equal to 1 criterion had a sensitivity of 81.8%, specificity of 35.9% (AUC 64.9%), positive LR of 1.3, and negative LR of 0.5. Morning stiffness was irrelevant as a parameter indicating axSpA in primary care. These data indicate which parameters could be useful for identifying patients with axSpA, AS, and nonradiographic SpA in primary care settings.

INFLAMMATORY VERSUS NONINFLAMMATORY MECHANICAL BP

The differentiation of IBP from noninflammatory mechanical BP is often difficult, particularly in the community, primary care clinics, and certain age groups, specifically children and adolescents and older people. As discussed previously, the classification and diagnosis of BP according to IBP criteria depend on the number of items met by an individual with BP. None of the IBP criteria existing thus far[18,21–23,27] have proposed a list of clinical situations that may exclude the classification and diagnosis of IBP.

Box 4
Case ascertainment tool for ankylosing spondylitis[a]

What is your gender?

Have you experienced pain or stiffness that lasted for at least 3 months?

Approximately how old were you when you first had pain or stiffness in your back that lasted for at least 3 months?

Approximately how long have you had BP or stiffness?

Have you felt numbness or tingling that spread into or down you leg(s) that you think or have been told might have been caused by your back or stiffness?

Is the pain or stiffness due to fall, sprain, or other incidents, such as twisting or lifting?

How does exercise affect the pain or stiffness in your lower back or buttocks?

How does daily physical activity affect the pain or stiffness in you lower back or buttocks?

Do you take any nonsteroidal antinflammatory drug(s)?

Have you been diagnosed with iritis?

[a] Please see Weisman and colleagues[23] for response categories and scoring algorithm.

Weisman and colleagues[23] approached that problem by including 2 answers related to noninflammatory BP. Alternatively, some studies, including one recently performed in primary care, found low negative LR, suggesting good performance of the criteria.[21–23,27]

Overlap of inflammatory and noninflammatory mechanical BP symptoms occurs and the lack of exclusion criteria might favor the number of false-positive IBP individuals. A survey in an industrial complex found BP in 1880 (65%) employees,[25] identifying 491 (26.1%) fulfilling greater than or equal to 4 of 5 of Calin and colleagues'[18] criteria but only 12 cases with AS.

Walker and Williamson[28] conducted a survey among both orthopedically and neurosurgically trained spine surgeons, rheumatologists, medical practitioners with a special interest in musculoskeletal medicine, chiropractors, and manipulative physiotherapists to determine the signs and symptoms that could differentiate inflammatory and mechanical LBP. Participants had to rate 27 signs and symptoms (26 generated by the investigators) on an 11-point semantic differential scale from strongly disagree (0) to strongly agree[10] regarding their association with mechanical or inflammatory LBP. The item, morning pain on waking, had the highest level of agreement as an indicator of ILBP, whereas constant pain, pain that wakes, and stiffness after resting showed moderate agreement. Regarding mechanical LBP, pain when lifting showed the highest level of agreement whereas intermittent pain during the day, pain that develops later in the day, pain on standing for a while, pain bending forward a little, pain on trunk flexion or extension, pain doing a sit-up, pain when driving long distances, pain getting out of a chair, and pain on repetitive bending, running, coughing or sneezing were considered moderate indicators of mechanical LBP. Based on such questions, Riksman and colleagues[29] developed the Mechanical and Inflammatory Low Back Pain Scale to distinguish the 2 conditions. Tested in LBP patients attending chiropractic clinics, the scale distinguished 6 patients with inflammatory LBP, 5 with mechanical LBP, and 39 (78%) with mixed symptoms. A community-based study of the prevalence of AS in Norway[30] showed that most patients with AS gave positive responses to 3 questions related to IBP (2 on BP chronicity and 1 stiffness), yet several non-AS individuals responded in the same way. Based on such findings, Gran[25] identified the clinical features—mostly related to IBP—allowing differentiation of patients with AS from non-AS individuals, but he did not calculated their sensitivity and specificity.

Overlaps of IBP and non-IBP symptoms may also occur in specific age-group populations. The identification of IBP in adolescents with SpAs complaining of BP is often difficult.[31] Most patients have both inflammatory and mechanical signs and symptoms at some time during the course of the disease. Many of these patients report pain relief with both spinal exercises and rest; alternatively, they often deny having pain at night but only some spinal stiffness when waking up. Alternatively, 2 recent studies in the US[32,33] have reported a high prevalence of IBP and SpAs, according to different sets of criteria, in individuals between 50 and 69 years. The prevalence rates of IBP in 1915 individuals in that age group (representing 37.5% of the total sample) were 4.1% and 5.0%, according to Calin and colleagues'[18] and the ESSG criteria,[17] respectively. The age at IBP onset in 258 (26.6%) individuals of 980 with IBP occurred at greater than 45 years of age. The prevalence of SpAs in the same age group was 1.5% and 1.4% according to Amor and colleagues[16] and the ESSG[17] criteria. None of these studies analyzed the characteristics of IBP according to age. More importantly, none of them searched for alternative conditions, specifically noninflammatory mechanical conditions affecting the spine or sacroiliac joints in those age groups. It is in these situations in which clear methods to distinguish IBP from non-IBP are needed.

THE VALUE OF IBP IN THE CLASSIFICATION AND DIAGNOSIS OF AXSPA

Today, some studies suggest that the recognition of AS and axSpA through the identification of IBP is less important than previously thought. Retrospective studies of patients with undifferentiated SpA have shown that most patients evolving to AS have not isolated axial involvement but peripheral signs and symptoms either accompanied or not by spondylitis and sacroiliitis.[34–43] Peripheral involvement is more notorious in juvenile-onset patients[31,44–52] and patients with late-onset SpA.[53–56]

In contrast, prospective studies include a predominant proportion of patients with axial symptoms. This is a selection bias because most cohorts focused on early disease include patients with IBP, chronic BP, axSpA, and preradiographic AS. In brief, the Maastricht Early Spondyloarthritis Clinic (ESPAC)[57] included patients with IBP,[18] Brandt and colleagues'[58] study included patients younger than 45 years with chronic BP, the Leeds IBP clinic[59] included patients with IBP,[18] the German Spondyloarthritis Inception Cohort (GESPIC)[60] included patients with axSpA (nonradiographic SpA or radiographic sacroiliitis grades 0 or 1) whose disease duration was 2.6 ± 1.7 years and all patients had IBP, the DEvenir des Spondylarthropathies Indifférenciées Récentes (DESIR)[61] cohort included patients with IBP for greater than 3 months and less than 3 years, and the SPondyloArthritis Caught Early (SPACE) cohort[61] included patients with (almost daily) BP for greater than or equal to 3 months. Except for GESPIC[60] and DESIR,[62] other clinics[57,60,62] included patients with a maximum of 2 years of symptoms. As expected, a variable proportion of patients in each of those cohorts had AS at entry or developed AS throughout follow-up. Several predictors of axSpA and AS, however, were also found in some of such studies.[57–59,61,63–65] Prospective cohorts of patients with SpAs, according to Amor and colleagues[16] or the ESSG[17] criteria, show a variable proportion of patients with IBP.[66–68] The diagnostic value of IBP in patients without peripheral arthritis should be higher than in those patients presenting peripheral symptoms.

This information is coincident with that from some studies in regards to the importance given to IBP in the algorithm for the diagnosis of axSpA. Originally, Rudwaleit and colleagues[69] set the level of IBP just below BP and above all other clinical data of SpAs in an algorithm for the diagnosis of axSpA. The information needed to develop such an algorithm came from the literature. In the ASAS axSpA criteria,[19] IBP is neither an entry nor a major criterion. IBP is placed at the same level of most SpA characteristics. The rationale for that change was the low sensitivity level of such a parameter in the ASAS axSpA criteria development study.[70] This finding was later confirmed with data from the SPACE and ASAS cohorts.[61] When chronic BP, instead of IBP, was considered an obligatory entry criterion and the latter was only implemented as an additional SpA feature, the sensitivity of the Berlin algorithm for the diagnosis of axSpA[69] increased up to 78.5% and 79.6% in the SPACE and ASAS cohorts whereas the specificity levels remained at 79.6% and 75.6%.[61] This measure could increase the recognition of axSpA in young individuals with chronic BP in the absence of IBP.

THE ROLE AND PREVALENCE OF IBP IN THE COMMUNITY

In community studies, the identification of individuals with BP and then of those with IBP usually precedes the recognition of AS and SpAs (I. Pelaez-Ballestas and colleagues, 2012, unpublished data).[71–81] Thus, individuals with greater than or equal to 1 IBP feature are asked about the presence of additional clinical features and selected for radiographic studies of the sacroiliac joints and/or HLA-B27 testing. Variations on the prevalence of AS and SpAs among populations have been attributed to differences in the prevalence of HLA-B27 and methodologic approaches. Less attention, however, has been given to the methodology followed to identify individuals with IBP (ie, How was a specific set of criteria and each of its parameters investigated and rated?) and to exclude other causes of BP. It seems that the approach of IBP in most studies depends on the straight administration of a specific a questionnaire by trained personal. The role of an expert in assessing BP and recognizing IBP was part of the rationale of ASAS when developing the latest classification criteria for IBP.[21] The expert has to judge the presence or absence of IBP based on the information given by the patient as well as an expert's interpretation.

Data from a Mexican study on the prevalence of SpAs and IBP in the community support such an idea.[81] The expert assessment of 121 individuals with IBP diagnosed by general physicians and rheumatology fellows because of positive responses to the IBP Berlin questionnaire confirmed IBP in 52 (42.9%). Expert assessment included a careful investigation of the clinical signs and symptoms of BP and each of the Berlin criteria.[22] Although an experienced rheumatologist, questioned, discussed, and interpreted the information provided by patients without setting and time restrictions, general physicians and rheumatology fellows relied on straight questions and answers. The value of expert assessment in that study was the identification of IBP false-positive individuals in the community. Consequently, the prevalence of SpAs was lower but closer to reality. Weisman and colleagues[33] studied the prevalence of IBP in the United States with the same instrument and reported higher figures in Mexican-Americans than the Mexican study.[81] The diagnosis of IBP in the study performed by Weisman and colleagues[33] was based on the responses to the questionnaire administered by trained interviewers but not verified by any physician or experienced rheumatologist.

Regarding the prevalence of IBP in the community, Pelaez-Ballestas and colleagues (83) found 52 individuals with IBP among 4059 individuals, representing a prevalence of 1.3% (95% CI, 1.0%, 1.7%) in the Mexican population. The mean (SD) age was 39.9 (12.6) years and 51% of such individuals were men. Twenty-eight individuals had SpAs according to ESSG[17] criteria and 4 had AS.[15] The prevalence of IBP in the United States[32] was 5.0% (95% CI, 4.2%–5.8%) according to Calin and colleagues,[18] 5.6% (95% CI, 4.7%–6.5%) accorcing to ESSG,[17] and 6.0% (95% CI, 4.9%–7.1%) according to the Berlin[22] criteria. There were slightly more women (51.6%) than men (48.4%) as well as some variations according to age and ethnicity.

COROLLARY

IBP is a concept that has been defined by different sets of criteria throughout the years. The original rationale was early identification of patients with AS and today it is of axSpA. Along with the chronic nature of the complaint and the young age at onset, however, some basic items are part of all criteria sets proposed: improvement by movement and waking up at the second half of the night. The localization in the buttock is likely to differ according to gender and disease duration.

Several studies of referral strategies have indicated that the diagnostic tool for IBP has a different value for general practitioners and orthopedic surgeons than for rheumatologists—this is due to the different pretest likelihood of having axSpA in a general practitioner's (approximately 5%) versus a rheumatologist's office (25%). The only study that has directly compared various items indicative of IBP and axSpA has included a younger age at onset (<35 years) and improvement by NSAIDs. The inclusion of HLA-B27, however, in the analysis seems to change the performance of the clinical criteria (Braun, 2012, unpublished data submitted).

Box 5
Criteria for the recognition of axial spondyloarthritis in primary care[a]

1. Age at onset ≤35 years
2. Waking up in the second half of the night
3. Alternating buttock pain
4. Improvement by NSAIDs within 48 hours or no NSAIDs
5. Improvement by movement, not rest

[a] See Braun and colleagues[27] for each item's diagnostic values.

The term, *screening*, is inappropriate for early identification of patients with axSpA because it is not the normal population without symptoms that is being examined but patients with chronic BP. Thus, the management task is good referral strategies for young patients with chronic BP. One of the major questions is whether HLA-B27, instead of MRI should be determined in primary care in a more systematic way. The interpretation of radiographs and MRI of the sacroiliac joints, which are helpful diagnostic procedures,[81] should rely on the expertise of the physician in charge. Alternatively, using the new ASAS criteria, there is a possibility of false-positive classification (not all HLA-B27 positive patients with BP have axSpA). Low negative LRs, however, have been calculated, for example, for HLA-B27 patients with negative imaging results **Box 5**.

IBP is a valuable diagnostic tool with a different value in primary and secondary or tertiary care, rheumatologist needs a complete history of the patient (the more clinical items suggestive of SpA the more likely is the diagnosis) as well as imaging methods, mainly conventional radiographs, but also MRI, and in some cases computed tomography.

REFERENCES

1. Hart LG, Deyo RA, Cherkin DC. Physician office visits for low back pain. Frequency, clinical evaluation, and treatment patterns from a U.S. national survey. Spine 1995;20:11–9.
2. Deyo RA, Mirza SK, Martin BI. Back pain prevalence and visit rates: estimates from U.S. national surveys, 2002. Spine 2006;31:2724–7.
3. Walker BF. The prevalence of low back pain. A systematic review of the literature from 1966 to 1998. J Spinal Disord 2000;13:205–17.
4. Walker B, Muller R, Grant W. Low back pain in Australian adults. Prevalence and associated disability. J Manipulative Physiol Ther 2004;27:236–44.
5. Pengel LH, Herbert RD, Maher CG, et al. Acute low back pain: systematic review of its prognosis. BMJ 2003;327:323.
6. Deyo R, Rainville J, Kent D. What can the history and physical examination tell us about low back pain. JAMA 1992;268:760–5.
7. White AA, Gordon SL. Synopsis: workshop on idiopathic low-back pain. Spine 1982;7:141–9.
8. Nachemson A. The lumbar spine: an orthopedic challenge. Spine 1976;1:59–71.
9. Diamond S, Borenstein D. Chronic low back pain in a working-age adult [Review]. Best Pract Res Clin Rheumatol 2006;20:707–20.
10. Hart FD, Robinson KC, Allchin FM, et al. Ankylosing spondylitis. Q J Med 1949; 18:217–34.

11. Blumberg B, Ragan C. The natural history of rheumatoid spondylitis. Medicine (Baltimore) 1956;35:1–31.
12. Wilkinson M, Bywaters EG. Clinical features and course of ankylosing spondylitis; as seen in a follow-up of 222 hospital referred cases. Ann Rheum Dis 1958;17: 209–28.
13. Kellgren JH, Jeffrey MR, Ball J. The epidemiology of chronic rheumatism, vol. I. Oxford: Blackwell Scientific Publications; 1963. p. 326–7.
14. Bennett PH, Burch TA. Population studies of the rheumatic diseases. Amsterdam: Excerpta Medica Foundation; 1968. p. 456–7.
15. van der Linden S, Valkenburg HA, Cats A. Evaluation of diagnostic criteria for ankylosing spondylitis. A proposal for modification of the New York criteria. Arthritis Rheum 1984;27:361–8.
16. Amor B, Dougados M, Mijiyawa M. Critères des classification des spondylartropaties. Rev Rhum Mal Osteoartic 1990;57:85–9 [in French].
17. Dougados M, van der Linden S, Juhlin R, et al. The European spondylarthropathy study group preliminary criteria for the classification of spondylarthropathy. Arthritis Rheum 1991;34:1218–27.
18. Calin A, Porta J, Fries JF, et al. Clinical history as a screening test for ankylosing spondylitis. JAMA 1977;237:2613–4.
19. Rudwaleit M, van der Heijde D, Landewe R, et al. The development of assessment of spondyloarthritis international society classification criteria for axial spondyloarthritis (part II): validation and final selection. Ann Rheum Dis 2009;68(6):777–83.
20. Rudwaleit M, van der Heijde D, Landewe R, et al. The assessment of spondyloarthritis international society classification criteria for peripheral spondyloarthritis and for spondyloarthritis in general. Ann Rheum Dis 2011;70(1):25–31.
21. Sieper J, van der Heijde DM, Landewé RB, et al. New criteria for inflammatory back pain in patients with chronic back pain: a real patient exercise of the Assessment of SpondyloArthritis international Society (ASAS). Ann Rheum Dis 2009;68:784–8.
22. Rudwaleit M, Metter A, Listing J, et al. Inflammatory back pain in ankylosing spondylitis: a reassessment of the clinical history for application as classification and diagnostic criteria. Arthritis Rheum 2006;54:569–78.
23. Weisman MH, Chen L, Clegg DO, et al. Development and validation of a case ascertainment tool for ankylosing spondylitis. Arthritis Care Res (Hoboken) 2010;62(1):19–27, 2.
24. Calin A, Kaye B, Sternberg M, et al. The prevalence and nature of back pain in an industrial complex: a questionnaire and radiographic and HLA analysis. Spine 1980;5:201–5.
25. Gran JT. An epidemiological survey of the signs and symptoms of ankylosing spondylitis. Clin Rheumatol 1985;4:161–9.
26. Van der Linden SM, Fahrer H. Occurrence of spinal pain syndromes in a group of apparently healthy and physically fit sportsmen (orienteers). Scand J Rheumatol 1988;17:475–81.
27. Braun A, Saracbasi E, Grifka J, et al. Identifying patients with axial spondyloarthritis in primary care: how useful are items indicative. of inflammatory back pain? Ann Rheum Dis 2011;70:1782–7.
28. Walker BF, Williamson OD. Mechanical or inflammatory low back pain. What are the potential signs and symptoms? Man Ther 2009;14:314–20.
29. Riksman JS, Williamson OD, Walker BF. Delineating inflammatory and mechanical sub-types of low back pain: a pilot survey of fifty low back pain patients in a chiropractic setting. Chiropr Man Therap 2011;19:5.

30. Gran JT, Husby G, Hordvik M. Prevalence of ankylosing spondylitis in males and females in a young middle-aged population of Tromsø, northern Norway. Ann Rheum Dis 1985;44:359–67.
31. Burgos-Vargas R, Vázquez-Mellado J. The early clinical recognition of juvenile-onset ankylosing spondylitis and its differentiation from juvenile rheumatoid arthritis. Arthritis Rheum 1995;38:835–44.
32. Reveille JD, Witter JP, Weisman MH. Prevalence of axial spondylarthritis in the United States: estimates from a cross-sectional survey. Arthritis Care Res (Hoboken) 2012;64:905–10.
33. Weisman MH, Witter JP, Reveille JD. The prevalence of inflammatory back pain: population-based estimates from the US National Health and Nutrition Examination Survey, 2009-10. Ann Rheum Dis 2012. [Epub ahead of print].
34. Sany J, Rosenberg F, Panis G, et al. Unclassified HLA-B27 inflammatory rheumatic diseases: followup of 23 patients. Arthritis Rheum 1980;23:258–9.
35. Sambrook P, McGuigan L, Champion D, et al. Clinical features and followup study of HLA-B27 positive patients presenting with peripheral arthritis. J Rheumatol 1985;12:526–8.
36. Schattenkirchner M, Krüger K. Natural course and prognosis of HLA-B27-positive oligoarthritis. Clin Rheumatol 1987;6(Suppl 2):83–6.
37. Mau W, Zeidler H, Mau R, et al. Clinical features and prognosis of patients with possible ankylosing spondylitis. Results of a 10-year followup. J Rheumatol 1988;15:1109–14.
38. Collantes E, Veroz R, Escudero A, et al. Can some cases of 'possible' spondyloarthropathy be classified as 'definite' or 'undifferentiated' spondyloarthropathy? Value of criteria for spondyloarthropathies. Spanish Spondyloarthropathy study group. Joint Bone Spine 2000;67:516–20.
39. Kumar A, Bansal M, Srivastava DN, et al. Long-term outcome of undifferentiated spondylarthropathy. Rheumatol Int 2001;20:221–4.
40. Sampaio-Barros PD, Bertolo MB, Kraemer MH, et al. Undifferentiated spondyloarthropathies: a 2-year follow-up study. Clin Rheumatol 2001;20:201–6.
41. Huerta-Sil G, Casasola-Vargas JC, Londoño JD, et al. Low grade radiographic sacroiliitis as prognostic factor in patients with undifferentiated spondyloarthritis fulfilling diagnostic criteria for ankylosing spondylitis throughout follow up. Ann Rheum Dis 2006;65:642–6.
42. Sampaio-Barros P, Bortoluzzo AB, Conde RA, et al. Undifferentiated spondyloarthritis: a long-term follow-up. J Rheumatol 2010;37:1195–9.
43. Burgos-Vargas R, Casasola-Vargas JC. From retrospective analysis of patients with undifferentiated spondyloarthritis (SpA) to analysis of prospective cohorts and detection of axial and peripheral SpA. J Rheumatol 2010;37:1091–5.
44. Jacobs JC, Johnston AD, Berdon WE. HLA-B27 associated spondyloarthritis and enthesopathy in childhood: clinical, pathologic and radiographic observations in 58 patients. J Pediatr 1982;100:521–8.
45. Rosenberg AM, Petty RE. A syndrome of seronegative enthesopathy and arthropathy in children. Arthritis Rheum 1982;25:1041–7.
46. Hall MA, Burgos-Vargas R, Ansell BM. Sacroiliitis in juvenile chronic arthritis: a 10 year follow-up. Clin Exp Rheumatol 1987;5(Suppl):65–7.
47. Sheerin KA, Giannini EH, Brewer EJ. HLA-B27-associated arthropathy in childhood: long-term clinical and diagnostic outcome. Arthritis Rheum 1988;31:1165–70.
48. Burgos-Vargas R, Clark P. Axial involvement in the seronegative enthesopathy and arthropathy syndrome and its progression to ankylosing spondylitis. J Rheumatol 1989;16:192–7.

49. Cabral DA, Oen KG, Petty RE. SEA syndrome revisited: a long term followup of children with a syndrome of seronegative enthesopathy and arthropathy. J Rheumatol 1992;19:1282–5.
50. Olivieri I, Foto M, Ruju GP. Low frequency of axial involvement in caucasian pediatric patients with seronegative enthesopathy and arthropathy syndrome after 5 years of disease. J Rheumatol 1992;19(3):469–75.
51. Flato B, Smerdel A, Johnston V. The influence of patient characteristics, disease variables, and HLA alleles on the development of radiographically evident sacroiliitis in juvenile idiopathic arthritis. Arthritis Rheum 2002;46:986–94.
52. Burgos-Vargas R. The assessment of the spondyloarthritis international society concept and criteria for the classification of axial spondyloarthritis and peripheral spondyloarthritis: a critical appraisal for the pediatric rheumatologist. Pediatr Rheumatol Online J 2012;10:14.
53. Dubost JJ, Sauvezie B. Late onset peripheral spondyloarthropathy. J Rheumatol 1989;16:1214–7.
54. Olivieri I, Padula A, Pierro A, et al. Late onset undifferentiated seronegative spondyloarthropathy. J Rheumatol 1995;22:899–903.
55. Caplanne D, Tubach F, Le Parc JM. Late onset spondylarthropathy: clinical and biological comparison with early onset patients. Ann Rheum Dis 1997;56:176–9.
56. Olivieri I, Salvarani C, Cantini F, et al. Ankylosing spondylitis and undifferentiated spondyloarthropathies: a clinical review and description of a disease subset with older age at onset. Curr Opin Rheumatol 2001;13:280–4, 10.
57. Heuft-Dorenbosch L, Landewé R, Weijers R, et al. Performance of various criteria sets in patients with inflammatory back pain of short duration; the maastricht early spondyloarthritis clinic. Ann Rheum Dis 2007;66:92–8.
58. Brandt HC, Spiller I, Song IH, et al. Performance of referral recommendations in patients with chronic back pain and suspected axial spondyloarthritis. Ann Rheum Dis 2007;66:1479–84.
59. Bennett AN, McGonagle D, O'Connor P, et al. Severity of baseline magnetic resonance imaging-evident sacroiliitis and HLA-B27 status in early inflammatory back pain predict radiographically evident ankylosing spondylitis at eight years. Arthritis Rheum 2008;58:3413–8.
60. Rudwaleit M, Haibel H, Baraliakos X, et al. The early disease stage in axial spondylarthritis: results from the German spondyloarthritis inception cohort. Arthritis Rheum 2009;60:717–27.
61. van den Berg R, de Hooge M, Rudwaleit M, et al. Proposal for a modification of the Berlin Algorithm for diagnosing axial spondyloarthritis: results from the spondyloarthritis caught early (SPACE)-cohort and from the assessment of spondyloarthritis international society (ASAS)-cohort. Ann Rheum Dis (in press).
62. Dougados M, d'Agostino MA, Benessiano J, et al. The DESIR cohort: a 10-year follow-up of early inflammatory back pain in France: study design and baseline characteristics of the 708 recruited patients. Joint Bone Spine 2011;78:598–603.
63. Chung HY, Machado P, van der Heijde D, et al. HLA-B27 positive patients differ from HLA-B27 negative patients in clinical presentation and imaging: results from the DESIR cohort of patients with recent onset axial spondyloarthritis. Ann Rheum Dis 2011;70:1930–6.
64. Chung HY, Machado P, van der Heijde D, et al. Smokers in early axial spondyloarthritis have earlier disease onset, more disease activity, inflammation and damage, and poorer function and health-related quality of life: results from the DESIR cohort. Ann Rheum Dis 2012;71:809–16.

65. Poddubnyy D, Haibel H, Listing J, et al. Baseline radiographic damage, elevated acute-phase reactant levels, and cigarette smoking status predict spinal radiographic progression in early axial spondylarthritis. Arthritis Rheum 2012;64: 1388–98.
66. Muñoz-Fernández S, de Miguel E, Cobo-Ibáñez T, et al, ESPIDEP Study Group. Early spondyloarthritis: results from the pilot registry ESPIDEP. Clin Exp Rheumatol 2010;28:498–503.
67. Rojas-Vargas M, Muñoz-Gomariz E, Escudero A, et al, Registro Español de Espondiloartritis de la Sociedad Española de Reumatología Working Group. First signs and symptoms of spondyloarthritis—data from an inception cohort with a disease course of two years or less (REGISPONSER-Early). Rheumatology 2009;48:404–9.
68. Vazquez-Mellado J, Font P, Azevedo V, et al. Disease patterns in patients with spondyloarthropathies (SpA) from Iberoamérica (IBA): the respondia group report [abstract]. Ann Rheum Dis 2008;67(Suppl II):627.
69. Rudwaleit M, van der Heijde D, Khan MA, et al. How to diagnose axial spondyloarthritis early. Ann Rheum Dis 2004;63:535–43.
70. Rudwaleit M, Landewe R, van der Heijde D, et al. The development of assessment of spondyloarthritis international society classification criteria for axial spondyloarthritis (part I): classification of paper patients by expert opinion including uncertainty appraisal. Ann Rheum Dis 2009;68:770–6.
71. Saraux A, Guedes C, Allain J, et al. Prevalence of rheumatoid arthritis and spondyloarthropathy in Brittany, France. Société de Rhumatologie de l'Ouest. J Rheumatol 1999;26:2622–7.
72. Hukuda S, Minami M, Saito T, et al. Spondyloarthropathies in Japan: nationwide questionnaire survey performed by the Japan ankylosing spondylitis society. J Rheumatol 2001;28:554–9.
73. Bruges-Armas J, Lima C, Peixoto MJ, et al. Prevalence of spondyloarthritis in Terceira, Azores: a population based study. Ann Rheum Dis 2002;61:551–3.
74. Trontzas P, Andrianakos A, Miyakis S, et al, ESORDIG study group. Seronegative spondyloarthropathies in Greece: a population-based study of prevalence, clinical pattern, and management. The ESORDIG study. Clin Rheumatol 2005;24: 583–9.
75. Ng SC, Liao Z, Yu DT, et al. Epidemiology of spondyloarthritis in the People's Republic of China: review of the literature and commentary. Semin Arthritis Rheum 2007;37:39–47.
76. Onen F, Akar S, Birlik M, et al. Prevalence of ankylosing spondylitis and related spondyloarthritides in an urban area of Izmir, Turkey. J Rheumatol 2008;35:305–9.
77. Adomaviciute D, Pileckyte M, Baranauskaite A, et al. Prevalence survey of rheumatoid arthritis and spondyloarthropathy in Lithuania. Scand J Rheumatol 2008; 37:113–9.
78. Liao ZT, Pan YF, Huang JL, et al. An epidemiological survey of low back pain and axial spondyloarthritis in a Chinese Han population. Scand J Rheumatol 2009;38: 455–9.
79. Burgos-Vargas R, Peláez-Ballestas I. Epidemiology of spondyloarthritis in México. Am J Med Sci 2011;341:298–300.
80. Haglund E, Bremander AB, Petersson IF, et al. Prevalence of spondyloarthritis and its subtypes in southern Sweden. Ann Rheum Dis 2011;70:943–8.
81. Braun J, Inman R. Clinical significance of inflammatory back pain for diagnosis and screening of patients with axial spondyloarthritis. Ann Rheum Dis 2010;69: 1264–8.

Inflammatory Back Pain

The United States Perspective

Michael H. Weisman, MD

KEYWORDS

- Back pain • Inflammatory back pain • Ankylosing spondylitis
- Spondyloarthropathies

KEY POINTS

- In theory, IBP is assumed to be characterized by inflammation in the sacroiliac joints and the lumbar spine.
- The generally accepted primary features of IBP are young age of onset, pain lasting continuously for more than 3 months, morning stiffness, and pain improved by activity or exercise.
- According to population based studies in the USA, IBP is present in 6% of the population whereas back pain itself is present in 20% of the population.
- IBP performs well as a case ascertainment tool to enrich a population of patients who come to seek medical care for back pain for further studies.
- The frequency of IPB of 6% and SpA of 1% present a challenge to determine what constitutes this gap; more studies are needed.

INTRODUCTION

Inflammatory back pain (IBP) is a relatively recent and well-accepted concept whose precise definition remains elusive. The first clinical description appeared in 1949, at which time Hart and colleagues provided the following account of ankylosing spondylitis (AS) patients:

> *A frequent feature of the pain and stiffness was the aggravation caused by immobility. Waking in the morning stiff and in pain, the patient gradually became more supple during the day, feeling at his best from the afternoon until bedtime. One patient noted that by frequent exercise, his condition was kept in check, but confinement to bed for any cause made him worse. Another woke himself up [every 2 hours] throughout the night to exercise his spine as otherwise, he suffered unduly in the morning*
>
> *(Hart as quoted in Rudwaleit and colleagues, 2006[1])*

Division of Rheumatology, Cedars-Sinai Medical Center, 8700 Beverly Boulevard, Los Angeles, CA 90048, USA
E-mail address: michael.weisman@cshs.org

Rheum Dis Clin N Am 38 (2012) 501–512
http://dx.doi.org/10.1016/j.rdc.2012.09.002 **rheumatic.theclinics.com**
0889-857X/12/$ – see front matter

Subsequent efforts to articulate an improved definition of IBP have become intertwined with the development of criteria sets to operationalize its measurement; its definition has become subsumed under the rubric of features of IBP used to distinguish back pain seen in the spondyloarthropathies (SpA) from mechanical back pain. In principle, IBP is a condition assumed to be related to inflammation of the sacroiliac joints and lower spine, and is frequently seen in patients with AS. Its primary features include: (1) relatively young age at onset, usually before the age of 40 or 45; (2) morning stiffness; (3) back pain present for at least 3 months or more, and (4) pain relieved by movement.[2] The characteristic pattern of IBP may occur in patients with AS as well as other chronic axial pain disorders such as undifferentiated SpA, reactive arthritis, inflammatory bowel diseases, and psoriasis.[3] Although the concept of IBP has been most frequently used within the context of AS and SpA, the presence of IBP clinical features does not equate to a diagnosis of either of these conditions.[3]

Although Hart and colleagues provided the first clinical description of IBP, it was not until Calin and colleagues[4] proposed classification criteria for IBP that the study of IBP was brought to the forefront.[2] As demonstrated herein, the definition of IBP varies by criteria set, as does its sensitivity and specificity regarding screening and case ascertainment in various clinical or epidemiologic settings. The purpose of this article is to review the history of efforts to define IBP, particularly the criteria sets that have been built around its measurement, to describe assessment of IBP in the clinical setting, and to illustrate how IBP has been used in epidemiologic and clinical research.

IBP CLINICAL ASSESSMENT CRITERIA SETS

Several criteria sets have been developed that either measure IBP or incorporate indicators of IBP into more detailed clinical assessments of AS and other SpA. In chronologic order, these criteria sets include: Calin,[4] modified New York criteria for ankylosing spondylitis,[5] Amor,[6] European Spondyloarthropathy Study Group,[7] Berlin criteria (2006),[1] and Assessment of SpondyloArthritis international Society (ASAS) (2009).[8,9] These classification criteria are intended to be applied to confirm a diagnosis in patients who fulfill criteria[10]; they were not meant for diagnostic purposes, although they may have been used as such in the absence of diagnostic criteria and, more recently, by nonrheumatologists. The development of each of these criteria sets is discussed in turn.

Calin Criteria

In 1977, Calin and colleagues[4] developed criteria to measure differences in symptoms between patients with back pain of an inflammatory nature (specifically, AS) and patients with mechanical or nonspecific back pain. In this study, a 17-item questionnaire (**Box 1**) was administered to 3 groups of patients: 42 HLA-B27–positive AS patients, 21 HLA-B27–negative patients seen in an orthopedic clinic but with normal sacroiliac joints on radiography, and 75 controls.

Analysis of the results reported by Calin and colleagues showed that 5 of the 17 questions were able to detect AS with a sensitivity of 60% and specificity of 97%. The 5 questions were discomfort for 3 months or more, back stiffness in the morning, age of onset younger than 40 years, insidious onset, and discomfort relieved by exercise. Furthermore, using 4 of these 5 characteristics differentiates AS from nonspecific back pain, with 95% sensitivity and 85% specificity in this test population. In comparing the 5 most discriminating items from the Calin questions to the 4 criteria for IBP (age of onset before age 40 or 45, morning stiffness, duration of back pain for at least 3 or more months, and pain relieved by movement), one sees that with

Box 1
Calin criteria

1. Have you ever had trouble with your back (excluding neck)?

If yes, please answer the following:

2. Have you had any discomfort (pain and/or stiffness) in your back today?
3. Have you had any discomfort in the last 3 months?
4. Has the discomfort ever gone on for 3 months or more?
5. Was the discomfort caused by an injury?
6. Has the discomfort extended below the knee?
7. With the discomfort, has there been numbness or tingling in a leg?
8. Has the back been stiff, especially in the morning?
9. Has the discomfort awakened you at night?
10. Have you seen a physician for the back trouble?
11. Have x-ray films been taken of your back?
12. At what age did you discover your back discomfort (years)?
13. Did the problem begin suddenly or (14)
14. Slowly?
15. Has the discomfort been improved by rest or (16)
16. Exercise?
17. Have any members of your family had persistent back pain (include only immediate family members)?

Answers were either "yes" or "no" except where indicated.

the exception of insidious onset, most all of the later classification criteria for AS, SpA, and IBP are almost identical. Thus, it is understandable how the criteria for IBP and AS have become so intertwined. In fact, subsequent criteria sets are much more focused on the assessment of AS and other types of SpA than on the measurement of IBP itself. That said, though, each of the subsequent criteria sets retains one or more elements of the definition of IBP.

Modified New York Criteria for Ankylosing Spondylitis

The modified New York criteria for ankylosing spondylitis (**Box 2**) were developed in response to an evaluation of the sensitivity and specificity of the Rome criteria for AS proposed in 1961 and the New York clinical criteria for AS formulated in 1966.[5] van der Linden and colleagues[5] studied 20 HLA-B27–positive AS probands and 102 first-degree relatives 15 years of age and older as well as 14 HLA-B27–negative probands and 74 first-degree relatives. Analysis of the Rome criteria and the New York criteria indicated that the history or presence of pain at the dorsolumbar junction or in the lumbar spine (one of the New York criteria) was not useful in discriminating between patients with AS and those without AS. In its place, the investigators recommended that the original Rome criterion for IBP, "low back pain and stiffness for more than 3 months which is not relieved by rest," be modified to "low back pain and stiffness for more than 3 months which improves with exercise, but is not relieved by rest."

Box 2
Modified New York criteria for ankylosing spondylitis

Clinical Criteria

- Low back pain and stiffness for more than 3 months that improves with exercise, but is not relieved by rest
- Limitation of motion of the lumbar spine in both the sagittal and frontal plans
- Limitation of chest expansion relative to normal values correlated for age and sex

Radiological Criterion

- Sacroiliitis grade 2 or more bilaterally or grade 3 to 4 unilaterally

Definite AS if the radiological criterion is associated with at least one clinical criterion.

Thus, the modified New York criteria for AS replace the original New York pain criteria with the modification of the Rome pain criteria.

The modified New York criteria for AS represent an important departure from the Calin criteria in that the focus is not exclusively on IBP. Rather, IBP is one of several clinical criteria used to characterize patients with AS. Also noteworthy is the fact that at this juncture in the development of IBP-related clinical assessments, the use of radiologic findings is introduced as a criterion for AS.

Amor Criteria

The Amor criteria (**Table 1**) were designed to distinguish patients with SpA from patients without SpA. The Amor criteria were developed using a 5-step process that included 1376 patients: 1219 subjects with SpA, and 157 controls.[6] The 1219 subjects with SpA were divided into 3 study groups: 250 were included in a retrospective review, 890 were recruited from a multicenter collaboration, and 79 were reviewed prospectively. The final criteria proposed by Amor had a sensitivity of 90% and a specificity of 86.6%.

As may be seen by examining these criteria, however, IBP is not well defined[10] and elements of IBP have been relegated to relatively minor importance in favor of other clinical factors, radiologic findings, and genetic history. These fairly wide-ranging clinical criteria, while not emphasizing IBP, are nevertheless important to an understanding of the history of the development of IBP and SpA criteria sets.

European Spondyloarthropathy Study Group

The European Spondyloarthropathy Study Group (ESSG) sought to overcome the limitations of earlier criteria sets by proposing classification criteria that would encompass the entire panoply of the spondyloarthropathies.[7] To meet the goal of being able to detect a range of SpA patients, the clinical variables included for evaluation in this study were diverse and encompassed far more than just definitional criteria for IBP. Data on 183 variables was collected from a total of 1077 patients (403 with spondyloarthropathy and 674 controls with other rheumatologic conditions). The information from these 183 variables was evaluated by an expert panel that reduced the number of candidate criteria variables to 25 (**Box 3**). The specificity for these 25 variables ranged from 28.8% to 98.1% while the sensitivity ranged from 5.5% to 84.9%. Statistical analysis further reduced these 25 variables to the set that ultimately became known as the ESSG criteria. The ESSG criteria for the classification of spondyloarthropathy require the presence of inflammatory spinal pain or synovitis (either asymmetric or

Table 1
Amor criteria for spondyloarthritis

Criterion	Points
Clinical Symptoms or History:	
Lumbar or dorsal pain during the night, or morning stiffness of lumbar or dorsal spine	1
Asymmetric oligoarthritis	2
Buttock pain	1
If affecting alternately the right or the left buttock	2
Sausage-like toe or digit (dactylitis)[a]	2
Heel pain or any other well-defined enthesiopathy (enthesitis)[a]	2
Iritis	2
Nongonococcal urethritis or cervicitis accompanying, or within 1 mo before, the onset of arthritis	1
Acute diarrhea accompanying, or within 1 mo before, the onset of arthritis	1
Presence or history psoriasis, balanitis, or inflammatory bowel disease (ulcerative colitis or Crohn disease)	2
Radiological Finding:	
Sacroiliitis (grade ≥2 if bilateral; grade ≥3 if unilateral)	3
Genetic Background:	
Presence of HLA-B27, or familial history of ankylosing spondylitis, Reiter syndrome, uveitis, psoriasis, or chronic enterocolopathies	2
Good response to NSAIDs in less than 48 h, or relapse of the pain in less than 48 h if NSAIDs discontinued	2

A patient is considered to have spondyloarthritis if the sum of the point counts is 6 or more. A total point count of 5 or more classifies for probably spondyloarthritis.

Abbreviation: NSAID, nonsteroidal anti-inflammatory drug.

[a] Terms were added by the authors for clarification, not in the original publication.

From Sieper J, Rudwaleit M, Baraliakos X, et al. The Assessment of SpondyloArthritis international Society (ASAS) handbook: a guide to assess spondyloarthritis. Ann Rheum Dis 2009;68(Suppl II): ii1–44; with permission.

predominantly in the lower limbs) and one or more of the following: positive family history; psoriasis; inflammatory bowel disease, urethritis, cervicitis, or acute diarrhea within 1 month before arthritis; buttock pain alternating between right and left gluteal areas; enthesopathy; or sacroiliitis. Similar to the preceding criteria sets, the ESSG criteria illustrate that IBP remains an important, but not an exclusive, element in these criteria sets.

Berlin Criteria

The Berlin criteria are an outgrowth of a study specifically designed to assess the individual components of IBP, test various combinations of these features, and compare them with each other with the ultimate worthwhile goal of identifying and studying AS patients ahead of progressive but not reversible damage and disability.[1] A total of 213 patients (101 with AS and 112 with mechanical low back pain [MLBP]) younger than 50 years and with low back pain for at least 3 months were included in the study. Patients were queried about age at onset of back pain, time period of onset of back pain before evaluation, preceding events (eg, trauma, infection, mental/emotional stress), duration of morning stiffness, improvement in back pain, buttock pain, and awakening at night

Box 3
Candidate variables of the European Spondyloarthropathy Study Group criteria

1. Spinal pain
2. Inflammatory spinal pain
3. Anterior chest wall pain
4. Buttock pain
5. Buttock pain alternating between right and left gluteal areas
6. Buttock pain, unilateral, without radiation below the knee
7. Chest expansion greater than 2.5 cm
8. Reduction in spinal mobility
9. Synovitis, predominantly in the lower limbs
10. Asymmetric synovitis
11. Mono- or oligo- versus polyarticular involvement
12. Dactylitis
13. Enthesopathy at any site
14. Heel pain
15. Conjunctivitis
16. Uveitis (acute, anterior)
17. Psoriasis
18. Mucosal ulcerations
19. Acute diarrhea (1 month before arthritis)
20. Inflammatory bowel disease
21. Nongonococcal urethritis or cervicitis (1 month before arthritis)
22. HLA-B27
23. Family history of either ankylosing spondylitis, reactive arthritis, psoriasis, uveitis, or inflammatory bowel disease
24. Sacroiliitis (on radiography)
25. Positive effect of nonsteroidal anti-inflammatory drugs

because of back pain. Statistical analyses were used to identify variables that discriminated between patients with AS and patients with MLBP. The following 3 sets of 4 variable combinations were similar in their ability to distinguish between AS and MLBP patients:

Set 8c: morning stiffness of greater than 30 minutes' duration, improvement in back pain with exercise but not with rest, alternating buttock pain, and age at onset of back pain less than 30 years (sensitivity 78.1%; specificity 66.1%).

Set 7a: morning stiffness of greater than 30 minutes' duration, improvement in back pain with exercise but not with rest, awakening because of back pain during the second half of the night only, and age at onset of back pain less than 30 years (sensitivity 82.2%; specificity 59.9%).

Set 8a: morning stiffness greater than 30 minutes' duration, improvement in back pain with exercise but not with rest, alternating buttock pain, and awakening because of back pain during the second half of the night only (sensitivity 70.3%; specificity 81.2%).

The authors express a preference for Set 8a, noting that it performed slightly better than Calin criteria and is easy to administer in a clinical setting.

Assessment of SpondyloArthritis International Society (ASAS)

The Assessment of SpondyloArthritis international Society (ASAS) convened a 2-day workshop in Berlin with 13 international experts in AS/SpA from 9 countries in Europe and North America to develop new classification criteria for axial and peripheral SpA.[9] During the workshop, these 13 experts evaluated the clinical history of, and performed examination on, 20 patients with chronic back pain and suspected axial SpA, resulting in a total of 124 clinical judgments on IBP. There were 4 to 7 judgments for each patient and each IBP parameter. Analysis of the concordance among experts and logistic regression resulted in the ASAS IBP according to experts' criteria (**Box 4**) so named because, in contrast to previous IBP criteria that were developed by comparing AS patients with patients with other types of back pain, these new IBP criteria were based on the judgment of experts. These criteria do not significantly differ from other IBP criteria, but rather represent a synthesis of previous work. In fact, 3 of the items (disease onset <40 years, insidious onset, and improvement with exercise) are included in the Calin criteria.

VALUE OF IBP FOR DIAGNOSTIC, CLASSIFICATION, AND SCREENING PURPOSES

The value of IBP with respect to diagnosis, classification, and identification of patients with SpA in the primary care setting has recently been called into question.[2] Thus far, there is limited evidence as to the value of IBP as a screening criterion in the primary care setting. This lack of evidence is not surprising, given that the construct of IBP has been incorporated into various sets and algorithms mostly for classification purposes as well as for case ascertainment in fairly limited and somewhat artificially constructed study populations.

Brandt and colleagues[11] investigated the value of proposed IBP screening parameters when used by primary care physicians and orthopedists for the detection of AS in patients with chronic back pain. Physicians participating in the study (114 orthopedists and 130 primary care physicians) were asked to refer patients to an outpatient rheumatology clinic if they possessed low back pain greater than 3 months' duration and onset before age 45 years. In addition, patients were required to meet at least 1 of the 3 criteria: (1) IBP defined as morning stiffness longer than 30 minutes, pain at night

Box 4
IBP parameters according to ASAS experts

1. Age at onset younger than 40 years
2. Insidious onset
3. Improvement with exercise
4. No improvement with rest
5. Pain at night (with improvement on getting up)

Sensitivity 77.0% and specificity 91.7% if at least 4 out of 5 parameters are present. Note that sensitivity and specificity refer to the presence of IBP, not to diagnosis.

or early morning with improvement by exercise; (2) positive HLA-B27 test; or (3) sacroiliitis detected by imaging. A total of 350 patients were referred by orthopedists and primary care physicians to the rheumatology clinic. Slightly more than 50% of the 350 patients were referred to the rheumatology clinic because of evidence of IBP, which was confirmed by the rheumatologist in 76.8% of these patients. A diagnosis of axial SpA could be made in 62.6% of patients when more than one of the referral criteria was positive. This study suggests that the use of IBP is useful in the primary care setting when it is used as one component of a triad of referral parameters.

Solmaz and colleagues[12] evaluated the sensitivity and specificity of the ASAS criteria for IBP relative to the Calin and Berlin criteria. In this study of 214 patients with axial SpA and 44 patients with MLBP, sensitivity was highest with Calin criteria (92%) and specificity was best with the Berlin criteria (84%). Sensitivity and specificity for the ASAS were 77% and 72%, respectively.

Most recently, Braun and colleagues[13] analyzed selected clinical parameters of IBP for diagnosing axial SpA patients with chronic back pain. Similar to the Brandt study, orthopedists were asked to refer patients to a rheumatologist if the patient had the onset of back pain between the ages of 16 and 45 years with chronic back pain lasting longer than 2 months, but less than 10 years. Patients were randomized to a rheumatologist based on 4 prespecified key questions: (1) morning stiffness lasting longer than 30 minutes; (2) pain improved by movement but not by rest; (3) waking up in the second half of the night because of back pain; and (4) improvement within 48 hours with nonsteroidal anti-inflammatory drugs (NSAIDs). A total of 950 patients were screened, with 670 being referred to a rheumatologist. Complete data were available on 322 patients; 133 of these 322 referred patients were diagnosed with some form of axial SpA based on rheumatologists' expert opinion. Although no single parameter alone was useful in diagnosing patients with axial SpA, combinations of selected parameters performed quite well, and the investigators state that "no single item was predictive, but $\geq$3 items proved useful for good sensitivity and specificity by receiver operating characteristic modeling."[13] It certainly seems clear from these recent data as well as others that performance of these criteria will vary, depending on whether the outcome reflects different case definitions of disease such as fully developed AS or earlier forms of the disease, or perhaps even for different subsets of SpA. The investigators do state with conviction that the definitions of primary care practices will differ from country to country and results using the same ascertainment tools might vary according to the setting.[13]

DETERMINING THE PREVALENCE OF IBP/AXIAL SPA IN THE GENERAL POPULATION

IBP and associated criteria sets were developed in well-defined health care settings and can be easily administered by general practitioners, rheumatologists, and orthopedic surgeons to determine whether a patient's IBP may indicate axial SpA. However, what is known about the prevalence of IBP in the general population? Can the aforementioned criteria sets be used in epidemiologic studies to generate prevalence estimates?

The National Health and Nutrition Examination Survey (NHANES) is an ongoing program of studies combining interviews and physical examinations that assess the health and nutritional status of adults and children in the United States. Data are collected from a cross-sectional, nationally representative survey of the civilian, noninstitutionalized population. The US prevalence of IBP by Berlin Criteria was estimated using data from NHANES II (1981–1975) for adults 25 to 49 years of age. At that time, the prevalence of IBP was 6.7% among those who reported having had a back pain episode for at least 4 months, and 0.8% of the overall adult US population.[14] The authors recently had an opportunity to develop an IBP questionnaire specifically for the NHANES III 2009-2010[15] survey to provide population-based prevalence estimates for 4 published IBP classification criteria: Calin, ESSG, and Berlin criteria sets 8a and 7b.[3] **Table 2** provides an overview of the variables from each of the criteria sets included in this analysis. The ASAS criteria were not included in this study because they were published after the development of the NHANES IBP/SpA questionnaire. The NHANES IBP/SpA instrument used a spinal pain diagram to identify history of chronic pain, aching, or stiffness at 1 of 5 specific axial locations (neck, upper, mid and lower back, and sacroiliac joint area; **Fig. 1**). For those with axial pain at any of these sites, additional detail was obtained: age at onset of symptoms, timing of development of symptoms, temporal pattern of pain variation, duration of symptoms of the longest pain episode (6 weeks and/or 3 months), history of pain, aching, and/or stiffness at the particular site, pattern of the onset of the pain, course of pain over a typical day, morning stiffness, history of rest pain, whether pain results in wakening from sleep, pain response to exercise, and history of alternating buttock pain.

A total of 980 out of 5103 (19.2%) individuals in the NHANES 2009-2010 survey had a history of pain from at least 1 axial site on the pain diagram for less than 3 months. Thus, it appears that back pain (from multiple sites, not just low back) is a very prevalent condition in the US population. IBP prevalence estimates were then constructed

Table 2
Inflammatory back pain case definition criteria

IBP Criterion	NHANES 2009–2010	Calin et al	ESSG	Berlin Set 8a	Berlin Set 7b
Spinal pain location	ARQ010; ARQ020	"Back"	Neck/dorsal/ back	Low back	Low back
Current age	RIDAGEYR	Any age	Any age	<50 y	<50 y
Duration of back pain (3 mo)	ARQ024	✔	✔	✔	✔
"Insidious" onset of back pain	ARQ025	✔	✔		
Age-at-onset back pain (years)	ARQ023	<40	<45		<30
Morning stiffness >30 min	ARQ040	✔[a]	✔[a]	✔	✔
Pain improves with exercise or activity	ARQ080	✔	✔		
Pain improves with activity/ not with rest	ARQ060; ARQ080			✔	✔
Pain awakens second half of night	ARQ073; ARQ077			✔	
Alternating buttock pain	ARQ100			✔	

Abbreviations: ARQ, NHANES 2009–2010 Arthritis Questionnaire; ✔ or highlighted, mandatory IBP case definition criteria.

[a] Duration of morning stiffness not specified in Calin and ESSG criteria.

Berlin criteria sets *From* Rudwaleit M, Metter A, Listing J, et al. Inflammatory back pain in ankylosing spondylitis: a reassessment of the clinical history for application as classification and diagnostic criteria. Arthritis Rheum 2006;54:569–78.

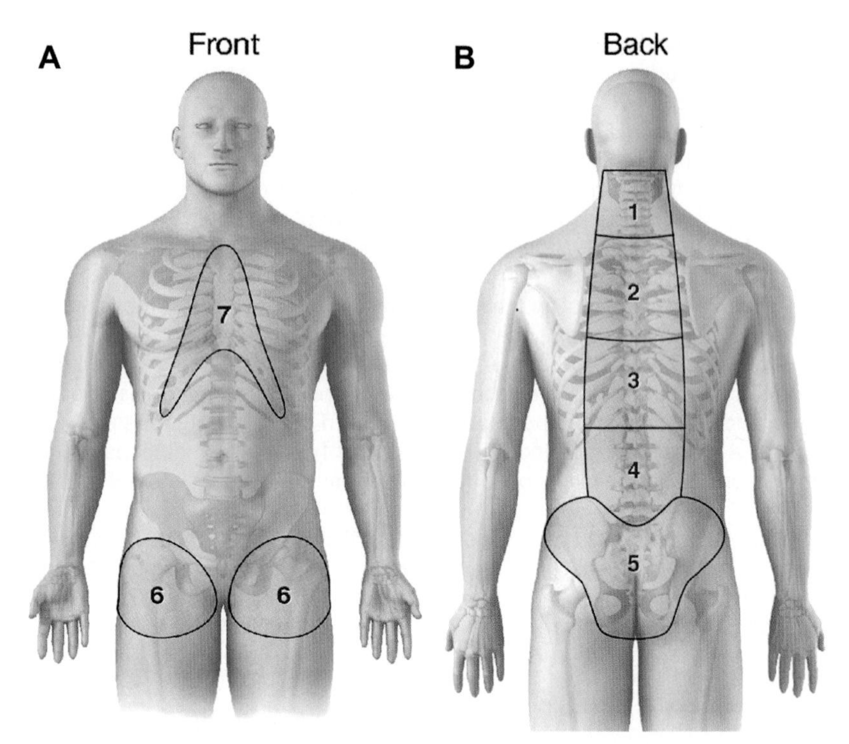

Fig. 1. (*A, B*). The NHANES IBP/SpA instrument used a spinal pain diagram to identify history of chronic pain, aching, or stiffness at 1 of 5 specific axial locations.

using accepted and validated criteria, revealing 5% by Calin, 5.6% by ESSG, 5.8% by Berlin criteria 8a, and 6.0% by Berlin criteria 7b. Because the Berlin criteria were only validated for adults younger than 50 years, the NHANES 2009-2010 prevalence estimates are for the subgroup of participants who were 20 to 49 years of age at the time of the survey (n = 3188).

In a companion study, the authors used the NHANES 2009-2010 survey to estimate the prevalence of SpA in the United States using the Amor criteria and the ESSG criteria (**Table 3**). The NHANES 2009-2010 questionnaire provided sufficient data for ESSG inflammatory spinal pain and captured 4 of the 7 additional ESSG SpA criteria elements. Several items could not be used to measure Amor back pain/stiffness.

Of 6684 persons aged 20 to 69 years who were screened for participation, 5103 complete arthritis interview records were available for analysis. The age-adjusted prevalence of definite and probable SpA by Amor criteria was 0.9% and 1.4% by ESSG criteria. These data compare quite favorably with estimates of 0.35% to 1.3% published by the US National Arthritis Data Workgroup. It does appear that 1% of the US population does suffer from some form of SpA, a figure that places this condition at a higher prevalence than quoted for rheumatoid arthritis,[16] although the ascertainment methodologies are different for each of these conditions.

UNANSWERED QUESTIONS AND FUTURE DIRECTIONS

IBP is one of the defining characteristics of AS and SpA, but does IBP constitute a separate nosologic entity? According to the NHANES surveys quoted here, there is a gap between estimates of SpA (1%) and the estimates of IBP by accepted criteria

Table 3
The Amor and European Spondyloarthritis Study Group case definitions for spondyloarthritis

Amor et al SpA Criteria Elements	Score	NHANES	ESSG SpA Criteria Elements	NHANES
Nocturnal spinal pain or morning stiffness[a]	1	Yes	Inflammatory spinal pain	Yes
Buttock/alternating buttock pain	1 or 2	Yes[b]	Alternating buttock pain	Yes
Heel pain/enthesiopathy	2	Yes	Enthesopathy	Yes
Acute diarrhea at or before SpA onset	1	No	Urethritis, cervicitis, diarrhea	No
Radiologic sacroiliitis	3	No	Radiologic sacroiliitis	No
HLA-B27+ or family/genetic background	2	No	Positive family history	No
Psoriasis, balanitis, inflammatory bowel disease	2	Yes[c]	Psoriasis	Yes
Iritis	2	Yes	Inflammatory bowel disease	Yes
Positive response to NSAIDs	2	Yes		
Asymmetric oligoarthritis	2	No		
Dactylitis	2	No		

Probable SpA is an Amor score of 5, definite SpA is a score of 6; the ESSG criteria for SpA is a history of inflammatory Spinal pain plus one other ESSG SpA criteria element.

Abbreviations: ESSG, European Spondyloarthritis Study Group; SpA, spondyloarthritis.

[a] Lumbar or dorsal pain during the night, or morning stiffness of lumbar or dorsal spine.

[b] Buttock pain = 1; history of alternating buttock pain = 2.

[c] NHANES did not collect a history of balanitis.

(5%–6%). What remains in this gap? The authors accept the notion that classification of disease can be based on etiology, known pathogenetic mechanisms, symptoms alone, and, nowadays, genetics. AS classification remains a struggle because these various criteria are not clear cut in themselves, and the concept of SpA suffers even more because several of these features are even less well defined. Whether SpA is a precursor to AS or perhaps even a different entity is at the debating stage. IBP is the next hurdle to overcome: is it something in and of itself or is it a precursor for SpA or AS?

The value of the concept of IBP in the primary care setting is straightforward: it does define a group at risk for SpA or AS and it can defend further diagnostic testing such as advanced imaging or genetic testing. However, if these tests are negative, does IBP in and of itself justify anti-inflammatory therapy or even biological drug intervention in an attempt to treat symptoms or potentially to prevent later development of SpA or AS? As yet, these questions remain unanswered.

However, one important use of the concept of IBP appears to be in its role as a distinguishing feature in the criteria sets that have been developed to identify AS and SpA. In the 35 years since the Calin criteria were introduced, criteria sets have evolved from measurement of IBP to measurement of AS and/or SpA, and here it must be made clear that IBP is not the same clinical entity as AS or SpA. These criteria sets share several key clinical features, while diverging on others such as radiographic parameters and genetic indicators. The difference among these criteria sets leads to several considerations for future research. First, do patients classified as having IBP who do not go on to develop AS or SpA represent a valid subset of IBP or are they false positives in IBP classification? Second, what is the association between IBP, elevated markers of inflammation, and HLA-B27? Third, can these criteria sets be used to analyze response to therapy?[2] Finally, is it possible to develop a unified criteria set for IBP? Answers to these questions are awaited.

REFERENCES

1. Rudwaleit M, Metter A, Listing J, et al. Inflammatory back pain in ankylosing spondylitis: a reassessment of the clinical history for application as classification and diagnostic criteria. Arthritis Rheum 2006;54:569–78.
2. Braun J, Inman R. Clinical significance of inflammatory back pain for diagnosis and screening of patients with axial spondyloarthritis. Ann Rheum Dis 2010;69:1264–8.
3. Weisman MH, Witter JP, Reveille JD. The prevalence of inflammatory back pain: population-based estimates from the US National Health and Nutrition Examination Survey, 2009-10. Ann Rheum Dis 2012. [Epub ahead of print].
4. Calin A, Porta J, Fries JF, et al. Clinical history as a screening test for ankylosing spondylitis. JAMA 1977;237:2613–4.
5. van der Linden S, Valkenburg HA, Cats A. Evaluation of diagnostic criteria for ankylosing spondylitis: a proposal for modification of the New York criteria. Arthritis Rheum 1984;27:361–8.
6. Amor B, Dougados M, Mijiyawa M. Criteria of the classification of spondyloarthropathies. Rev Rhum Mal Osteoartic 1990;57:85–9.
7. Dougados M, van der Linden S, Juhlin R, et al. The European Spondyloarthropathy Study Group preliminary criteria for the classification of spondyloarthropathy. Arthritis Rheum 1991;34:1218–27.
8. Rudwaleit M, van der Heijde D, Landewé R, et al. The development of Assessment of SpondyloArthritis international Society classification criteria for axial spondyloarthritis (part II): validation and final selection. Ann Rheum Dis 2009; 68:777–83.
9. Sieper J, van der Heijde D, Landewé R, et al. New criteria for inflammatory back pain in patients with chronic back pain: a real patient exercise by experts from the Assessment of SpondyloArthritis international Society (ASAS). Ann Rheum Dis 2009;68:784–8.
10. Rudwaleit M, Khan MA, Sieper J. The challenge of diagnosis and classification in early ankylosing spondylitis. Do we need new criteria? Arthritis Rheum 2005;52: 1000–8.
11. Brandt HC, Spiller I, Song IH, et al. Performance of referral recommendations in patients with chronic back pain and suspected axial spondyloarthritis. Ann Rheum Dis 2007;66:1479–84.
12. Solmaz D, Akar S, Gunduz O, et al. Performance of different criteria sets for inflammatory back pain in patients with axial spondyloarthritis with and without radiographic sacroiliitis [abstract]. Arthritis Rheum 2010;62(Suppl 10):544.
13. Braun A, Saracbasi E, Grifka J, et al. Identifying patients with axial spondyloarthritis in primary care: how useful are items indicative of inflammatory back pain? Ann Rheum Dis 2011;70:1782–7.
14. Dillon CF, Hirsch R. The United States National Health and Nutrition Examination Survey and the epidemiology of ankylosing spondylitis. Am J Med Sci 2011;341:281–3.
15. National Health and Nutrition Examination Survey 2009-2010. Available at: http://www.cdc.gov/nchs/data/nhanes/nhanes_09_10/sp_handcards_0910.pdf. Accessed August 10, 2012.
16. Helmick CG, Felson DT, Lawrence RC, et al. Estimates of the prevalence of arthritis and other rheumatic conditions in the United States. Part I. Arthritis Rheum 2008;58:15–25.

Imaging in Axial Spondyloarthritis

Diagnostic Problems and Pitfalls

Xenofon Baraliakos, MD[a,*], Kay-Geert A. Hermann, MD[b], Jürgen Braun, MD[a]

KEYWORDS

- Pitfalls • Magnetic resonance imaging • Sacroiliac joints • Ankylosing spondylitis

KEY POINTS

- Magnetic resonance imaging (MRI) is considered the gold standard for assessment of inflammatory changes. Furthermore, there is increasing evidence that structural changes can also be detected by MRI.
- Computed tomography is currently the most precise imaging method to depict erosions, sclerosis, and ankylosis – however its use is limited due to relatively high radiation exposure.[1]
- Imaging is an important but not solitary tool for making a solid diagnosis in patients with inflammatory or degenerative diseases of the axial skeleton.

INTRODUCTION

The concept of axial spondyloarthritis (axSpA) includes 2 subgroups, ankylosing spondylitis (AS) and nonradiographic axial SpA (nr-axSpA),[2] which are differentiated on the basis of presence or absence of definite structural changes in the sacroiliac joints (SIJ) while no clear decision has been made regarding such changes in the spine. The disease that mainly affects the axial skeleton is characterized by inflammatory (sacroiliitis, spondylitis) and osteoproliferative changes (syndesmophytes, ankylosis). Sacroiliitis, spondylitis, and spondylodiscitis are considered almost pathognomonic for axSpA, because the main differential diagnosis is infection, which occurs relatively rarely in developed countries.[3] How inflammation and new bone formation are linked has remained a matter of debate for several years. Osteodestructive changes such as erosions in both the SIJ and the spine may also occur, although in the spine this is a rare event.[4]

[a] Rheumazentrum Ruhrgebiet, Landgrafenstr. 15, 44652 Herne, Germany; [b] Department of Radiology, Charité Medical School, Chariteplatz 1, 10117 Berlin, Germany
* Corresponding author.
E-mail address: baraliakos@me.com

Rheum Dis Clin N Am 38 (2012) 513–522
http://dx.doi.org/10.1016/j.rdc.2012.08.011 **rheumatic.theclinics.com**

Imaging of the axial skeleton is important for the diagnosis, classification, and monitoring of patients with axial SpA. Whereas structural changes are best identified by conventional radiographs,[3] magnetic resonance imaging (MRI) is considered the gold standard for the assessment of inflammatory changes. Furthermore, there is increasing evidence that structural changes can also be detected by MRI.[5,6] Computed tomography (CT) has also been used, especially for the SIJ, and is considered the gold standard for the assessment of structural changes in these joints.[1]

USE OF IMAGING FOR THE CLASSIFICATION OF AXIAL SPA

For several decades, conventional radiographs of the axial skeleton have been essential for the diagnosis and classification of AS, mainly because they are an essential feature of the modified New York criteria.[7] However, the complicated S-shaped anatomy of the SIJ but also the lack of ability of conventional radiographs to detect inflammation have caused problems for differentiation between positive and negative findings regarding a diagnosis of AS and axSpA. This quandary has contributed to the substantial delay in the diagnosis.[8] Another issue that may cause problems with the use of conventional radiographs is that with increasing age, degenerative changes in the axial skeleton become more prevalent.[9] Conventional radiographs are currently used in daily practice to detect structural changes but in the future, CT may also be increasingly used to better detect structural changes in the axial skeleton. In general, CT can be helpful in doubtful cases of chronic changes and for the differential diagnosis against other frequent spinal disorders such as diffuse idiopathic skeletal hyperostosis (DISH).

Scintigraphy has been widely used in the past to diagnose patients with axSpA. However, because of its low sensitivity and specificity,[10] scintigraphy is no longer recommended for routine use in such patients.

USE OF IMAGING FOR DIAGNOSING AXIAL SPA BY CONVENTIONAL RADIOGRAPHS

Conventional Radiographs of the Sacroiliac Joints

As already mentioned, quantification of structural changes is used in the modified New York criteria for the diagnosis of established AS (**Box 1**).

Differential Diagnoses and Pitfalls of Conventional Radiographs of the Sacroiliac Joints in Axial Spondyloarthritis

Examples of the most frequent clinical problems are provided here to illustrate the main difficulties and pitfalls in the diagnosis of axSpA.

Box 1
Modified New York criteria

- Grade 0: normal
- Grade 1: suspicious changes
- Grade 2: minimal changes: small localized areas with erosion or sclerosis, without involvement of the joint width
- Grade 3: definite changes: moderate or advanced sacroiliitis with 1 or more of: erosions, evidence of sclerosis, widening, narrowing, or partial ankylosis
- Grade 4: severe changes: total ankylosis

Extensive sclerosis and osteitis condensans ilii
Extensive sclerosis at the sacral or iliac side of the SIJ can lead to misdiagnosis of AS (**Fig. 1**). It is important that the joint margins are assessed for the occurrence of erosions and for joint width. Triangular-shaped sclerosis of the iliac side of the SIJ manifests as osteitis condensans ilii, especially in women after pregnancy, although the condition may also occur in men.

Diffuse idiopathic skeletal hyperostosis (DISH, Forestier disease)
The SIJ can be irregularly shaped, including some sclerosis mimicking sacroiliitis and also showing bony bridges crossing both sides of the joint (**Fig. 2**).

Differential Diagnoses and Pitfalls of Conventional Radiographs of the Spine in Axial Spondyloarthritis

Degenerative changes (spondylophytes/spondylosis deformans)
Bridging osteophytes that grow in a horizontal direction can be differentiated from new bone formation due to AS, which shows a more vertical growth (**Figs. 3** and **4**).[3] The former are considered degenerative and cannot always easily be differentiated from the latter, which are considered to be related to inflammation.

Degenerative changes (erosive osteochondrosis)
Degenerative changes associated with chronic back pain in patients of every age are frequently found (see **Fig. 4**). Typically seen on conventional radiographs are decreased disc height and reactive spondylophyte development. On MRI, typical findings of erosive osteochondrosis are the so-called Modic lesions (**Table 1**).

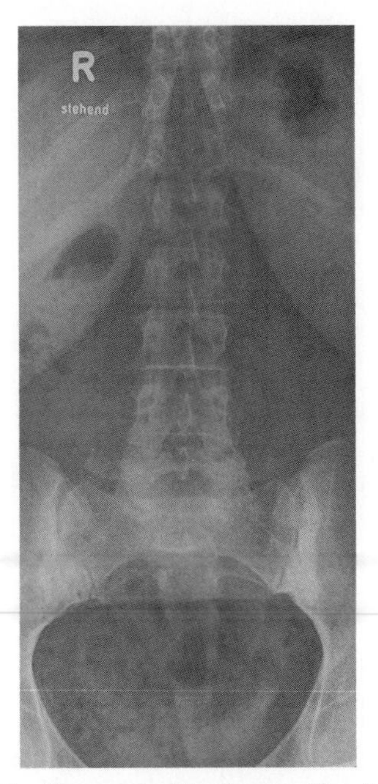

Fig. 1. Extensive sclerosis on the iliac part of both sacroiliac joints as a sign of osteitis condensans iliis (triangular hyperostosis) as a differential diagnosis of a bilateral sacroiliitis, in a 49-year-old woman with clinical signs of low back pain.

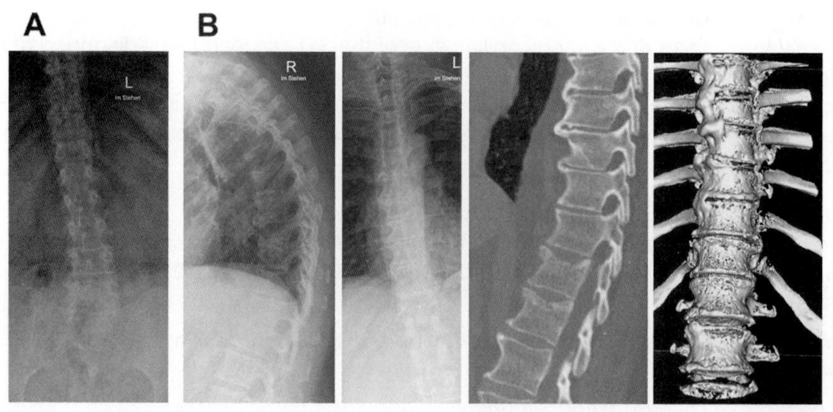

Fig. 2. (*A*) Sclerosis and bilateral bony bridging in a 46-year-old woman, mimicking sacroiliitis similar to advanced ankylosing spondylitis. This patient presented with chronic back pain not of inflammatory nature, negative HLA-B27, and no other clinical features of SpA, additional metabolic syndrome. (*B*) Conventional radiographs, CT, and 3-dimensional reconstruction of the thoracic spine of the same patient, showing the typical bridging osteophytes in typical formation.

Scheuermann disease

Uneven growth of vertebral borders (upper and lower), mainly with wedged-shaped vertebrae and irregularities in the upper or lower part of the vertebral body (**Fig. 5**), is apparent. The disease mainly starts in childhood and is associated with chronic back pain in adulthood.

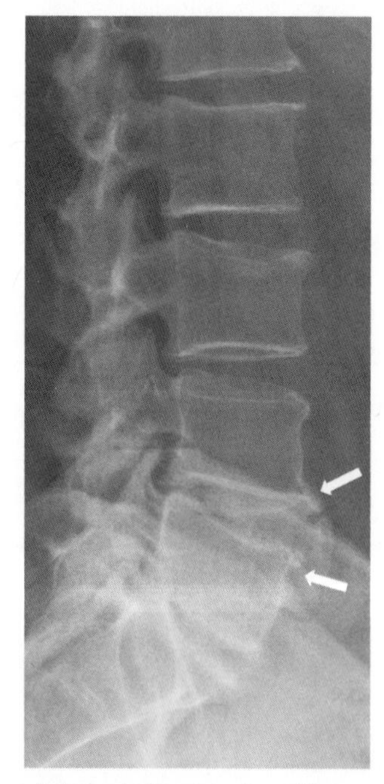

Fig. 3. Typical example of spondylosis deformans in a 60-year-old man. Initially, the growth of these findings is in a horizontal direction (*arrow*). Very frequently, these findings are seen in segments with disc degeneration.

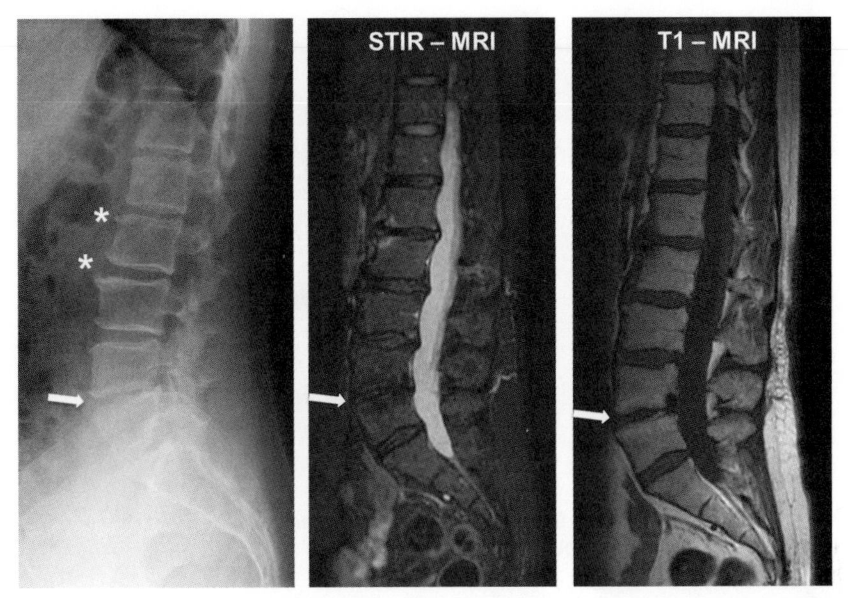

Fig. 4. Degenerative spondylophytes (*asterisks*) in a 60-year-old man with chronic back pain. On conventional radiographs erosive osteochondrosis can be assumed by the clinical symptoms, and advanced disc degeneration (here in L4/5, *arrow*) is confirmed by MRI (here Modic II lesion, see also **Table 1**).

Diffuse idiopathic skeletal hyperostosis (DISH, Forestier disease)

This condition is characterized by development of wide, bulky osteophytes, which extend along the course of the anterior longitudinal ligament (see **Fig. 2**).

USE OF IMAGING FOR DIAGNOSING AXIAL SPA BY MRI

MRI can be used for the depiction of acute inflammatory lesions and chronic/structural changes in both the SIJ and the spine. To date, only inflammatory lesions have been taken into account as pathognomonic signs for a "positive MRI" in the classification criteria of axial SpA according to the Assessment of SpondyloArthritis international Society (ASAS), while both lesion types have been used for the definition of a "positive MRI of the spine."[11]

There is international consensus[12] that a short-tau inversion recovery (STIR) or fat-saturated T2-weighted turbo spin-echo sequence with a high resolution (image matrix of 512 pixels, slice thickness of 3 mm or 4 mm) and with a field strength of 1.0 or 1.5 T

Table 1
Definition of Modic lesions according to the signal intensity of the bone marrow surrounding an intervertebral disc on one spinal segment on MRI

	MRI Signal	
Stage	**STIR**	**T1**
Modic I	Hyperintense	Hypointense
Modic II	Hypointense	Hyperintense
Modic III	Hypointense	Hypointense

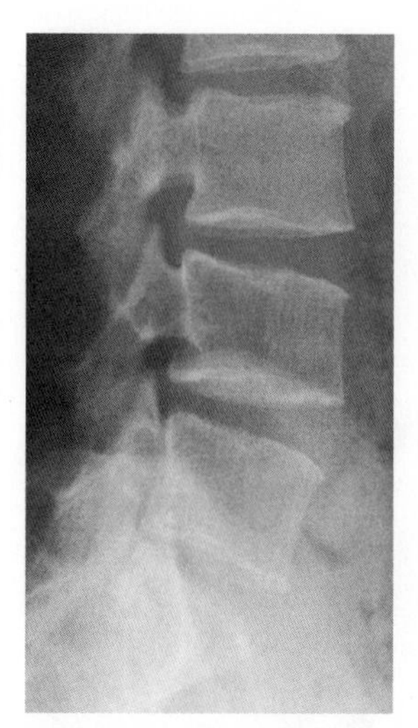

Fig. 5. Typical example of Scheuermann disease with a wedge-shaped vertebra and irregularities in the upper or lower part of the vertebral body.

should be used in routine clinical practice for the detection of bone marrow edema. For structural (chronic) changes, T1-weighted turbo spin-echo sequences are recommended.

According to the definition of sacroiliitis in SpA, the inflammation of bone marrow should be preferably located in the periarticular location. Regarding the amount of signal required for definition of a positive MRI of the SIJ in patients with axial SpA, more than 1 lesion on 1 MRI slice are needed, whereas if there is 1 lesion only, this should be present on at least 2 slices.[12]

Differential Diagnoses and Pitfalls of MRI of the Sacroiliac Joints in Axial Spondyloarthritis

Insufficiency fracture

Similar to inflammation due to sacroiliitis, bone marrow edema is characteristic for this finding. These patients complain about similar symptoms to those of axial SpA, such as low back pain **Fig. 6**.

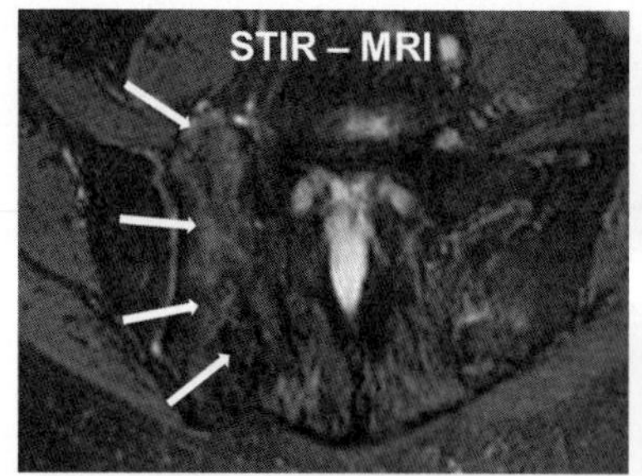

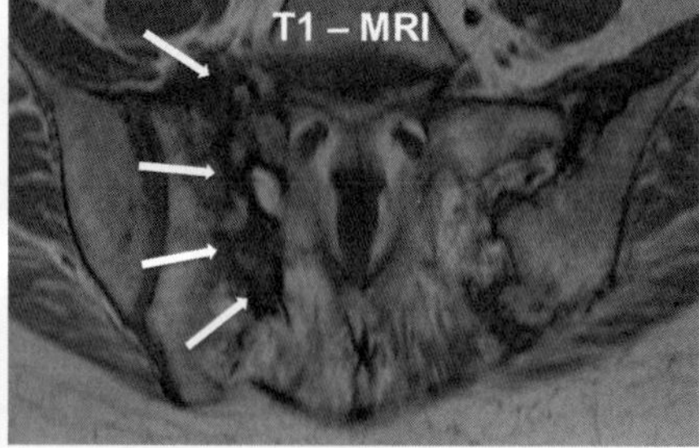

Fig. 6. Insufficiency fracture in a 35-year-old woman after a minor accident. The MRI findings imitate sacroiliitis, with bone marrow edema seen as hyperintense signal on short-tau inversion recovery (STIR) and hypointense signal on T1-weighted MRI (*arrows*). Anatomically there is disruption of the bone, which is better seen on the T1 sequence.

Infectious sacroiliitis
These lesions cross the anatomic borders and frequently extend to the surrounding soft tissue (see similar image for the spine in **Fig. 7**).

Coil effect
The coil effect refers to false-positive signals in STIR MRI, seen especially in older MRI machines (**Fig. 8**). These findings are mainly seen outside of the periarticular region, but may extend into the sacral bone. This effect is seen on STIR but not on contrast-enhanced T1-weighted fat-saturated MRI.

Differential Diagnoses and Pitfalls of MRI of the Spine in Axial Spondyloarthritis

Blood vessels
The typical shape and position of hyperintense signal on STIR and hypointense signal on T1-weighted MRI for a blood vessel, in the middle of the vertebral body, from the posterior to the anterior part, is shown in **Fig. 9**.

Hemangioma
Accumulation of vessels, typically located within the vertebral body, is seen as a hyperintense signal on STIR sequences and as either a hypointense or isointense signal on T1 sequences, sometimes also with some hyperintensity caused by fat metaplasia of the hemangioma cavity (see **Fig. 9**).

Bacterial (infectious) spondylodiscitis
This condition is similar to the lesions in the SIJ. Anatomic borders are blurry and disrupted (see **Fig. 7**).

Degenerative lesions/erosive osteochondrosis
These lesions show a hyperintense signal in the bone marrow around the intervertebral disc in STIR, in addition to a hypointense/hyperintense signal on T1 as a typical sign of

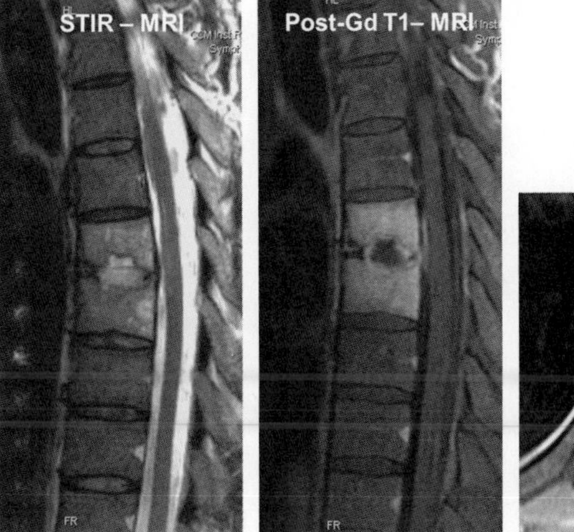

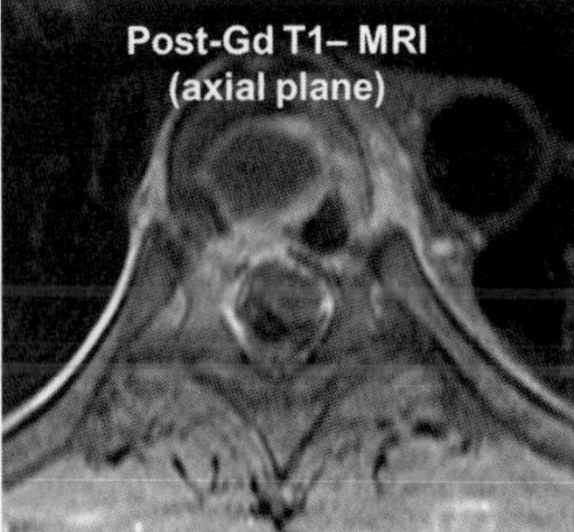

Fig. 7. Bacterial (infectious) spondylodiscitis with hyperintense signal on STIR and on postgadolinium T1-weighted MRI. The anatomic borders are not more extended (also seen in the axial plane). Bacterial invasion is preserved not only for the bone but also for the intervertebral disc.

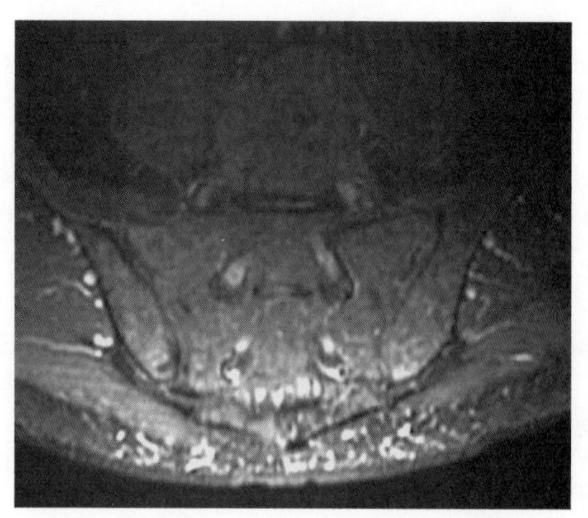

Fig. 8. False-positive signs on STIR MRI of the sacroiliac joint, not periarticularly located and mimicking sacroiliitis, with hyperintense signal as a sign of bone marrow edema.

a Modic I/II lesion. MRI is not able to give the final diagnosis in many of these patients, because MR images can be dubious in some cases (see **Fig. 4**, **Table 1**). Information should be obtained on the patient's history, former and present clinical symptoms for inflammatory versus mechanical low back pain, and laboratory results.

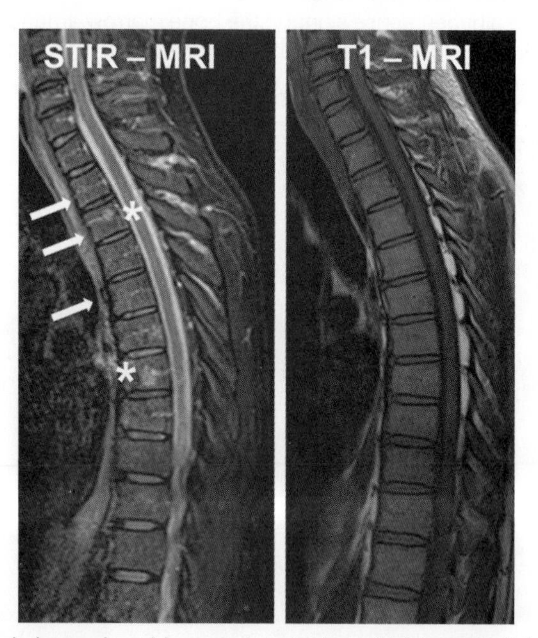

Fig. 9. Blood vessels (*arrows*) and hemangiomata (*asterisks*) in typical shape and position within the vertebral bodies. Despite the hyperintense signal on the STIR sequence and the hypointense signal on the T1 sequence, these finding represent physiologic findings and not inflammatory changes.

SUMMARY

Imaging of the axial skeleton, which includes both the SIJ and the 3 spinal segments, is an important tool to be considered for a diagnosis of axSpA. Thus, imaging of the SIJ is a major criterion for the classification of axSpA according to the 2009 ASAS classification criteria.[13] Imaging is also essential to differentiate between AS and nr-axSpA. Although the existing definitions for a positive MRI of the SIJ[12] and the spine[11] are still valid, it must be stressed that such predefined lesions may also be seen in other conditions, representing pitfalls and false-positive conclusions in patients with similar clinical symptoms who, however, do not have axSpA. Thus, imaging is an important but not solitary tool for making a solid diagnosis in patients with inflammatory or degenerative diseases of the axial skeleton. For a diagnosis of axSpA, a combination of clinical, laboratory, and imaging findings is usually required.

REFERENCES

1. van Tubergen A, Heuft-Dorenbosch L, Schulpen G, et al. Radiographic assessment of sacroiliitis by radiologists and rheumatologists: does training improve quality? Ann Rheum Dis 2003;62(6):519–25.
2. Rudwaleit M, van der Heijde D, Landewe R, et al. The development of Assessment of SpondyloArthritis international Society classification criteria for axial spondyloarthritis (part II): validation and final selection. Ann Rheum Dis 2009; 68(6):777–83.
3. Baraliakos X, Listing J, Rudwaleit M, et al. Progression of radiographic damage in patients with ankylosing spondylitis: defining the central role of syndesmophytes. Ann Rheum Dis 2007;66(7):910–5.
4. Braun J, van der Heijde D. Imaging and scoring in ankylosing spondylitis. Best Pract Res Clin Rheumatol 2002;16(4):573–604.
5. Braun J, Baraliakos X, Golder W, et al. Analysing chronic spinal changes in ankylosing spondylitis: a systematic comparison of conventional x rays with magnetic resonance imaging using established and new scoring systems. Ann Rheum Dis 2004;63(9):1046–55.
6. Bennett AN, Rehman A, Hensor EM, et al. Evaluation of the diagnostic utility of spinal magnetic resonance imaging in axial spondyloarthritis. Arthritis Rheum 2009;60(5):1331–41.
7. van der Linden S, Valkenburg HA, Cats A. Evaluation of diagnostic criteria for ankylosing spondylitis. A proposal for modification of the New York criteria. Arthritis Rheum 1984;27(4):361–8.
8. Feldtkeller E, Bruckel J, Khan MA. Scientific contributions of ankylosing spondylitis patient advocacy groups. Curr Opin Rheumatol 2000;12(4):239–47.
9. Vosse D, van der Heijde D, Landewe R, et al. Determinants of hyperkyphosis in patients with ankylosing spondylitis. Ann Rheum Dis 2006;65(6):770–4.
10. Song IH, Carrasco-Fernandez J, Rudwaleit M, et al. The diagnostic value of scintigraphy in assessing sacroiliitis in ankylosing spondylitis: a systematic literature research. Ann Rheum Dis 2008;67(11):1535–40.
11. Hermann KG, Baraliakos X, van der Heijde D, et al. Descriptions of spinal magnetic resonance imaging (MRI) lesions and definition of a positive MRI of the spine in axial spondyloarthritis (SpA)—a consensual approach by the ASAS/OMERACT MRI Study Group. Ann Rheum Dis 2012;71(8):1278–88.
12. Rudwaleit M, Jurik AG, Hermann KG, et al. Defining active sacroiliitis on magnetic resonance imaging (MRI) for classification of axial spondyloarthritis: a consensual

approach by the ASAS/OMERACT MRI group. Ann Rheum Dis 2009;68(10): 1520–7.

13. Sieper J, Rudwaleit M, Baraliakos X, et al. The Assessment of SpondyloArthritis international Society (ASAS) handbook: a guide to assess spondyloarthritis. Ann Rheum Dis 2009;68(Suppl 2):ii1–44.

Comorbidities in Patients with Spondyloarthritis

Irene E. van der Horst-Bruinsma, MD, PhD[a,b,*], Michael T. Nurmohamed, MD, PhD[a,b,c], Robert B.M. Landewé, MD[d]

KEYWORDS

- Ankylosing spondylitis • Spondyloarthritis • Uveitis • Psoriasis
- Inflammatory bowel disease • Cardiovascular disease • Myocardial infarction
- Cardiovascular risk management

KEY POINTS

- Extra-articular manifestations (EAMs) contribute significantly to the burden of disease in ankylosing spondylitis (AS).
- The manifestation of EAMs has consequences for the choice of treatment.
- Patients with AS have an approximately doubled risk for cardiovascular (CV) disease.
- AS is a new, independent, CV risk factor.
- The inflammatory process contributes significantly to the increased CV risk.
- CV risk management is necessary and should focus on traditional CV risk factors and tight disease control.

INTRODUCTION

Spondyloarthritis (SpA) is a group of rheumatic diseases that includes ankylosing spondylitis (AS), inflammatory back pain, asymmetrical synovitis (eg, psoriatic arthritis), arthritis accompanying inflammatory bowel disease (IBD) (eg, Crohn disease and ulcerative colitis), and reactive arthritis.

SpA can be dominated by spinal symptoms, which can be classified as axial SpA,[1] or by peripheral arthritis, which is classified as peripheral SpA.[2] Axial SpA is subdivided in two types: (1) AS, which requires radiographic changes of the sacroiliac

[a] Department of Rheumatology, VU University Medical Center, P.O. Box 7057, 1007 MB Amsterdam, The Netherlands; [b] Department of Rheumatology, Jan van Breemen Research Institute, Reade Jan van Breemenstraat 2, 1056 AB Amsterdam, The Netherlands; [c] Department of Internal Medicine, VU University Medical Center, P.O. Box 7057, 1007 MB, Amsterdam, The Netherlands; [d] Academic Medical Center University of Amsterdam, Meibergdreef 9, 1105AZ Amsterdam, The Netherlands
* Corresponding author. VU University Medical Center, Room 3A-64, P.O. Box 7057, 1007 MB Amsterdam, The Netherlands.
E-mail address: ie.vanderhorst@vumc.nl

Rheum Dis Clin N Am 38 (2012) 523–538
http://dx.doi.org/10.1016/j.rdc.2012.08.010 rheumatic.theclinics.com
0889-857X/12/$ – see front matter

joints (according to the Modified New York Criteria),[3] and (2) the nonradiographic axial SpA, which is mainly based on a combination of clinical symptoms, the presence of HLA-B27 antigen, and signs of sacroiliitis on MRI. The nonradiographic axial SpA can progress toward AS within a couple of years. The clinical symptoms of axial SpA include inflammatory back pain during at least 3 months with onset before 45 years of age and at least one of the other SpA-features: arthritis, enthesitis (heel), uveitis, dactylitis, psoriasis, Crohn disease or ulcerative colitis, good response to nonsteroidal antiinflammatory drugs (NSAIDs), family history of SpA, and elevated C-reactive protein.[1]

Peripheral SpA requires peripheral arthritis compatible with SpA (usually asymmetric and/or predominant involvement of the lower limb), enthesitis or dactylitis, and at least one of the other SpA features (see above).[2]

AS is the most common type of SpA and presents with low-back pain and morning stiffness, due to a chronic inflammation of the sacroiliac joints and vertebral spine. This inflammatory process can result in calcification of the spinal ligaments, additional bone formation (syndesmophytes), and destruction of the vertebral spine leading to postural deformities, such as ankylosis of the cervical spine and kyphosis of the thoracic spine. AS is associated with the HLA-B27 antigen, starts at a relatively young age (15–40 years), and predominantly occurs in males, with a male/female ratio of 3:1. The diagnosis of AS is defined by the modified New York criteria[3] and depends, among other factors, on the presence of sacroiliitis on the radiograph. The prevalence of SpA, including AS, is estimated at 0.9% in the white population, which equals the prevalence of rheumatoid arthritis.[4]

Peripheral arthritis occurs in 30% of patients with SpA and, at onset, shows a predominately asymmetrical and oligoarticular pattern involving large joints of the lower limbs (ie, knees, hips, and ankles), shoulders, or smaller joints (dactylitis). Symmetric polyarthritis may develop later during the disease. Arthritis might result in joint destruction that sometimes necessitates joint replacement of the hip or knee. Enthesitis is a common manifestation in SpA that occurs in 25% to 40% of the patients and is caused by a local inflammatory reaction at the bony adherence of the tendon. The sites most often involved are the Achilles tendons, plantar fascia, costosternal junctions, spinous processes, iliac crests, great trochanters, ischial tuberosities, and tibial tubercles.[5] Evaluation of the enthesitis lesions can be performed with the Maastricht AS Enthesis Score (MASES)[6] or the Spondyloarthritis Research Consortium of Canada (SPARCC) Enthesitis Index.[7]

Next to the spinal symptoms and peripheral arthritis, several extra-articular manifestations (EAMs) often occur in SpA, such as uveitis, psoriasis, and IBD, as well as comorbidities, such as osteoporosis and cardiovascular (CV) disease.

Acute anterior uveitis, previously called iridocyclitis, occurs in 25% to 30% of patients with AS and can be the first presenting symptom of the disease. Psoriasis develops in 10% to 25% of patients with SpA and IBD develops in only 5% to 10%.

Osteoporosis of the spine frequently occurs and can lead to vertebral fractures at a young age.[8] Because of the rigidity of the ankylosed spine, minor trauma can also cause vertebral fractures and should be considered if the pattern of pain and mobility are changed after an accident. The use of CT scan can help to detect these fractures,[9] which may be missed with conventional radiography. The changes in bone formation in SpA will be discussed in more detail in elsewhere in this issue.

CV manifestations, particularly conduction disturbances and aortic insufficiency, occur in 1% to 10% of patients with long-standing disease and the risk of atherosclerotic events is approximately doubled. Pulmonary complications are infrequent and can be caused by rigidity of the chest wall and apical pulmonary fibrosis.[10] Renal involvement was encountered in severe AS in the past (amyloidosis), but seem to be less common in the current SpA population.[10]

It is important to realize the impact and prevalence of these EAMs and comorbidities because they might interfere with the efficacy of the commonly used drugs in SpA or, worse, some can be a contraindication for these drugs.

NSAIDs, as well as selective cyclooxygenase-2 (COX-2)–inhibitors (eg, celecoxib and etoricoxib), are very effective in reducing pain and morning stiffness, and for the treatment of arthritis and enthesitis.[11–15] However, the presence of IBD or severe CV disease can be a relative contraindication for these drugs.

Tumor necrosis factor (TNF)-blocking agents made possible a substantial improvement of the treatment of SpA. Up to now, large placebo-controlled trials have demonstrated the efficacy of infliximab, etanercept, adalimumab, and golimumab in 60% to 70% of subjects with SpA.[16–23] but other biologicals are not very effective in SpA so far.[24–28] Next to clinical improvement, a decrease of inflammation was observed on MRI of the sacroiliac joints and vertebral spine.[29–36] However, some of these TNF-blocking agents seem to be more effective in the treatment of EAMs, such as colitis, compared with other drugs of this group.

Interestingly, patients with SpA with comorbidities, such as osteoporosis, seem to show improvement of this manifestation because bone mineral density rises during anti-TNF treatment in most patients with SpA.[37]

EAMS OF SPA

Uveitis

Acute anterior uveitis is an acute attack with inflammation of the uvea and can be the first presenting symptom of the disease. In a study of 433 subjects with different types of uveitis, 44 cases (almost 10%) of SpA were detected, whereas other studies showed a percentage up to 50% of previously undiagnosed cases of SpA among subjects with uveitis.[38–40]

The occurrence of acute anterior uveitis is increased in the HLA-B27 positive population, with a lifetime cumulative incidence of 0.2% in the general population compared with 1% in the HLA-B27 positive population.[41]

The attacks of uveitis are usually recurrent and unilateral. The symptoms are sudden ocular pain with redness and photophobia. Inflammation can lead to debris, which accumulates in the anterior chamber and may cause papillary and lens dysfunction with blurring of vision. In some cases, glaucoma and severe visual impairment occurs if adequate treatment is delayed, but usually the uveitis subsides spontaneously within 3 months.

In patients with SpA who have sudden symptoms of a painful red eye it is recommended to refer the patient to the ophthalmologist as soon as possible. In most cases, acute uveitis can be treated successfully by the ophthalmologist with local corticosteroids and mydriatics. Sometimes an intraocular injection with corticosteroids or a high oral dosage of prednisone (up to 60 mg daily) is necessary to treat the inflammation. In most cases there is no residual visual impairment.

NSAIDs seem to show efficacy for uveitis. There is some evidence that the use of sulfasalazine reduces the recurrence rate of uveitis.[42,43] Other immunosuppressive drugs used by the ophthalmologists to treat refractory uveitis, such as azathioprine and methotrexate, do not have much efficacy on the disease activity of SpA.

Some TNF-blocking agents can be used for indications of and active SpA disease, as well as refractory uveitis. Infliximab, an adequate treatment of SpA, decreases the recurrence rate of uveitis and is effective in refractory uveitis.[44,45] The efficacy of etanercept on uveitis is uncertain because etanercept does not seem to prevent a relapse in combination with methotrexate[46] and it was suggested that etanercept might even trigger an attack of uveitis.[47] However, a comparison of three randomized studies with etanercept in AS showed a lower number of cases with uveitis in subjects treated with etanercept compared with placebo,[48] indicating that etanercept inhibits the recurrence of uveitis.

An analysis of four placebo-controlled studies and three open-label studies with TNF agents in AS showed a frequency of flares of anterior uveitis in the placebo-group of 15.6 per 100 patient-years, compared with 7.9 per 100 patient-years in etanercept group and 3.4 per 100 patient-years in the subjects treated with infliximab.[45] The attacks of uveitis during these studies were reported by the subjects and no follow-up studies or ophthalmologic controls were performed.

Reports on the efficacy of adalimumab on uveitis are mainly based on retrospective analysis of placebo-controlled trials, which show beneficial results.[49] In a prospective study, subjects with AS were treated with adalimumab because of their high disease activity and screened by an ophthalmologist on uveitis. This study demonstrates a significant decrease (73%) of the recurrence rate of uveitis during adalimumab treatment.[50]

Data on the efficacy of golimumab on the recurrence rate of anterior uveitis are lacking. It can be concluded that, in most cases, attacks of anterior uveitis respond very well to (local) treatment by the ophthalmologist. In cases with refractory uveitis or a high uveitis recurrence rate, treatment with TNF-blocking agents can be successful, especially if the treatment is indicated for high disease activity of SpA. Adalimumab and infliximab seem to be more effective in lowering the recurrence rate of uveitis compared with etanercept.

Psoriasis

Psoriasis is a common skin disease with plaque lesions and nail deformities. Psoriatic arthritis occurs in 5% to 20% of people with psoriasis and can present as a symmetric polyarthritis, resembling rheumatoid arthritis, but with additional involvement of the distal interphalangeal joints.[51] Axial disease occurs in about 5% of patients with psoriasis, asymmetrical sacroiliitis occurs in one-third of the cases, and spondylitis without sacroiliitis occurs in the rest. Enthesitis and dactylitis are common, especially in the oligoarticular form of the disease. In SpA, patients with psoriatic arthritis excluded, psoriasis occurs in approximately 5% to10%.

In case of scaling skin lesions or nail changes suspicious for psoriasis in SpA it is recommended to refer the patient to a dermatologist. Skin manifestations of psoriasis respond to local corticosteroids or psoralen plus ultraviolet A (PUVA) therapy.

In case of psoriatic arthritis, NSAIDs and intra-articular injections with corticosteroid are effective in monoarthritis or oligoarthritis.[52] Methotrexate and leflunomide are effective in both psoriasis and peripheral arthritis, but show efficacy for the axial manifestations of SpA,[53] whereas TNF-α blockers, such as infliximab, etanercept, adalimumab, and golimumab, are efficacious on psoriasis as well as the axial manifestations of SpA.[52] In some cases, treatment of SpA with TNF-blocking agents can result in controversial reactions, including as new manifestations of psoriasis such as palmoplantar pustulosis.[54]

IBD

IBD includes Crohn disease and ulcerative colitis. Approximately 10% of patients with IBD develop SpA. On the other hand, the chance of patients with SpA developing IBD is 5% to10%. Asymptomatic IBD is described in a high percentage (60%) of patients with SpA and can be detected by endoscopy of the colon and terminal ileum.[55] During follow-up studies, it seemed that up to 6% of subjects with SpA who had chronic gut inflammation eventually developed Crohn disease.[56]

Another indication that diseases such as SpA and IBD show some overlap is a study on serologic markers of IBD. In this study, a high percentage (55%) of subjects with AS without abdominal complaints had positive tests for perinuclear antineutrophil cytoplasmic autoantibody (pANCA), ANCA, or outer membrane porin C *Saccharomyces cerevisiae* IgG and IgA (Omp-C ASCA).[57]

In case of persistent or frequently recurring diarrhea and/or blood or mucus production with the stools, it is advised to refer the patient with SpA to a gastroenterologist to perform a colonoscopy.

Treatment of IBD by a gastroenterologist is based on immunosuppressive drugs and anti-TNF. The use of NSAIDs can worsen the colitis manifestation; therefore it is advised to minimize the use of these drugs by patients with SpA who have IBD, except for celecoxib, which does not seem to increase the risk at exacerbation of the IBD.[58] The use of sulfasalazine can be beneficial for SpA and !BD. In most cases, the efficacy of other immunosuppressive drugs used in IBD has no proven efficacy in SpA.[59] Among the TNF-blocking agents, only infliximab and adalimumab are effective in SpA and IBD. Golimumab is effective in SpA, but not yet registered for IBD.[60–64] Etanercept works well for spinal symptoms in SpA but not on IBD and, even worse, new manifestations of IBD might occur during etanercept treatment.[65,66]

Therefore, in patients with SpA who have IBD, the use of NSAIDs should be minimized except for celecoxib, sulfasalazine might be beneficial for both indications, and the first choice of anti-TNF is infliximab or adalimumab.

CV COMORBIDITIES—RECENT INSIGHTS

It has been clearly established that patients with AS suffer from an increased CV risk in comparison with the general population. This increased risk is due to atherosclerotic diseases, such as myocardial and cerebral infarction, and the so-called AS-specific cardiac manifestations.

The traditional CV risk factors, as well as the underlying chronic inflammatory process, are important for the increased atherosclerotic risk in AS.[67] In addition, inflammation also seems important for the development of AS-specific cardiac manifestations.

Mortality

Two recent mortality studies indicated a 60% to 90% increased mortality in comparison to the general population (**Table 1**).[68,69] Most important, the causes of death were circulatory (40%), malignancies (27%), and infections (23%)[68]; or were 17%, 17%, and 29%, respectively.[69]

Table 1
Mortality in AS

Study	Study Design	Comparison Group	Number of Patients	Time Period	Findings
Bakland et al,[68] 2011	Hospital-based	General population	677	1977–2009	SMR[a]: 1.61 (1.29–1.93)
Mok et al,[69] 2011	Hospital-based	General population	2332	1999–2008	SMR: 1.87 (1.61–2.13)

[a] SMR: Standardized mortality ratio.

These figures are similar to the standardized mortality ratio in older studies,[70,71] indicating that there was no decline of mortality during the last decades. Predictors of mortality may include increased C-reactive protein levels and infrequent or non-NSAID use.[68]

CV Comorbidity

A population-based cohort investigation in almost 5400 men, demonstrated a 40% increased risk for myocardial infarction,[72] that was age-dependent and peaked at age 60–64 (hazard ratio = 2.4; 95% CI: 1.3–4.5). The largest study comprised more than 8.600 subjects with AS and prevalence ratios ranged from 1.25 for cerebrovascular disease to 1.37 for ischemic heart disease, with the greater excess risk in younger subjects.[73]

However, an almost threefold increased prevalence of myocardial infarction was reported in a questionnaire-based study of 400 subjects with AS,[74] and a doubled prevalence of ischemic heart disease was reported in a Swedish population study (**Table 2**).[75]

It is important to realize that patients with AS might also suffer from an increased risk for hemorrhagic stroke as a recent population-based investigation revealed a standardized incidence ratio of 8.1 for hemorrhagic stroke after hospitalization for AS.[76]

PRECLINICAL ATHEROSCLEROSIS

Carotid artery intima media thickness (cIMT) is a valid instrument to assess preclinical, atherosclerosis and an important predictor for future CV disease. Thus far, several small scale studies demonstrated cIMT increases ranging from 0.07 mm and 0.12 mm, respectively.[77,78] This indicates only a 10% to 15% % increased CV risk and is much lower than the expected, approximately double, CV risk demonstrated in the studies mentioned above. This might indicate that, in AS, atherosclerotic plaques have an increased tendency to rupture (unstable plaques) in comparison to the general population; this needs further investigation.

AS-RELATED CARDIAC MANIFESTATIONS

Several studies indicated that AS is also associated with non-atherosclerotic CV manifestations and it is hypothesized that inflammation affects different structures of the heart leading to these complications. Whereas aortitis was reported often in the older literature, now this complication is rare, and contemporary prevalence data are not available.

Aortic Regurgitation, Aortic and Mitral Valve Thickening

The prevalence of aortic regurgitation ranges from 1%–10% and increases with age, disease duration, and presence of arthritis[79]; and is increased in comparison with the general population (albeit that some studies could not confirm this).[80] This discrepancy could come from different disease duration between the studies. In a recent investigation, aortic and mitral valve thickening without regurgitation was seen in subjects with early AS.[81]

Aortic regurgitation is still relevant because patients with AS have a 60% higher chance of hospitalization with aortic valve disease in comparison with the general population.[73]

Table 2
CV atherosclerotic comorbidities in AS

Study	Population Studied	Study Design	Number of AS Patients	Outcome Measures and Findings
Symmons et al,[72] 2004	UK	Community-based AS cohort vs general population	5392	First myocardial infarction, hazard ratio: 1.4 (95% CI: 1.2–1.8)
Han et al,[88] 2006	US	PharMetrics Patient Centric database (US) Cross-sectional vs 4 matched controls	1843	Prevalence ratio: • Ischemic heart disease: 1.2 (95% CI 1.0–1.5) • Peripheral vascular disease: 1.6 (95% CI 1.2–2.2) • Congestive heart failure 1.8 (95% CI 1.2–2.6) • Cerebrovascular disease: 1.7 (95% CI 1.3–2.3)
Peters et al,[74] 2010	Netherlands	Referral based two-center study vs general population	383	Odds ratio: 3.1 (95% CI 1.9–5.1)
Szabo et al,[73] 2011	Canada	Population-based cohort compared with general population	8616	Prevalence ratio: • Ischemic heart disease: 1.37 (95% CI 1.31–1.91) • Peripheral vascular disease: 1.6 (95% CI 1.2–2.2) • Cerebrovascular disease: 1.25 (95% CI 1.15–1.35)
Bremander et al,[75] 2011	Sweden	Population-based cohort study	935	Ischemic heart disease SMR[a]: 2.20 (95% CI 1.77–2.70)

[a] SMR: Standardized mortality ratio.

Conduction Disturbances

The older literature reports prevalence of conduction disturbances ranging from 1% to 33% and the presence of the HLA-B27 antigen increases this risk.[82,83] However, two out of three more recent studies[80,84,85] did not show an increased rate in comparison to general population.[80,84]

It is not known if and to what extent conduction disturbances are increased in AS. Again, large scale prospective studies are needed to determine the prevalence of conduction disturbances in AS and its clinical relevance.

Left Ventricular Dysfunction

In a controlled study in 88 subjects with AS and 33 age-matched controls, significantly higher left ventricular end-diastolic and stroke volumes,[84] indicating a decreased left ventricular function, were seen in the subjects with AS versus the controls. Another controlled study found an impaired coronary flow reserve.[86] Left ventricular wall motion abnormalities were seen in a study of 22 subjects with AS using gated technetium-99m methoxyisobutylisonitrile (Tc 99m-MIBI) myocardial perfusion single-photon emission computed tomography (SPECT).[87]

CV RISK FACTORS

Several large scale studies have demonstrated significantly higher, increased up to twofold, prevalence of hypertension[75,88,89] and dyslipidemia.[88] Dyslipidemia in AS is related to disease activity and, in active disease, characterized by lowered total and HDL-cholesterol concentrations.[90,91]

There are also some indications that subjects with AS smoke much more than non–AS controls.[91,92]

THE EFFECTS OF ANTIRHEUMATIC TREATMENT

Because atherosclerosis is in essence an inflammation of the artery,[93] one would expect that effective antirheumatic (ie, antiinflammatory), therapy would have a favorable impact on the CV risk in patients with AS. In rheumatoid arthritis there is increasing evidence from observational studies that TNF-blocking agents reduce the CV risk (albeit CV endpoint trials have not been conducted).

Because large-scale placebo-controlled CV endpoint studies with TNF blocking agents are not feasible anymore, several investigators have looked at the effect of TNF-blockers in AS on cIMT because this is a validated surrogate endpoint for atherosclerosis. A small-scale controlled study showed a decreased cIMT progression in 12 subjects with AS who were treated with anti-TNF.[94]

In addition, anti-TNF seems to improve microvascular and macrovascular function.[95–97] This is important because endothelial dysfunction is the initiating step of atherogenesis.

The effect of TNF-blocking therapy on conduction disturbances was studied in 21 subjects with AS in whom TNF-blocking therapy was initiated and revealed a favorable effect (ie, shortening of the QT interval),[98] thereby underscoring the causal role of inflammation in conduction disturbances.

The effects of TNF blockade on the lipid profile in AS are mixed, showing only minor or no improvement.[99–101] Hence, the favorable effects TNF-blockade on the CV risk are not mediated by effects on the lipid profile.

However, when looking at HDL-cholesterol protein composition, it seems that in an inflammatory situation HDL-cholesterol loses its antiatherogenic capacity because the

HDL-apolipoprotein A-I is replaced by serum amyloid A and, thus, a different pattern emerges. With surface-enhanced laser desorption/ionization time-of flight (SELDI-TOF) techniques it was found that during anti-TNF treatment the concentrations of serum amyloid A within the HDL-cholesterol particles decreased, thereby restoring the atheroprotective capacity of HDL-cholesterol.[102]

Altogether, most (albeit small-scale) studies suggest that effective antirheumatic treatment has beneficial effects on markers of preclinical atherosclerosis and CV risk factors, but whether the CV risk is ultimately reduced remains to be assessed.

UNDERTREATMENT OF CV COMORBIDITY

Generally comorbidity is undertreated in patients with chronic diseases[103]; however, AS-specific data are lacking.

Particularly in AS, the identification of specific CV problems could be masked in patients with AS. For example, chest pain can be misinterpreted as musculoskeletal rather than originating from the heart.

CV RISK MANAGEMENT

AS should be regarded as a new, independent CV risk factor for which CV risk management should be considered. In 2009, the European League Against Rheumatism (EULAR) recommended CV risk management in patients with inflammatory arthritis, including AS,[104] consisting of yearly CV risk screening (and treatment, if necessary) and effective treatment of the underlying inflammation. This was confirmed by the 2010 update of the Assessment of Spondyloarthritis International Society (ASAS)-EULAR recommendations for the management of AS.[105]

SUMMARY

SpA is a chronic inflammatory disease with either predominantly axial symptoms of the spine and sacroiliac joints (axial SpA, including ankylosing spondylitis) or predominantly arthritis (peripheral SpA). Many patients with SpA also suffer from EAMs, including anterior uveitis, psoriasis or IBD, and cardiovascular manifestations. Peripheral arthritis occurs in approximately 30% of the patients, especially in large joints and shows an asymmetrical, oligoarticular pattern. Other common joint complaints are due to enthesitis, which manifest as extra-articular bony tenderness in areas such as the Achilles tendon. Acute anterior uveitis presents with acute pain, loss of vision and redness in one eye that usually subsides spontaneously after several weeks. Rapid treatment by an ophthalmologist is required to prevent synechiae formation, which could ultimately result in glaucoma and blindness. Although less common, organ involvement in SpA can also be located in the heart, lungs, or kidneys. Treatment of SpA includes physical exercise, NSAIDs, and, in case of peripheral arthritis, sulfasalazine. In case of insufficient response to NSAIDs, TNF-blockers (especially infliximab, etanercept, adalimumab, and golimumab) are effective. These drugs work well on the axial manifestations and on arthritis, enthesitis, and psoriasis. However, their efficacy differs in several EAMs, such as uveitis and IBD. Anterior uveitis can be treated adequately by an ophthalmologist but, in refractory uveitis or a with a high recurrence rate, treatment with adalimumab and infliximab seems to be more effective compared with etanercept. In case of IBD in SpA, the use of NSAIDs should be minimized; however, celecoxib can be used if needed. The choice of anti-TNF therapy in SpA with IBD is in favor of infliximab and adalimumab instead of etanercept. Overall, it is important to realize that EAMs do occur frequently in SpA and should be taken into account in the choice of treatment. Patients with AS also suffer from comorbidities, such as osteoporosis. They also have an increased CV risk due to atherosclerotic diseases, such as myocardial and cerebral infarction, as well as the so-called AS-specific cardiac manifestations (albeit that the exact contribution of these AS-specific manifestations, such as myocardial dysfunction, still needs to be assessed). Additional studies are mandatory in view of the potential clinical consequences, including routine echocardiographic examination of AS patients. The traditional CV risk factors, as well as the underlying chronic inflammatory process, are important for the increased atherosclerotic risk in AS. In addition, inflammation seems important for the development of the AS-specific cardiac manifestations. CV risk management is mandatory for patients with AS and this consists of assessment, and treatment if necessary, of the traditional CV risk factors, as well as effective treatment of the underlying inflammation. EAMs occur frequently in AS and increase the burden of the disease. Therefore, physicians should be aware of these manifestations and refer patients to the ophthalmologist or gastroenterologist if uveitis or IBD is suspected. The manifestation of EAMs is an important factor in the choice of treatment, especially in case of NSAIDs and the selection of a TNF-blocking agent. There is accumulating evidence for a significantly increased CV risk in patients with AS originating from atherosclerotic disease as well as AS-specific cardiac manifestations. However, the precise magnitude of the AS-specific cardiac manifestations is not known. Therefore, the results of large epidemiological studies should be awaited before routine echocardiographic screening can be recommended for every patient with AS. In contrast, because increased atherosclerotic risk has been well established, CV risk management should not be withheld.

REFERENCES

1. Rudwaleit M, van der Heijde D, Landewé R, et al. The development of assessment of spondyloarthritis international society classification criteria for axial spondyloarthritis (part II): validation and final selection. Ann Rheum Dis 2009;68:777–83.
2. Rudwaleit M, van der Heijde D, Landewé R, et al. The assessment of Spondyloarthritis International Society Classification criteria for peripheral spondyloarthritis and for spondyloarthritis in general. Ann Rheum Dis 2011;70:25–31.
3. Van der Linden S, Valkenburg HA, Cats A. Evaluation of the diagnostic criteria for ankylosing spondylitis; a proposal for the modification of the New York criteria. Arthritis Rheum 1984;27:361–8.
4. Braun J, Bollow M, Remlinger G, et al. Prevalence of spondylarthropathies in HLA-B27 positive and negative blood donors. Arthritis Rheum 1998;41:58–67.
5. McGonagle D, Khan MA, Marzo-Ortega H, et al. Enthesitis in ankylosing spondylitis and related spondylarthropathies. Curr Opin Rheumatol 1999;11:244–50.
6. Heuft-Dorenbosch L, Spoorenberg A, Tubergen A, et al. Assessment of enthesitis in ankylosing spondylitis. Ann Rheum Dis 2003;62:127–32.
7. Maksymowych WP, Mallon C, Morrow S, et al. Development and validation of the Spondyloarthritis Research Consortium of Canada (SPARCC) Enthesitis Index. Ann Rheum Dis 2009;68(6):948–53.
8. van der Weijden MA, Claushuis TA, Nazari T, et al. High prevalence of low bone mineral density in patients within 10 years of onset of ankylosing spondylitis: a systematic review. Clin Rheumatol 2012. [Epub ahead of print].
9. van der Weijden MA, van der Horst-Bruinsma IE, van Denderen JC, et al. High frequency of vertebral fractures in early spondylarthropathies. Osteoporos Int 2012;23(6):1683–90.

10. El Maghraoui A. Extra-articular manifestations of ankylosing spondylitis: prevalence, characteristics and therapeutic implications. Eur J Intern Med 2011; 22(6):554–60.
11. Dougados M, Behier JM, Jolchine I, et al. Efficacy of celecoxib, a cycloogynase-2-specific inhibitor, in the treatment of ankylosing spondylitis. Arthritis Rheum 2001;44:180–5.
12. van der Heijde D, Baraf HS, Ramos-Remus C, et al. Evaluation of the efficacy of etoricoxib in ankylosing spondylitis: results of a fifty-two-week, randomized, controlled study. Arthritis Rheum 2005;52:1205–15.
13. Wanders A, Heijde D, Landewe R, et al. Nonsteroidal antiinflammatory drugs reduce radiographic progression in patients with ankylosing spondylitis: a randomized clinical trial. Arthritis Rheum 2005;52:1756–65.
14. Poddubnyy D, Rudwaleit M, Haibel H, et al. Effect of non-steroidal anti-inflammatory drugs on radiographic spinal progression in patients with axial spondyloarthritis: results from the German spondyloarthritis inception cohort. Ann Rheum Dis 2012. [Epub ahead of print].
15. Zochling J, van der Heijde D, Dougados M, et al. Current evidence for the management of ankylosing spondylitis: a systematic literature review for the ASAS/EULAR management recommendations in ankylosing spondylitis. Ann Rheum Dis 2006;65(4):423–32.
16. Braun J, van der Horst-Bruinsma IE, Huang F, et al. Clinical efficacy and safety of etanercept versus sulfasalazine in patients with ankylosing spondylitis: a randomized, double-blind trial. Arthritis Rheum 2011;63(6):1543–51.
17. Song IH, Hermann K, Haibel H, et al. Effects of etanercept versus sulfasalazine in early axial spondyloarthritis on active inflammatory lesions as detected by whole-body MRI (ESTHER): a 48-week randomised controlled trial [Erratum in Ann Rheum Dis 2011;70(7):1350]. Ann Rheum Dis 2011;70(4):590–6.
18. van der Heijde D, Dijkmans B, Geusens P, et al, Ankylosing Spondylitis Study for the Evaluation of Recombinant Infliximab Therapy Study Group. Efficacy and safety of infliximab in patients with ankylosing spondylitis: results of a randomized, placebo-controlled trial (ASSERT). Arthritis Rheum 2005;52:582–91.
19. van der Heijde D, Da Silva JC, Dougados M, et al. Once-weekly 50-mg dosing of etanercept (Enbrel(R)) is as effective as 25-mg twice-weekly dosing in patients with ankylosing spondylitis. Ann Rheum Dis 2006; 65(12):1572–7.
20. Van der Heijde D, Kivitz A, Schiff MH, et al. Efficacy and safety of adalimumab in patients with ankylosing spondylitis. Results of a multicenter, randomized, double-blind, placebo-controlled trial. Arthritis Rheum 2006;54:2136–46.
21. Inman RD, Davis JC Jr, Heijde D, et al. Efficacy and safety of golimumab in patients with ankylosing spondylitis: results of a randomized, double-blind, placebo-controlled, phase III trial. Arthritis Rheum 2008;58:3402–12.
22. Brandt J, Khariouzov A, Listing J, et al. Successful short term treatment of patients with severe undifferentiated spondyloarthritis with the anti-tumor necrosis factor-alpha fusion receptor protein etanercept. J Rheumatol 2004; 31(3):531–8.
23. Baraliakos X, Listing J, Brandt J, et al. Clinical response to discontinuation of anti-TNF therapy in patients with ankylosing spondylitis after 3 years of continuous treatment with infliximab [Erratum in Arthritis Res Ther 2005;7(3):113]. Arthritis Res Ther 2005;7(3):R439–44.
24. Haibel H, Rudwaleit M, Listing J, et al. Open label trial of anakinra in active ankylosing spondylitis over 24 weeks. Ann Rheum Dis 2005;64(2):296–8.

25. Tan AL, Marzo-Ortega H, O'Connor P, et al. Efficacy of anakinra in active ankylosing spondylitis: a clinical and magnetic resonance imaging study. Ann Rheum Dis 2004;63(9):1041–5.
26. Song IH, Heldmann F, Rudwaleit M, et al. Different response to rituximab in tumor necrosis factor blocker-naive patients with active ankylosing spondylitis and in patients in whom tumor necrosis factor blockers have failed: a twenty-four-week clinical trial. Arthritis Rheum 2010;62(5):1290–7.
27. Lekpa FK, Farrenq V, Canouï-Poitrine F, et al. Lack of efficacy of abatacept in axial spondylarthropathies refractory to tumor-necrosis-factor inhibition. Joint Bone Spine 2012;79(1):47–50.
28. Song IH, Heldmann F, Rudwaleit M, et al. Treatment of active ankylosing spondylitis with abatacept: an open-label, 24-week pilot study. Ann Rheum Dis 2011;70(6):1108–10.
29. Braun J, Landewé R, Hermann KG, et al. Major reduction in spinal inflammation in patients with ankylosing spondylitis after treatment with infliximab: results of a multicenter, randomized, double-blind, placebo-controlled magnetic resonance imaging study. Arthritis Rheum 2006;54(5):1646–52.
30. Baraliakos X, Davis J, Tsuji W, et al. Magnetic resonance imaging examinations of the spine in patients with ankylosing spondylitis before and after therapy with the tumor necrosis factor alpha receptor fusion protein etanercept. Arthritis Rheum 2005;52(4):1216–23.
31. Lambert RG, Salonen D, Rahman P, et al. Adalimumab significantly reduces both spinal and sacroiliac joint inflammation in patients with ankylosing spondylitis: a multicenter randomized, double-blind, placebo-controlled study. Arthritis Rheum 2007;56(12):4005–14.
32. Braun J, Baraliakos X, Hermann KG, et al. Golimumab reduces spinal inflammation in ankylosing spondylitis: MRI results of the randomised, placebo-controlled GO-RAISE study. Ann Rheum Dis 2012;71(6):878–84.
33. Rudwaleit M, Claudepierre P, Wordsworth P, et al. Effectiveness, safety, and predictors of good clinical response in 1250 patients treated with adalimumab for active ankylosing spondylitis. J Rheumatol 2009;36(4):801–8.
34. Vastesaeger N, van der Heijde D, Inman RD, et al. Predicting the outcome of ankylosing spondylitis therapy. Ann Rheum Dis 2011;70(6):973–81.
35. Haibel H, Rudwaleit M, Listing J, et al. Efficacy of adalimumab in the treatment of axial spondyloarthritis without radiographically defined sacroiliitis. Arthritis Rheum 2008;58:1981–91.
36. Barkham N, Keen HI, Coates LC, et al. Clinical and imaging efficacy of infliximab in HLA-B27-Positive patients with magnetic resonance imaging-determined early sacroiliitis [Erratum in Arthritis Rheum 2010;62(10):3005]. Arthritis Rheum 2009;60(4):946–54.
37. Barnabe C, Hanley DA. Effect of tumor necrosis factor alpha inhibition on bone density and turnover markers in patients with rheumatoid arthritis and spondyloarthropathy. Semin Arthritis Rheum 2009;39(2):116–22.
38. Linder R, Hoffmann A, Brunner R. Prevalence of the spondyloarthritides in patients with uveitis. J Rheumatol 2004;31(11):2226–9.
39. Monnet D, Breban M, Hudry C, et al. Ophthalmic findings and frequency of extraocular manifestations in patients with HLA-B27 uveitis: a study of 175 cases. Ophthalmology 2004;111(4):802–9.
40. Pato E, Banares A, Jover JA, et al. Undiagnosed spondyloarthropathy in patients presenting with anterior uveitis. J Rheumatol 2000;27(9):2198–202.

41. Linssen A, Rothova A, Valkenburg HA, et al. The lifetime cumulative incidence of acute anterior uveitis in a normal population and its relation to ankylosing spondylitis and histocompatibility antigen HLA-B27. Invest Ophthalmol Vis Sci 1991; 32(9):2568–78.
42. Munoz-Fernandez S, Hidalgo V, Fernandez-Melon J, et al. Sulfasalazine reduces the number of flares of acute anterior uveitis over a one-year period. J Rheumatol 2003;30(6):1277–9.
43. Wakefield D, Chang JH, Amjadi S, et al. What is new HLA-B27 acute anterior uveitis? Ocul Immunol Inflamm 2011;19(2):139–44.
44. El-Shabrawi Y, Hermann J. Anti-tumor necrosis factor-alpha therapy with infliximab as an alternative to corticosteroids in the treatment of human leukocyte antigen B27-associated acute anterior uveitis. Ophthalmology 2002;109(12):2342–6.
45. Braun J, Baraliakos X, Listing J, et al. Decreased incidence of anterior uveitis in patients with ankylosing spondylitis treated with the anti-tumor necrosis factor agents infliximab and etanercept. Arthritis Rheum 2005;52(8):2447–51.
46. Foster CS, Tufail F, Waheed NK, et al. Efficacy of etanercept in preventing relapse of uveitis controlled by methotrexate. Arch Ophthalmol 2003;121(4):437–40.
47. Rosenbaum JT. Effect of etanercept on iritis in patients with ankylosing spondylitis. Arthritis Rheum 2004;50(11):3736–7.
48. Sieper J, Koenig A, Baumgartner S, et al. Analysis of uveitis rates across all etanercept ankylosing spondylitis clinical trials. Ann Rheum Dis 2010;69(1):226–9.
49. Rudwaleit M, Rødevand E, Holck P, et al. Adalimumab effectively reduces the rate of anterior uveitis flares in patients with active ankylosing spondylitis: results of a prospective open-label study. Ann Rheum Dis 2009;68(5):696–701.
50. van der Horst-Bruinsma IE, van Denderen JC, Visman I, et al. Decreased recurrence rate of uveitis in ankylosing spondylitis treated with adalimumab-an interim analysis. Clin Exp Rheumatol 2010;28:630.
51. Khan MA. Clinical features of ankylosing spondylitis. In: Hochberg MC, Silman AJ, Weinblatt ME, et al, editors. Rheumatology, vol. 2. Edinburg (TX): Mosby; 2003. p. 1161–81.
52. Gossec L, Smolen JS, Gaujoux-Viala C, et al, European League Against Rheumatism. European League Against Rheumatism recommendations for the management of psoriatic arthritis with pharmacological therapies. Ann Rheum Dis 2012;71(1):4–12.
53. Nash P, Thaçi D, Behrens F, et al. Leflunomide improves psoriasis in patients with psoriatic arthritis: an in-depth analysis of data from the TOPAS study. Dermatology 2006;212(3):238–49.
54. Kary S, Worm M, Audring H, et al. New onset or exacerbation of psoriatic skin lesions in patients with definite rheumatoid arthritis receiving tumour necrosis factor alpha antagonists. Ann Rheum Dis 2006;65(3):405–7.
55. Mielants H, Veys EM, Cuvelier C, et al. Ileocolonoscopy and spondarthritis. Br J Rheumatol 1988;27(2):163–4.
56. Mielants H, Veys EM, Goemaere S, et al. Gut inflammation in the spondyloarthropathies: clinical, radiologic, biologic, and genetic features in relation to the type of histology. A prospective study. J Rheumatol 1991;18(10):1542–51.
57. de Vries M, van der Horst-Bruinsma I, van Hoogstraten I, et al. pANCA, ASCA, and OmpC antibodies in patients with ankylosing spondylitis without inflammatory bowel disease. J Rheumatol 2010;37(11):2340–4.
58. Sandborn WJ, Stenson WF, Brynskov J, et al. Safety of celecoxib in patients with ulcerative colitis in remission: a randomized, placebo-controlled, pilot study. Clin Gastroenterol Hepatol 2006;4(2):203–11.

59. van der Horst-Bruinsma IE, Clegg DO, Dijkmans BA. Treatment of ankylosing spondylitis with disease modifying antirheumatic drugs. Clin Exp Rheumatol 2002;20:S67–70.
60. Braun J, Baraliakos X, Listing J, et al. Differences in the incidence of flares or new onset of inflammatory bowel diseases in patients with ankylosing spondylitis exposed to therapy with anti-tumor necrosis factor alpha agents. Arthritis Rheum 2007;57(4):639–47.
61. Hanauer SB, Feagan BG, Lichtenstein GR, et al. Maintenance infliximab for Crohn's disease: the ACCENT I randomised trial. Lancet 2002;359(9317):1541–9.
62. Rutgeerts P, Sandborn WJ, Feagan BG, et al. Infliximab for induction and maintenance therapy for ulcerative colitis [Erratum in N Engl J Med 2006 18;354(20):2200]. N Engl J Med 2005;353(23):2462–76.
63. Sandborn WJ, Rutgeerts P, Enns R, et al. Adalimumab induction therapy for Crohn disease previously treated with infliximab: a randomized trial. Ann Intern Med 2007;146(12):829–38.
64. Sandborn WJ, Hanauer SB, Rutgeerts P, et al. Adalimumab for maintenance treatment of Crohn's disease: results of the CLASSIC II trial. Gut 2007;56(9): 1232–9.
65. Sandborn WJ, Hanauer SB, Katz S, et al. Etanercept for active Crohn's disease: a randomized, double-blind, placebo-controlled trial. Gastroenterology 2001; 121(5):1088–94.
66. Song IH, Appel H, Haibel H, et al. New onset of Crohn's disease during treatment of active ankylosing spondylitis with etanercept [Erratum in J Rheumatol 2008;35(4):729]. J Rheumatol 2008;35(3):532–6.
67. Hahn BH, Grossman J, Chen W, et al. The pathogenesis of atherosclerosis in autoimmune rheumatic diseases: roles of inflammation and dyslipidemia. J Autoimmun 2007;28:69–75.
68. Bakland G, Gran JT, Nossent JC. Increased mortality in ankylosing spondylitis is related to disease activity. Ann Rheum Dis 2011;70:1921–5.
69. Mok CC, Kwok CL, Ho LY, et al. Life expectancy, standardized mortality ratios, and causes of death in six rheumatic diseases in Hong Kong, China. Arthritis Rheum 2011;63:1182–9.
70. Peters MJ, van der Horst-Bruinsma IE, Dijkmans BA, et al. Cardiovascular risk profile of patients with spondylarthropathies, particularly ankylosing spondylitis and psoriatic arthritis. Semin Arthritis Rheum 2004;34:585–92.
71. Zochling J, Braun J. Mortality in rheumatoid arthritis and ankylosing spondylitis. Clin Exp Rheumatol 2009;27(4 Suppl 55):S127–30.
72. Symmons DP, Goodson NJ, Cook MN, et al. Men with ankylosing spondylitis have an increased risk of myocardial infarction. Arthritis Rheum 2004; 50(Suppl):S477.
73. Szabo SM, Levy AR, Rao SR, et al. Increased risk of cardiovascular and cerebrovascular disease in individuals with ankylosing spondylitis: a population-based study. Arthritis Rheum 2011;63:3294–304.
74. Peters MJ, Visman I, Nielen MM. Ankylosing spondylitis; a risk factor for myocardial infarction? Ann Rheum Dis 2010;69:579–81.
75. Bremander A, Petersson IF, Bergman S, et al. Population-based estimates of common comorbidities and cardiovascular disease in ankylosing spondylitis. Arthritis Care Res 2011;63:550–6.
76. Zöller B, Li X, Sundquist J, et al. Risk of subsequent ischemic and hemorrhagic stroke in patients hospitalized for immune-mediated diseases: a nationwide follow-up study from Sweden. BMC Neurol 2012;12(1):41.

77. Gonzalez-Juanatey C, Vazquez-Rodriguez TR, Miranda-Filloy JA, et al. The high prevalence of subclinical atherosclerosis in patients with ankylosing spondylitis without clinically evident cardiovascular disease. Medicine (Baltimore) 2009;88: 358–65.
78. Hamdi W, Chelli Bouaziz M, Zouch I, et al. Assessment of preclinical atherosclerosis in patients with ankylosing spondylitis. J Rheumatol 2012;9:322–6.
79. Palazzi C, Salvarani C, D'Angelo S, et al. Aortitis and periaortitis in ankylosing spondylitis. Joint Bone Spine 2011;78:451–5.
80. Brunner F, Kunz A, Weber U, et al. Ankylosing spondylitis and heart abnormalities: do cardiac conduction disorders, valve regurgitation and diastolic dysfunction occur more often in male patients with diagnosed ankylosing spondylitis for over 15 years than in the normal population? Clin Rheumatol 2006;25:24–9.
81. Park SH, Sohn IS, Joe BH, et al. Early cardiac valvular changes in ankylosing spondylitis: a transesophageal echocardiography study. J Cardiovasc Ultrasound 2012;20(1):30–6.
82. Youssef W, Russell AS. Cardiac, ocular, and renal manifestations of seronegative spondylarthropathies. Curr Opin Rheumatol 1990;2:582–5.
83. Peeters AJ, ten Wolde S, Sedney MI, et al. Heart conduction disturbance: an HLA-B27 associated disease. Ann Rheum Dis 1991;50:348–50.
84. Yildirir A, Aksoyek S, Calguneri M, et al. Echocardiographic evidence of cardiac involvement in ankylosing spondylitis. Clin Rheumatol 2002;21:129–34.
85. Dik VK, Peters MJ, Dijkmans PA, et al. The relationship between disease-related characteristics and conduction disturbances in ankylosing spondylitis. Scand J Rheumatol 2010;39:38–41.
86. Caliskan M, Erdogan D, Gullu H, et al. Impaired coronary microvascular and left ventricular diastolic functions in patients with ankylosing spondylitis. Atherosclerosis 2008;196:306–12.
87. Yalcin H, Guler H, Gunay E, et al. Left ventricular wall function abnormalities in patients with ankylosing spondylitis evaluated by gated myocardial perfusion scintigraphy. Rev Esp Med Nucl 2011;30:292–6.
88. Han C, Robinson DW, Hackett MV, et al. Cardiovascular disease and risk factors in patients with rheumatoid arthritis, psoriatic arthritis, and ankylosing spondylitis. J Rheumatol 2006;33:2167–72.
89. Kang JH, Chen YH, Lin HC. Comorbidity profiles among patients with ankylosing spondylitis: a nationwide population-based study. Ann Rheum Dis 2010;69:1165–8.
90. Mathieu S, Gossec L, Dougados M, et al. Cardiovascular profile in ankylosing spondylitis: a systematic review and meta-analysis. Arthritis Care Res 2011; 63:557–63.
91. Divecha H, Sattar N, Rumley A, et al. Cardiovascular risk parameters in men with ankylosing spondylitis in comparison with non-inflammatory control subjects: relevance of systemic inflammation. Clin Sci 2005;109:171–6.
92. Papadakis JA, Sidiropoulos PI, Karvounaris SA, et al. High prevalence of metabolic syndrome and cardiovascular risk factors in men with ankylosing spondylitis on anti-TNF alpha treatment: correlation with disease activity. Clin Exp Rheumatol 2009;27:292–8.
93. Hansson GK. Inflammation, atherosclerosis, and coronary artery disease. N Engl J Med 2005;352:1685–95.
94. Angel K, Provan SA, Gulseth HL, et al. Tumor necrosis factor-alpha antagonists improve aortic stiffness in patients with inflammatory arthropathies: a controlled study. Hypertension 2010;55:333–8.

95. Angel K, Provan SA, Fagerhol MK, et al. Effect of 1-Year anti-TNF-α therapy on aortic stiffness, carotid atherosclerosis, and calprotectin in inflammatory arthropathies: a controlled study. Am J Hypertens 2012;25(6):644–50.
96. van Eijk IC, Peters MJ, Serné EH, et al. Microvascular function is impaired in ankylosing spondylitis and improves after tumour necrosis factor alpha blockade. Ann Rheum Dis 2009;68:362–6.
97. Syngle A, Vohra K, Sharma A, et al. Endothelial dysfunction in ankylosing spondylitis improves after tumor necrosis factor-alpha blockade. Clin Rheumatol 2010;29:763–70.
98. Senel S, Cobankara V, Taskoylu O, et al. Effect of infliximab treatment on QT intervals in patients with ankylosing spondylitis. J Investig Med 2011;59:1273–5.
99. Spanakis E, Sidiropoulos P, Papadakis J, et al. Modest but sustained increase of serum high density lipoprotein cholesterol levels in patients with inflammatory arthritides treated with infliximab. J Rheumatol 2006;33:2440–6.
100. Kiortsis DN, Mavridis AK, Filippatos TD, et al. Effects of infliximab treatment on lipoprotein profile in patients with rheumatoid arthritis and ankylosing spondylitis. J Rheumatol 2006;33:921–3.
101. Mathieu S, Dubost JJ, Tournadre A, et al. Effects of 14 weeks of TNF alpha blockade treatment on lipid profile in ankylosing spondylitis. Joint Bone Spine 2010;77:50–2.
102. van Eijk I, de Vries MK, Levels JH, et al. Improvement of lipid profile is accompanied by atheroprotective alterations in high-density lipoprotein composition upon tumor necrosis factor blockade: a prospective cohort study in ankylosing spondylitis. Arthritis Rheum 2009;60:1324–30.
103. Redelmeier DA, Tan SH, Booth GL. The treatment of unrelated disorders in patients with chronic medical diseases. N Engl J Med 1998;338:1516–20.
104. Peters MJ, Symmons DP, McCarey D, et al. EULAR evidence-based recommendations for cardiovascular risk management in patients with rheumatoid arthritis and other forms of inflammatory arthritis. Ann Rheum Dis 2010;69:325–31.
105. Braun J, vd Berg R, Baraliakos X, et al. 2010 update of the ASAS/EULAR recommendations for the management of ankylosing spondylitis. Ann Rheum Dis 2011;70:896–904.

The Genetics of Ankylosing Spondylitis and Axial Spondyloarthritis

Philip C. Robinson, MBChB, FRACP,
Matthew A. Brown, MBBS, MD, FRACP*

KEYWORDS

• Genetics • Genomics • Ankylosing spondylitis • Axial spondyloarthritis • Arthritis • *HLA-B27* • *ERAP1*

KEY POINTS

- Ankylosing spondylitis is a polygenic disease with a strong association with *HLA-B27*.
- Thirteen non-MHC loci are now also associated with ankylosing spondylitis.
- The MHC class I presentation, IL-23, and tumor necrosis factor pathways are implicated in the cause of AS.
- The carriage rate of *HLA-B27* is lower in cohorts of axial spondyloarthritis compared with cohorts of ankylosing spondylitis.

INTRODUCTION

The spondyloarthropathies (SpA) share characteristic clinical and histopathologic manifestations, and have long been thought to share genetic causes, including *HLA-B27* and non-B27 genes. As more is learned about the genetics of ankylosing spondylitis (AS), inflammatory bowel disease (IBD), and psoriasis, the known extent of this sharing is expanding. This article outlines what is known about the genetics of AS and related SpA and diseases.

GENETIC EPIDEMIOLOGY

AS is a highly heritable polygenic disease, in which environmental factors in developed countries play only a minor role in determining risk of developing the disease. The prevalence of AS varies according to some genetic and as yet undescribed

---

Conflict of interest: The University of Queensland has applied for patents related to the genetic findings in AS.
University of Queensland Diamantina Institute, Princess Alexandra Hospital, Ipswich Road, Brisbane, Woolloongabba, Queensland 4102, Australia
* Corresponding author.
E-mail address: matt.brown@uq.edu.au

Rheum Dis Clin N Am 38 (2012) 539–553
http://dx.doi.org/10.1016/j.rdc.2012.08.018 **rheumatic.theclinics.com**
0889-857X/12/$ – see front matter

environmental factors. Differences in *HLA-B27* prevalence drives most of the variation in prevalence seen worldwide.[1] For example, the carriage rate of *HLA-B27* is approximately 8% to 10% in white European populations and the prevalence of AS is estimated at 0.1% to 1%.[2] When the *HLA-B27* carriage rate is increased, then SpA prevalence rises accordingly. For example, in the Canadian Haida Indians the *HLA-B27* carriage rate is around 50% and the SpA prevalence is 5% to 6%.[3]

There has been gene-phenotype discordance reported, for example in the Fula ethnic group, which inhabit The Gambia in Africa.[4] Although in most African ethnicities *HLA-B27* is rare, among the Fula *HLA-B27* carriage was 6%, yet no cases of AS were found or have been reported. Cases of AS have been reported in American Africans carrying the European *HLA-B27* subtype B*2705, and the African subtype B*2703, indicating that the paucity of AS in *HLA-B27*–positive Africans is likely not caused by protective genetic effects. Rather, this suggests that although AS has a high heritability, environmental factors do play a role in determining susceptibility in some populations.

MAJOR HISTOCOMPATIBILITY COMPLEX GENES

HLA-B Alleles

The association of *HLA-B27* with AS was described in 1973, and remains one of the strongest genetic associations with any common human disease. Nonetheless, only a minority (likely <5%) of B27-positive individuals develop AS. The discovery that allelic variation of HLA-DRB1*01 and *04 influenced the risk of rheumatoid arthritis stimulated research into variation in *HLA-B27* itself. There are now known to be more than 90 subtypes of *HLA-B*27*, which have arisen from the common ancestral subtype, HLA-B*2705. Unlike the situation in rheumatoid arthritis, for the most part in AS B*27 subtype variation plays little role in influencing disease risk. There is strong evidence to suggest that HLA-B*2706 (found in east Asian populations) and B*2709 (found in Sardinia) have reduced strength of association with AS. The common white European subtypes, B*2705 and B*2702, are equally strongly associated with AS. The primarily Asian subtype B*2704 is at least as strongly associated with AS as B*2705 in the same populations, with some studies suggesting that it may be more strongly associated. B*2707, also mainly found in Asians, seems equally strongly associated with AS as B*2705. Although AS cases have been reported carrying many other B27 subtypes, for most alleles the number of cases reported is too few to definitely comment on their relative strength of association with the disease.

There are currently four main theories as to how *HLA-B27* is involved in AS etiopathogenesis. The arthritogenic peptide hypothesis proposes that HLA-B27 presents a pathogenic peptide that initiates disease. This hypothesis is consistent with the antigen presentation function of HLA-B27, and also is consistent with the gene-gene interaction (epistasis) seen with *ERAP1* (discussed later). Despite extensive efforts, no definitive "arthritogenic peptide" has been identified. There are many potential explanations for this including that the peptide may only be present at particular phases in the disease pathogenesis or at particular sites, that it may only represent a small fraction of HLA class I presented peptides, or that more than one peptide may be involved. Because the arthritogenic peptide is proposed to be presented to CD8 T-lymphocytes, the finding that in the *HLA-B27* transgenic rat model of SpA disease is independent of CD8 cells is inconsistent with this hypothesis.[5] However, no animal model perfectly captures human AS, and the relevance of this finding to human AS is not entirely certain.

It has been shown that *HLA-B27* heavy chains, either alone or as heavy chain homodimers, can form on the cell surface and then interact with antigen-presenting cells carrying receptors, such as killer-cell immunoglobulin-like receptors.[6,7] These antigen-presenting cells can then initiate a pathogenic T-helper 17 (Th17) response. These homodimers are thought to occur when unstable HLA-B27:peptide complexes dissociate on the cell surface.[8] ERAP1-deficient cells have more unstable HLA-peptide complexes on the cell surface, which one would expect to promote cell surface homodimer formation, but the AS-protective alleles of the *ERAP1* variants are associated with decreased function, which is inconsistent with this hypothesis.[9,10]

Endoplasmic reticulum (ER) stress, which occurs when misfolding leads to accumulation of HLA-B27 heavy chains in the ER, precipitates a stress response called the unfolded protein response. The unfolded protein response is a homeostatic mechanism that the cell initiates to clear the misfolded proteins and return the ER environment to normal. ER stress has been shown to be present in the HLA-B27 transgenic rat model of SpA,[11] and has been shown to induce interleukin (IL)-23 production,[12] providing a potent link between HLA-B27 and AS.

Finally, *HLA-B27* may tag a nearby disease-causative gene, the association of *HLA-B27* with AS being caused by linkage disequilibrium with this nearby "linked gene." This theory was made much less likely by the findings of the Australian-Anglo-American (TASC) genomewide association study (GWAS) that confirmed the highest association with AS was with *HLA-B27* and not a linked gene.[10]

There are mixed reports on whether homozygosity for *HLA-B27* influences clinical manifestations,[13,14] and although some reports have suggested an increased risk of AS among *HLA-B27* homozygotes, the sample sizes involved in these studies were not sufficient to produce definitive results either way.[15,16] An association with *HLA-B60* has also been described in HLA-B27–positive and HLA-B27–negative individuals,[17–19] although the strength of association reported was not definitive.

The huge volume of genetic information produced by GWASs has allowed researchers to examine further questions of interest relating to heritability of disease and disease-genotype correlations. If one considers the known AS associations, there is not a higher burden of genetic associations in familial AS than sporadic AS, except for *HLA-B27*.[20]

HLA-B27–negative AS makes up only about 10% of AS cohorts, but does demonstrate that an essentially identical disease can be evident without the major genetic risk factor being present. *HLA-B27*–negative AS is less likely to be familial, has a later disease onset, and is less likely to respond to anti–tumor necrosis factor (TNF) treatment,[21–23] but controlling for disease duration has similar disease severity (measured by the Bath Ankylosing Spondylitis Functional Index), activity (measured by the Bath Ankylosing Spondylitis Disease Activity Index),[16] and radiographic severity (measured by the modified Stoke Ankylosing Spondylitis Severity Score).[24] *HLA-B27*–negative AS has been shown to have similar, although not identical, genetic associations with *HLA-B27*–positive AS,[10] the main exception being the association with *ERAP1*, which is restricted to *HLA-B27*–positive AS.

HLA-B27 Typing for Clinical Practice

Accurate HLA-typing is technically challenging and difficult to establish as a high throughput method. This has reduced enthusiasm for the use of HLA-B27 in population screening for risk of AS. Recently, an major histocompatibility complex (MHC) tag single nucleotide polymorphism (SNP) rs4349859 was shown to be able to identify HLA-B27 in those of European descent with a sensitivity of 98% and a specificity of 99%, within the likely boundaries of accuracy of direct HLA-B27 genotyping itself.[10] Another SNP, rs13202464, was then reported that showed high sensitivity and specificity in east Asian populations.[25] The use of these SNPs has significant advantages over the current methods for *HLA-B27* typing in cost and complexity. Further research incorporating other ethnic groups may lead to additional ethnicity-neutral *HLA-B27* tag SNPs. This discovery has implications for potential screening of high-risk cohorts either in the primary care or population-based settings. It may be able to be integrated into referral strategies, by taking advantage of point-of-care testing, which is currently being developed.[26]

NON-MHC GENES

Rapid progress has been made in identifying new non-MHC gene associations in recent years through GWAS. Several these are in genomic regions and involve pathways not thought to be associated with AS, and this further validates the hypothesis-free approach this type of study design affords. The contribution of the described associations to the heritability of AS, as calculated by the variance in liability method, is shown in **Table 1**.

Antigen-Presentation Genes

ERAP1 is a member of the MHC class I presentation pathway and trims peptides before presentation on MHC class I molecules, such as HLA-B27 (**Fig. 1**). *ERAP1* has been robustly associated with AS in multiple studies and populations including Europeans, Hungarians, Portuguese, Taiwanese, Han Chinese, and Koreans.[10,27–32] Recently, it has been demonstrated that the association of *ERAP1* with AS is restricted to *HLA-B27*–positive disease.[10] *ERAP1* is also associated with psoriasis, and the association in psoriasis is restricted to *HLA-Cw6* carriers.[33] The AS-protective SNPs in *ERAP1* result in reduced peptide trimming function of the ERAP1 enzyme.[10] It is not yet clear whether the protective variants of ERAP1 lead to just quantitative reductions in trimmed peptide availability, or if they also lead to qualitative changes in the peptides.[34]

Table 1
Contribution of genome-wide genetic associations to the heritability of AS in populations of white European descent

Gene/Region	Heritability %	Function
HLA-B27	23.3	Antigen presentation
2p15	0.54	Unknown
ERAP1	0.34	Antigen presentation
IL23R	0.31	IL-23/Th17 pathway
KIF21B	0.25	Possibly NF-κβ pathway
IL1R2	0.12	Innate immune responses
RUNX3	0.12	Antigen presentation
IL12B	0.11	IL-23/Th17 pathway
TNFRI/LTBR	0.08	TNF pathway
ANTXR2	0.05	Possibly skeletal involvement
PTGER4	0.05	Innate immune responses
TBKBP1/NPEPPS/TBX21	0.05	TNF pathway/antigen presentation/Th1
21q22	0.04	Unknown
CARD9	0.03	Innate immune responses

Data from Evans DM, Spencer CC, Pointon JJ, et al. Interaction between ERAP1 and HLA-B27 in ankylosing spondylitis implicates peptide handling in the mechanism for HLA-B27 in disease susceptibility. Nat Genet 2011;43:761–7; and Reveille JD, Sims AM, Danoy P, et al. Genome-wide association study of ankylosing spondylitis identifies non-MHC susceptibility loci. Nat Genet 2010;42:123–7.

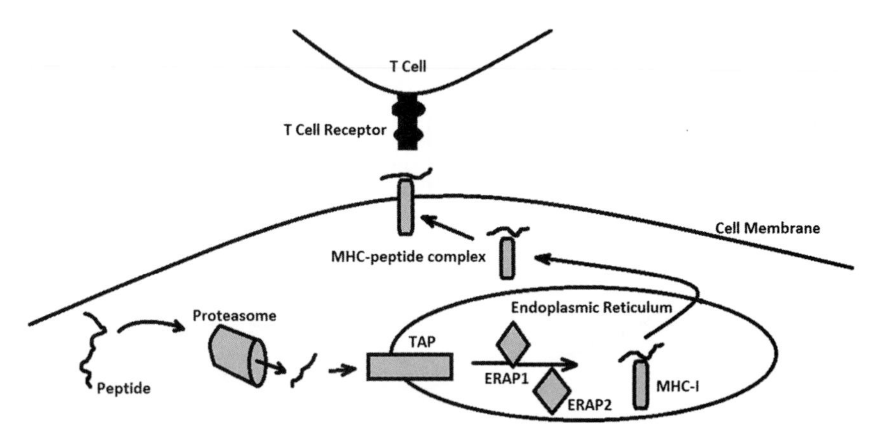

Fig. 1. The antigen presentation pathways with ERAP1 (and ERAP2) trimming the peptide before loading onto the MHC class I molecule.

The ERAP1 enzyme has also been described to have two other functions. First, it has been described to act as a sheddase to cleave cytokine receptors, such as IL-6, TNF, and IL-1β, from the cell surface.[35–37] Studies of ERAP1-deficient mice have demonstrated that the levels of TNF receptor and IL-6 receptor are no different to control animals and in patients with AS there is no difference in serum cytokines based on *ERAP1* genotypes.[10,38] Second, ERAP1 has also been described to be secreted from macrophages in response to interferon-γ and lipopolysaccharide and assists in phagocytosis.[39] Deficiency in phagocytosis could impair responses to commensal or invasive microbes and HLA-B27's restricted repertoire may interact to exacerbate this, or push it over a disease-causing threshold.

ERAP2 encodes an aminopeptidase, which is encoded at chromosome 5p15 immediately adjacent to *ERAP1*, and has also been shown to be associated with AS, although whether this is independent of the ERAP1 association is not clear.[28,40] An *ERAP2* association has been described with Crohn disease.[41] ERAP2 is an aminopeptidase similar to ERAP1, which also trims peptides in the ER before their MHC class I presentation on the cell surface. It has a different peptide preference from ERAP1 and has been shown to form heterodimers with ERAP1.[42,43]

T-Helper 17 Pathway Genes

The association of multiple genes in the pathogenic T-helper 17 (Th17) cell pathway, including *IL23R*, *STAT3*, and *IL12B*, suggests this is an important pathway in AS. The preliminary report of the effective use of anti–IL-17 therapy is also a pragmatic demonstration that clinically this is a pathway that deserves further attention.[44]

IL-23 is made up of two subunits, IL-23p19 and IL-12p40. IL-12p40 is encoded by *IL12B*. IL-23 signals through its receptor IL-23R, present on a wide range of cells, but importantly on gamma-delta T cells and Th17 cells.[45] This receptor, once activated, signals through STAT3 by promoting its phosphorylation. This STAT3 phosphorylation then promotes IL-17 production by Th17 cells.

In cells of the innate immune system and γσ T cells, pattern recognition receptors, such as dectin-1, signal through CARD9 after β-glucan stimulation (**Fig. 2**). The SKG mouse model develops an SpA phenotype when stimulated with β-glucan, characterized by axial and peripheral spondyloarthritis, IBD, and unilateral iritis.[46] After this pathway is activated this promotes the production of prostaglandin E_2.[47]

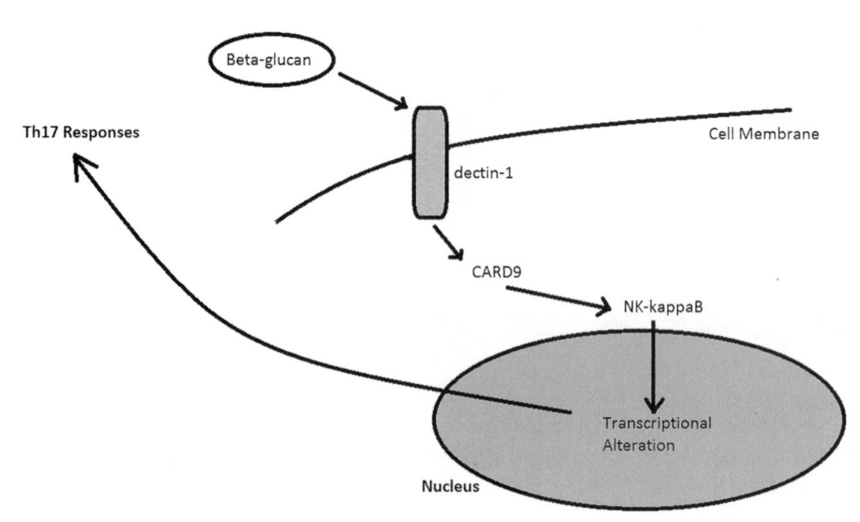

Fig. 2. The interaction of microbial β-glucan and dectin-1, which signals through CARD9 to promote pathogenic proinflammatory cytokines.

Prostaglandin E_2 is a proinflammatory mediator that can signal through the arachadonic acid pathway and promote inflammation. Prostaglandin E_2 can also upregulate IL-23 and IL-17 by signally through prostaglandin E receptor 4, subtype EP4 (PTGER4). This receptor has been associated with AS at genomewide levels of significance.[10] Nonsteroidal anti-inflammatory drugs inhibit cyclooxygenase enzymes and consequently the production of prostaglandins. The finding that nonsteroidal anti-inflammatory drugs retard radiographic progression in AS and that nonsteroidal anti-inflammatory drugs are used to reduce heterotopic ossification is a clinical demonstration of the importance of this pathway to bone formation and homeostasis.[48,49]

Potential Skeletal Structure and Mineralization Genes

ANTXR2, which encodes protein capillary morphogenesis protein 2, is an AS-associated gene with potential impacts on bone and the skeleton. Defects in this gene cause the human syndromes infantile systemic hyalinosis and juvenile hyaline fibromatosis.[50] How variants of this gene are involved in AS is unclear.

A recent GWAS in east Asians[25] found GWAS-significant associations in two loci harboring bone and cartilage related genes. The first associated locus harbors the genes *HAPLN1* and *EDIL3* ($P = 9 \times 10^{-10}$; odds ratio [OR] = 1.2). *HAPLN1* encodes hyaluronan and proteoglycan link protein 1, potentially relevant to AS etiology through bone effects. *EDIL3* encodes EGF-like repeats and discoidin I-like domains 3, which promotes endothelial cell adhesion. The second association lies in an intron of *ANO6* ($P = 2 \times 10^{-8}$; OR = 1.3), which encodes a transmembrane protein involved in phosphatidylserine regulation on the cell surface. Phosphatidylserine exposure is involved in macrophage phagocytosis of apoptotic cells, potentially mediating immune responses.[51] In addition, phosphatidylserine is involved in osteoclastogenesis.[52] It will be valuable to see if these loci replicate in other east Asian or European cohorts.

TNF-Associated Genes

Multiple genes in the TNF pathway have been associated with AS, consistent with this pathway playing a major role in AS etiopathogenesis. Association has been described at the 17q21 locus, which was attributed to *TBKBP1*, a member of the TNF signaling pathway. There are, however, two other plausible candidate genes at this locus include *NPEPPS*, an aminopeptidase similar to *ERAP1* and *ERAP2*, and *TBX21*, a Th1 transcription factor. Further follow-up studies are required to clarify the association at this locus.

Association has also been reported at chromosome 12p13 at a locus containing two TNF-receptors, *TNFRSF1A* and *LTBR*[27]. *LTBR* encodes the lymphotoxin beta receptor; lymphotoxin is a member of the TNF family. Further TNF genes that have been associated with AS include *TBKBP1*, which is a component of the TNF signaling pathway, and *TRADD*,[27,53] another TNF receptor protein has also been associated. An animal model of extreme supraphysiologic TNF overexpression causes an SpA phenotype; how this correlates to human SpA is not yet clear.[54] Several factors implicate this biologic pathway in AS including raised TNF-α in patients with AS and the effectiveness of therapies that block TNF, such as anti-TNF biologics and thalidomide.[55]

Other Genetic Associations

Two intergenic regions at 2p15 and 21q22 have now been robustly associated with AS at genomewide levels of significance.[10,27] Proteasome assembly chaperone 1 (*PSGM1*) gene is found near the 21q22 locus; the proteasome is part of the MHC class I presentation pathway. It is therefore plausible that the association operates through this gene. Against this, the association is not in close proximity to the gene. At chromosome 2p15 there is no nearby candidate gene. RNA-sequencing studies identified long noncoding RNA transcripts at both loci, and it may that the associations operate through *cis*- or *trans*-gene regulation, potentially through noncoding RNA (ncRNA).[27]

RUNX3 encodes Runt-related transcription factor 3, which has been shown to be expressed in thymocytes on signaling by IL-7.[56] These IL-7–stimulated CD4 and CD8 double-positive cells then differentiate into CD8 positive lymphocytes. Further evidence to support this finding is the moderate level of association found in the IL-7 receptor ($P = 8 \times 10^{-5}$) in the TASC AS GWAS.[10] Consistent with this it will be informative to examine other components of this pathway, such as the cytokine IL-7 itself, for association in future experiments.

IL1R2 encodes the IL-1 receptor 2, the biologic action of which is to inhibit IL-1 by acting as a decoy receptor. This protein exists in two forms, a long membrane-bound form and a shorter soluble form, which is produced by alternate splicing.[57] The longer membrane-bound form is the functionally active inhibitory molecule. IL-1β is stimulated by conserved microbial sequences, such as pathogen-associated molecular patterns or damage-associated molecular patterns. Inhibition of an appropriate response to microbial colonization or infection may be the mechanism by which this association acts.

KIF21B has been associated with AS and with other autoimmune disorders including multiple sclerosis,[58] Crohn disease,[59] and ulcerative colitis.[60] It is expressed in a variety of tissues, but best characterized in dendrites. It is involved in trafficking of components within the cell. It is also expressed in B cells, T cells, and natural killer cells.[61] Preliminary evidence suggests *KIF21B* and a nearby open reading frame C1orf106 at the 1q32 locus are involved in ER stress and the NF-$\kappa\beta$ pathway but further functional work is required.[62]

OVERLAP WITH OTHER DISEASES

There is overlap of important risk variants between AS and a whole host of other immune-mediated diseases including but not limited to psoriasis, IBD, multiple sclerosis, rheumatoid arthritis, and anterior uveitis (see **Table 1**).

Psoriasis is a chronic inflammatory autoimmune skin condition present in 3% to 4% of the general population; about 15% of patients with AS have psoriasis. Psoriasis has a major class I MHC association in *HLA-Cw6*, and in a directly analogous situation to AS, there is also an epistatic association with *ERAP1*.[33]

The IL-23 pathway is also a common component of several autoimmune diseases. Genetic associations with *IL23R*, *IL12B*, *PTGER4*, *CARD9*, *STAT3*, and *JAK2*, which have been reported variously with AS, psoriasis, and IBD, likely operate through effects on IL-23 signaling. Various components of this pathway have been described to be associated with psoriasis, IBD, ulcerative colitis, Crohn disease, and multiple sclerosis. The downstream mechanisms by which these associations operate, including the key cytokines involved (IL-17 or IL-22) and cell types (Th17 or noncanonical IL-17–expressing cells, such as gamma-delta cells, mast cells, neutrophils, or dendritic cells), are not clear. Nonetheless, blockade of the pathway including with anti–IL-12p40 and IL-17 antibodies is effective in these conditions (**Table 2**).

THE GENETICS OF AXIAL SPONDYLOARTHRITIS VERSUS AS

Consistent with the differences in the clinical phenotypes seen in patients with SpA there are differences in the genetics between AS and axial SpA. To date the only published data on the genetics of axial SpA is on *HLA-B27* carriage rate. A summary of the published cohorts of patients with SpA is presented in **Table 3**. One of the limitations of examining the *HLA-B27* carriage rate in cohorts of patients with axial SpA is the ascertainment bias that may result from recruiting patients based on their *HLA-B27* status, as would occur with the *HLA-B27* arm of the 2009 ASAS Axial SpA criteria.[63]

From these data it is clear that the *HLA-B27* carriage rate is lower is axial SpA than in AS cohorts, with a 58% to 75% carriage rate compared with 82% to 89% in AS cohorts. Because classification criteria for axial SpA include patients with AS, it is likely that there are significant genetic overlaps between axial SpA and AS.

GENETIC PREDICTORS OF RADIOGRAPHIC PROGRESSION

Studies on the heritability of radiographic change in AS have found that there is a good correlation ($r = 0.86$) between siblings, and the additive heritability of radiographic disease severity based on the Bath Ankylosing Spondylitis Radiographic Index (BASRI) is 0.62.[64,65]

Haroon and colleagues[66] genotyped 13 coding SNPs from antigen-presentation genes (*ERAP1*, *LMP2*, *LMP7*, *TAP1*, and *TAP2*) in the Spondyloarthritis Research Consortium of Canada cohort with the aim of investigating the genetic predictors of radiographic progression. In multivariate analysis allele G of rs17587 in large multifunctional peptidase 2 (*LMP2*) was associated with the baseline modified Stoke

Table 2
Shared genetic associations and pathways in multiple immune mediated

	Ankylosing Spondylitis	Psoriasis	Inflammatory Bowel Disease
MHC class I antigen processing	HLA-B27, ERAP1, ERAP2[a], RUNX3	HLA-Cw6, ERAP1	
IL-23 pathway	IL23R, IL12B, CARD9, PTGER4, STAT3[a]	IL12B, IL23R	IL12B, IL23R, CARD9, PTGER4, STAT3

[a] Suggestive level of association.

Table 3
HLA-B27 carriage rates in ankylosing spondylitis and axial spondyloarthritis patient cohorts

Cohort	SpA Definition	AS Definition	SpA HLA-B27 Rate %	AS HLA-B27 Rate %
GESPIC[78]	Modified ESSG	mNY	74.7	82.2
GESPIC[79]	Modified ESSG	mNY	72.6	84.3
Kiltz et al,[80] 2012	ASAS ASpA	mNY	86.4	89.1
ABILITY-1[75]	ASAS ASpA MRI Arm[a]	—	58.4	—
Haibel et al,[76] 2008	[b]	—	59	—

[a] MRI arm used solely because of the *HLA-B27* arm of the study being affected by ascertainment bias, because *HLA-B27* is part of the entry criteria for this part of the study.
[b] To be included patients had to have low back pain for greater than 3 months and a symptom onset before the age of 50 years and at least three of the following six criteria and at least two of criteria 1 to 3: 1. Inflammatory back pain; 2. Carry *HLA-B27;* 3. Active inflammation in the spine or sacroiliac joints demonstrated on MRI; 4. Good response to nonsteroidal anti-inflammatory drugs; 5. Current or past anterior uveitis, peripheral arthritis, or enthesitis; 6. A family history of spondyloarthritis. Patients who met the modified New York criteria for AS were excluded.

Ankylosing Spondylitis Spinal Score but not with progression. This result has not been replicated.

Bartolome and colleagues[67] investigated 384 SNPs from 190 genes and reported that SNPs in the *MHC*, *TAP2*, *NELL1*, and *ADRB1*, and clinical factors, such as gender and later age at disease onset, could be used to in a model to predict radiographic severity of AS. The predictive model had an area under the receiver operator curve of 0.76 (95% confidence interval, 0.71–0.80); this dropped to 0.68 (96% confidence interval, 0.63–0.73) when the SNPs were removed from the model. The MHC genes were in or near the classical alleles *HLA-DRB1*, *HLA-B*, and *HLA-DQA1*. *NELL1* is expressed in bone and promotes bone formation in animal models.[68] *ADRB1* is the gene that encodes the β1 adrenergic receptor. β-blockers have effects on bone mineral density and fracture risk, which supports this finding.[69,70] These data have not been replicated.

In contrast to the previously described studies, which examined the patient's radiographic progression over time, Ward and colleagues[71] examined the genetic predictors of the ratio of BASRI of the spine to disease duration as an indicator of disease progression in patients with disease duration of 20 years or more. They found HLA-B*4100 (OR = 12), HLA-DRB1*0804 (OR = 12), HLA-DQA1*0401 (OR = 5), HLA-DQB1*0603 (OR = 3), and HLA-DPB1*0202 (OR = 23) associated with more progressive disease. In this study HLA-DRB1*0801 was associated with protection from radiographic progression with an OR of 0.03.

In contrast to its important effects in disease onset *HLA-B27* has not been associated with radiographic change in multiple studies.[15,24,72]

FUTURE DEVELOPMENTS

The continuing development of genomics offers further potential for genetic discoveries in AS. Study design features likely to lead to further progress include the following:

1. Increase in sample sizes: Thus far the largest genetic study in AS involved a GWAS of 3023 cases, far fewer than have been studied for other autoimmune diseases of

similar population frequency, such as multiple sclerosis,[73] or even rheumatic diseases of much lower population frequency than AS, such as systemic lupus erythematosus. There is a clear link between sample size and productivity.[74] Much larger studies in AS are clearly indicated, and are likely to flow from international collaborative studies, such as the International Genetics of AS Consortium Immunochip study.
2. Transethnic studies: Most studies to date of AS genetics have been performed in white European populations, and little data are available about other important ethnic groups including east Asians and Indian Asians. These studies are likely to be beneficial particularly in localizing genetic effects, using differences in the linkage disequilibrium structure of the various populations studied.
3. Low-frequency and rare-variant studies: Early sequencing studies and studies using microarray genotyping targeting low-frequency variants have already been productive in AS-related diseases, notably in IBD.[77] These variants are not well detected by current GWAS microarrays, which target common variants. Although they will take large studies to identify, sequencing and low-frequency targeted microarray studies are likely to be productive in such diseases as AS, where a significant fraction of the disease's heritability remains unaccounted for.
4. Genetic studies of AS-disease manifestations: Very little is known about the genetics of disease severity in AS, or of associated features, such as the development of acute anterior uveitis. These are likely to have genetic determinants, and to be addressable by GWAS and other genetic studies.

The use of genetic prediction of those at risk of AS is likely to be one of the earliest genetic screens adopted for common conditions, because the high heritability of the disease suggests that genetic risk prediction will be informative. At this stage, however, more evidence regarding the benefit of early intervention is required before this approach can be recommended.

SUMMARY

Genetic discoveries in AS have identified associated pathways previously not considered important. These discoveries have enabled direct translation to clinical practice as agents to target the pathways have been developed with other uses in mind but are now being turned to treat AS. This is the exciting future for the genetics of AS, from the laboratory to the clinic, and in doing so improving the lives of patients.

REFERENCES

1. Reveille JD, Ball EJ, Khan MA. HLA-B27 and genetic predisposing factors in spondyloarthropathies. Curr Opin Rheumatol 2001;13:265–72.
2. van der Linden SM, Valkenburg HA, de Jongh BM, et al. The risk of developing ankylosing spondylitis in HLA-B27 positive individuals. A comparison of relatives of spondylitis patients with the general population. Arthritis Rheum 1984;27: 241–9.
3. Gofton JP, Robinson HS, Trueman GE. Ankylosing spondylitis in a Canadian Indian population. Ann Rheum Dis 1966;25:525–7.
4. Brown MA, Jepson A, Young A, et al. Ankylosing spondylitis in West Africans: evidence for a non-HLA-B27 protective effect. Ann Rheum Dis 1997;56:68–70.
5. May E, Dorris ML, Satumtira N, et al. CD8 alpha beta T cells are not essential to the pathogenesis of arthritis or colitis in HLA-B27 transgenic rats. J Immunol 2003;170:1099–105.

6. Bowness P, Ridley A, Shaw J, et al. Th17 cells expressing KIR3DL2+ and responsive to HLA-B27 homodimers are increased in ankylosing spondylitis. J Immunol 2011;186:2672–80.
7. Scrivo R, Morrone S, Spadaro A, et al. Evaluation of degranulation and cytokine production in natural killer cells from spondyloarthritis patients at single-cell level. Cytometry B Clin Cytom 2011;80:22–7.
8. McHugh K, Bowness P. The link between HLA-B27 and SpA–new ideas on an old problem. Rheumatology (Oxford) 2012;51(9):1529–39.
9. Hammer GE, Gonzalez F, Champsaur M, et al. The aminopeptidase ERAAP shapes the peptide repertoire displayed by major histocompatibility complex class I molecules. Nat Immunol 2006;7:103–12.
10. Evans DM, Spencer CC, Pointon JJ, et al. Interaction between ERAP1 and HLA-B27 in ankylosing spondylitis implicates peptide handling in the mechanism for HLA-B27 in disease susceptibility. Nat Genet 2011;43:761–7.
11. Turner MJ, Sowders DP, DeLay ML, et al. HLA-B27 misfolding in transgenic rats is associated with activation of the unfolded protein response. J Immunol 2005;175: 2438–48.
12. DeLay ML, Turner MJ, Klenk EI, et al. HLA-B27 misfolding and the unfolded protein response augment interleukin-23 production and are associated with Th17 activation in transgenic rats. Arthritis Rheum 2009;60:2633–43.
13. Arnett FC Jr, Schacter BZ, Hochberg MC, et al. Homozygosity for HLA-B27. Impact on rheumatic disease expression in two families. Arthritis Rheum 1977; 20:797–804.
14. Kim TJ, Na KS, Lee HJ, et al. HLA-B27 homozygosity has no influence on clinical manifestations and functional disability in ankylosing spondylitis. Clin Exp Rheumatol 2009;27:574–9.
15. Khan MA, Kushner I, Braun WE, et al. HLA–B27 homozygosity in ankylosing spondylitis: relationship to risk and severity. Tissue Antigens 1978;11:434–8.
16. Jaakkola E, Herzberg I, Laiho K, et al. Finnish HLA studies confirm the increased risk conferred by HLA-B27 homozygosity in ankylosing spondylitis. Ann Rheum Dis 2006;65:775–80.
17. Brown MA, Pile KD, Kennedy LG, et al. HLA class I associations of ankylosing spondylitis in the white population in the United Kingdom. Ann Rheum Dis 1996;55:268–70.
18. Robinson WP, van der Linden SM, Khan MA, et al. HLA-Bw60 increases susceptibility to ankylosing spondylitis in HLA-B27+ patients. Arthritis Rheum 1989;32: 1135–41.
19. Wei JC, Tsai WC, Lin HS, et al. HLA-B60 and B61 are strongly associated with ankylosing spondylitis in HLA-B27-negative Taiwan Chinese patients. Rheumatology (Oxford) 2004;43:839–42.
20. Joshi R, Reveille JD, Brown MA, et al. Is there a higher genetic load of susceptibility loci in familial ankylosing spondylitis? Arthritis Care Res (Hoboken) 2012;64: 780–4.
21. Rudwaleit M, Claudepierre P, Wordsworth P, et al. Effectiveness, safety, and predictors of good clinical response in 1250 patients treated with adalimumab for active ankylosing spondylitis. J Rheumatol 2009;36:801–8.
22. Saraux A, de Saint-Pierre V, Baron D, et al. The HLA B27 antigen-spondylarthropathy association. Impact on clinical expression. Rev Rhum Engl Ed 1995;62:487–91.
23. Feldtkeller E, Khan MA, van der Heijde D, et al. Age at disease onset and diagnosis delay in HLA-B27 negative vs. positive patients with ankylosing spondylitis. Rheumatol Int 2003;23:61–6.

24. Boonen A, vander Cruyssen B, de Vlam K, et al. Spinal radiographic changes in ankylosing spondylitis: association with clinical characteristics and functional outcome. J Rheumatol 2009;36:1249–55.
25. Lin Z, Bei JX, Shen M, et al. A genome-wide association study in Han Chinese identifies new susceptibility loci for ankylosing spondylitis. Nat Genet 2012;44: 73–7.
26. Rudwaleit M, Sieper J. Referral strategies for early diagnosis of axial spondyloarthritis. Nat Rev Rheumatol 2012;8:262–8.
27. Reveille JD, Sims AM, Danoy P, et al. Genome-wide association study of ankylosing spondylitis identifies non-MHC susceptibility loci. Nat Genet 2010;42: 123–7.
28. Burton PR, Clayton DG, Cardon LR, et al. Association scan of 14,500 nonsynonymous SNPs in four diseases identifies autoimmunity variants. Nat Genet 2007; 39:1329–37.
29. Li C, Lin Z, Xie Y, et al. ERAP1 is associated with ankylosing spondylitis in Han Chinese. J Rheumatol 2011;38:317–21.
30. Pazar B, Safrany E, Gergely P, et al. Association of ARTS1 gene polymorphisms with ankylosing spondylitis in the Hungarian population: the rs27044 variant is associated with HLA-B*2705 subtype in Hungarian patients with ankylosing spondylitis. J Rheumatol 2010;37:379–84.
31. Pimentel-Santos FM, Ligeiro D, Matos M, et al. Association of IL23R and ERAP1 genes with ankylosing spondylitis in a Portuguese population. Clin Exp Rheumatol 2009;27:800–6.
32. Szczypiorska M, Sanchez A, Bartolome N, et al. ERAP1 polymorphisms and haplotypes are associated with ankylosing spondylitis susceptibility and functional severity in a Spanish population. Rheumatology (Oxford) 2011;50:1969–75.
33. Strange A, Capon F, Spencer CC, et al. A genome-wide association study identifies new psoriasis susceptibility loci and an interaction between HLA-C and ERAP1. Nat Genet 2010;42:985–90.
34. York IA, Chang SC, Saric T, et al. The ER aminopeptidase ERAP1 enhances or limits antigen presentation by trimming epitopes to 8–9 residues. Nat Immunol 2002;3:1177–84.
35. Cui X, Hawari F, Alsaaty S, et al. Identification of ARTS-1 as a novel TNFR1-binding protein that promotes TNFR1 ectodomain shedding. J Clin Invest 2002; 110:515–26.
36. Cui X, Rouhani FN, Hawari F, et al. Shedding of the type II IL-1 decoy receptor requires a multifunctional aminopeptidase, aminopeptidase regulator of TNF receptor type 1 shedding. J Immunol 2003;171:6814–9.
37. Cui X, Rouhani FN, Hawari F, et al. An aminopeptidase, ARTS-1, is required for interleukin-6 receptor shedding. J Biol Chem 2003;278:28677–85.
38. Haroon N, Tsui FW, Chiu B, et al. Serum cytokine receptors in ankylosing spondylitis: relationship to inflammatory markers and endoplasmic reticulum aminopeptidase polymorphisms. J Rheumatol 2010;37:1907–10.
39. Goto Y, Ogawa K, Hattori A, et al. Secretion of endoplasmic reticulum aminopeptidase 1 is involved in the activation of macrophages induced by lipopolysaccharide and interferon-gamma. J Biol Chem 2011;286:21906–14.
40. Tsui FW, Haroon N, Reveille JD, et al. Association of an ERAP1 ERAP2 haplotype with familial ankylosing spondylitis. Ann Rheum Dis 2010;69:733–6.
41. Franke A, McGovern DP, Barrett JC, et al. Genome-wide meta-analysis increases to 71 the number of confirmed Crohn's disease susceptibility loci. Nat Genet 2010;42:1118–25.

42. Birtley JR, Saridakis E, Stratikos E, et al. The crystal structure of human endoplasmic reticulum aminopeptidase 2 reveals the atomic basis for distinct roles in antigen processing. Biochemistry 2012;51:286–95.
43. Saveanu L, Carroll O, Lindo V, et al. Concerted peptide trimming by human ERAP1 and ERAP2 aminopeptidase complexes in the endoplasmic reticulum. Nat Immunol 2005;6:689–97.
44. Baeten D, Sieper J, Emery P, et al. The anti-IL7A monoclonal antibody secukinumab (AIN457) showed good safety and efficacy in the treatment of active ankylosing spondylitis. Arthritis Rheum 2010;62:2840–1.
45. Kenna TJ, Davidson SI, Duan R, et al. Enrichment of circulating IL-17-secreting IL-23 receptor-positive gammadelta T cells in patients with active ankylosing spondylitis. Arthritis Rheum 2012;64:1420–9.
46. Ruutu M, Thomas G, Steck R, et al. beta-glucan triggers spondylarthritis and Crohn's disease-like ileitis in SKG mice. Arthritis Rheum 2012;64:2211–22.
47. Gagliardi MC, Teloni R, Mariotti S, et al. Endogenous PGE2 promotes the induction of human Th17 responses by fungal ss-glucan. J Leukoc Biol 2010;88:947–54.
48. Baird EO, Kang QK. Prophylaxis of heterotopic ossification - an updated review. J Orthop Surg Res 2009;4:12.
49. Poddubnyy D, Rudwaleit M, Haibel H, et al. Effect of non-steroidal anti-inflammatory drugs on radiographic spinal progression in patients with axial spondyloarthritis: results from the German spondyloarthritis inception cohort. Ann Rheum Dis 2012. [Epub ahead of print].
50. Dowling O, Difeo A, Ramirez MC, et al. Mutations in capillary morphogenesis gene-2 result in the allelic disorders juvenile hyaline fibromatosis and infantile systemic hyalinosis. Am J Hum Genet 2003;73:957–66.
51. Helming L, Gordon S. Molecular mediators of macrophage fusion. Trends Cell Biol 2009;19:514–22.
52. Wu Z, Ma HM, Kukita T, et al. Phosphatidylserine-containing liposomes inhibit the differentiation of osteoclasts and trabecular bone loss. J Immunol 2010;184:3191–201.
53. Pointon JJ, Harvey D, Karaderi T, et al. The chromosome 16q region associated with ankylosing spondylitis includes the candidate gene tumour necrosis factor receptor type 1-associated death domain (TRADD). Ann Rheum Dis 2010;69:1243–6.
54. Kontoyiannis D, Pasparakis M, Pizarro TT, et al. Impaired on/off regulation of TNF biosynthesis in mice lacking TNF AU-rich elements: implications for joint and gut-associated immunopathologies. Immunity 1999;10:387–98.
55. Braun J, Sieper J. Therapy of ankylosing spondylitis and other spondyloarthritides: established medical treatment, anti-TNF-alpha therapy and other novel approaches. Arthritis Res 2002;4:307–21.
56. Park JH, Adoro S, Guinter T, et al. Signaling by intrathymic cytokines, not T cell antigen receptors, specifies CD8 lineage choice and promotes the differentiation of cytotoxic-lineage T cells. Nat Immunol 2010;11:257–64.
57. Liu C, Hart RP, Liu XJ, et al. Cloning and characterization of an alternatively processed human type II interleukin-1 receptor mRNA. J Biol Chem 1996;271:20965–72.
58. Aulchenko YS, Hoppenbrouwers IA, Ramagopalan SV, et al. Genetic variation in the KIF1B locus influences susceptibility to multiple sclerosis. Nat Genet 2008;40:1402–3.
59. Barrett JC, Hansoul S, Nicolae DL, et al. Genome-wide association defines more than 30 distinct susceptibility loci for Crohn's disease. Nat Genet 2008;40:955–62.

60. Danoy P, Pryce K, Hadler J, et al. Association of variants at 1q32 and STAT3 with ankylosing spondylitis suggests genetic overlap with Crohn's disease. PLoS Genet 2010;6:e1001195.
61. Goris A, Boonen S, D'Hooghe MB, et al. Replication of KIF21B as a susceptibility locus for multiple sclerosis. J Med Genet 2010;47:775–6.
62. David G, Budarf M, Charron G, et al. Identification of putative causal genes for IBD in the 1q32 region: from genetics to biological mechanism. Presented at the 12th International Congress of Human Genetics/61st Annual Meeting of The American Society of Human Genetics. Montreal, 2011.
63. Rudwaleit M, van der Heijde D, Landewe R, et al. The development of assessment of spondyloarthritis international society classification criteria for axial spondyloarthritis (part II): validation and final selection. Ann Rheum Dis 2009;68: 777–83.
64. Brophy S, Hickey S, Menon A, et al. Concordance of disease severity among family members with ankylosing spondylitis? J Rheumatol 2004;31:1775–8.
65. Calin A, Elswood J. Relative role of genetic and environmental factors in disease expression: sib pair analysis in ankylosing spondylitis. Arthritis Rheum 1989;32: 77–81.
66. Haroon N, Maksymowych WP, Rahman P, et al. Radiographic severity of ankylosing spondylitis is associated with polymorphism of the large multifunctional peptidase 2 gene in the Spondyloarthritis Research Consortium of Canada cohort. Arthritis Rheum 2012;64:1119–26.
67. Bartolome N, Szczypiorska M, Sanchez A, et al. Genetic polymorphisms, inside and outside the MHC, improve prediction of AS radiographic severity in addition to clinical variables. Rheumatology (Oxford) 2012;51(8):1471–8.
68. Xue J, Peng J, Yuan M, et al. NELL1 promotes high-quality bone regeneration in rat femoral distraction osteogenesis model. Bone 2011;48:485–95.
69. Perez-Castrillon JL, Sanz-Cantalapiedra A, Duenas-Laita A. Beta-blockers: effects on bone mineral density and fracture risk. Curr Rheumatol Rev 2006;2: 353–7.
70. Turker S, Karatosun V, Gunal I. Beta-blockers increase bone mineral density. Clin Orthop Relat Res 2006;443:73–4.
71. Ward MM, Hendrey MR, Malley JD, et al. Clinical and immunogenetic prognostic factors for radiographic severity in ankylosing spondylitis. Arthritis Rheum 2009; 61:859–66.
72. Spencer DG, Hick HM, Dick WC. Ankylosing spondylitis: the role of HLA-B27 homozygosity. Tissue Antigens 1979;14:379–84.
73. Sawcer S, Hellenthal G, Pirinen M, et al. Genetic risk and a primary role for cell-mediated immune mechanisms in multiple sclerosis. Nature 2011;476:214–9.
74. Visscher PM, Brown MA, McCarthy MI, et al. Five years of GWAS discovery. Am J Hum Genet 2012;90:7–24.
75. Sieper J, Van der Heijde D, Dougados M, et al. Efficacy and safety of adalimumab in patients with non-radiographic axial spondyloarthritis: results from a phase 3 study. Arthritis Rheum 2011;63:S970, 2486A.
76. Haibel H, Rudwaleit M, Listing J, et al. Efficacy of adalimumab in the treatment of axial spondylarthritis without radiographically defined sacroiliitis: results of a twelve-week randomized, double-blind, placebo-controlled trial followed by an open-label extension up to week fifty-two. Arthritis Rheum 2008;58:1981–91.
77. Rivas MA, Beaudoin M, Gardet A, et al. Deep resequencing of GWAS loci identifies independent rare variants associated with inflammatory bowel disease. Nat Genet 2011;43:1066–73.

78. Rudwaleit M, Haibel H, Baraliakos X, et al. The early disease stage in axial spondylarthritis: results from the German Spondyloarthritis Inception cohort. Arthritis Rheum 2009;60:717–27.
79. Poddubnyy D, Rudwaleit M, Haibel H, et al. Rates and predictors of radiographic sacroiliitis progression over 2 years in patients with axial spondyloarthritis. Ann Rheum Dis 2011;70:1369–74.
80. Kiltz U, Baraliakos X, Karakostas P, et al. Patients with non-radiographic axial spondyloarthritis differ from patients with ankylosing spondylitis in several aspects. Arthritis Care Res (Hoboken) 2012. http://dx.doi.org/10.1002/acr.21688.

Pathophysiology of New Bone Formation and Ankylosis in Spondyloarthritis

Rik J.U. Lories, MD, PhD[a,b,*], Georg Schett, MD[c]

KEYWORDS

• Spondyloarthritis • Chronic inflammation • New bone formation • Ankylosis

KEY POINTS

- Chronic inflammation and new bone formation, specifically progressive ankylosis, determine the burden of disease and outcome of patients with spondyloarthritis.
- Insights into the cellular and molecular mechanisms that contribute to ankylosis in spondyloarthritis (SpA) are linked to better understanding of the key players in skeletal development and homeostasis.
- The paradox of concurrent ankylosis and osteoporosis in close proximity highlights the hypothesis that the mechanisms of new bone formation are different from those involved in the normal bone remodeling cycle.
- Different pathways, including bone morphogenetic proteins (BMPs), Wnt, and hedgehog proteins, have been studied in animal models and could become new therapeutic targets.
- Biomarkers for bone formation are potential tools for predicting structural bone changes in SpA but have specific challenges because changes in local as well as systemic bone homeostasis affect their serum levels.
- The relationship between inflammation and ankylosis remains controversial. Long-term data of therapeutic interventions as well as the effects of treatment in early disease stages may provide better insights into this matter.

INTRODUCTION

The iconic image of a fully ankylosed spine in patients with ankylosing spondylitis (AS) represents the final consequence of a chronic inflammatory process and the

---

Disclosure: R.J.U.L. has received consultancy or speaker's fees from Abbott, Pfizer, and Merck. Abbott and Pfizer have supported investigator-initiated research of R.J.U.L.

[a] Laboratory for Skeletal Development and Joint Disorders, Department of Development and Regeneration, Herestraat 49, B 3000 Leuven, Belgium; [b] Division of Rheumatology, University Hospitals Leuven, Herestraat 49, B 3000 Leuven, Belgium; [c] Department of Internal Medicine 3, Institute for Clinical Immunology, University of Erlangen-Nuremberg, Krankenhausstraße 12, Erlangen 91054, Germany

* Corresponding author. Division of Rheumatology, UZ Leuven, Herestraat 49, B3000 Leuven, Belgium.

E-mail address: Rik.Lories@uz.kuleuven.be

Rheum Dis Clin N Am 38 (2012) 555–567
http://dx.doi.org/10.1016/j.rdc.2012.08.003 **rheumatic.theclinics.com**
0889-857X/12/$ – see front matter

threatening prospect for patients who have recently been diagnosed with SpA. All subtypes of SpA, including AS, psoriatic arthritis, inflammatory bowel disease–associated arthritis, reactive arthritis, juvenile SpA, and undifferentiated SpA, are characterized by inflammation and structural damage to the skeleton.[1] Damage presents as new bone formation leading to bony fusion (ankylosis) of the sacroiliac joints, syndesmophyte formation eventually bridging the intervertebral spaces, and enthesophytes originating from tendon or ligament insertion sites in the peripheral skeleton (**Fig. 1**).

For most patients with SpA, the burden of disease results from a combination of inflammation and structural bone changes.[2] The inflammatory process manifests by osteitis, enthesitis, and synovitis and may clinically appear as pain, stiffness, local swelling, warmth, redness, and loss of function.[1,3] Structural bone changes not only affect patients by causing disability and permanent loss of function but also with secondary effects; thus, ankylosis changes the balance of loads and forces in the skeletal system, leading to muscle stiffness and accelerated degenerative spine disease. For instance, ankylosis of the sacroiliac joints has only a limited impact on the direct mobility of the pelvis but changes the biomechanical loads in the spine because vertical forces can no longer be translated toward the limbs in the optimal way.[4,5]

Clinicians and researchers face several challenges with respect to investigating the mechanism, kinetics, prediction, and impact of new bone formation and ankylosis in SpA. In general, ankylosis is a slow process but has a considerable and often underestimated individual variability.[6] Analyses of progression of ankylosis in cohort studies

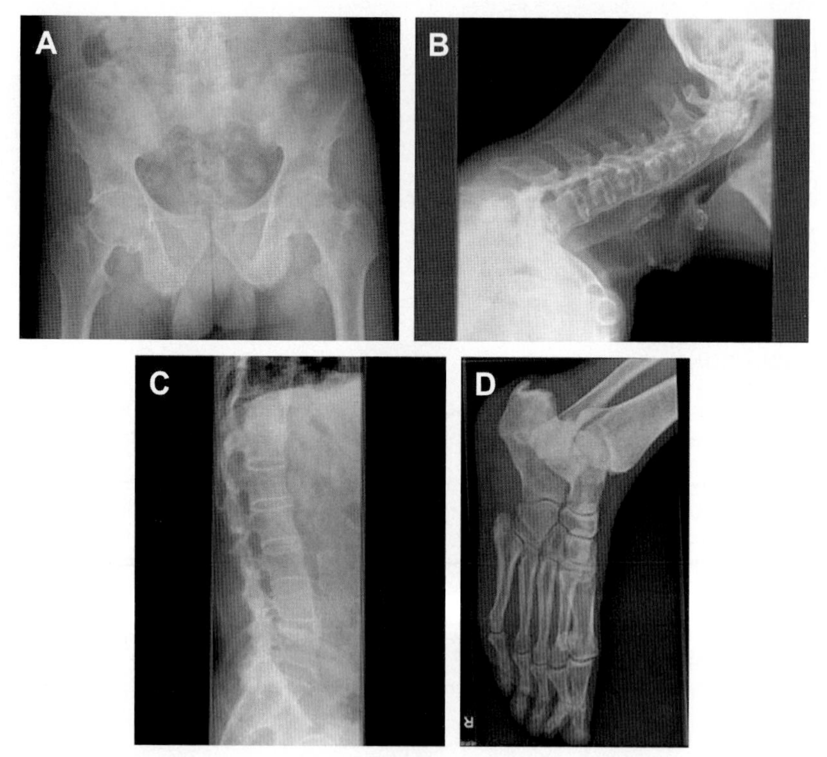

Fig. 1. Different aspects of bone formation in patients with spondyloarthritis. Progressive ankylosis of (*A*) the sacroiliac joints, (*B*) cervical spine, and (*C*) lumbar spine. (*D*) An example of new bone formation at the Achilles tendon insertion (enthesophytes).

and clinical trials, therefore, usually require long-term sequential observations. Also, the assessment of ankylosis is challenging due to the complexity of scoring systems and the challenge of whether such scoring systems detect not only statistically but also clinically meaningful changes.[7,8] In addition, access to human tissue from the spine for pathology studies is limited. As discussed later, different animal and in vitro models have been used to understand cellular and molecular events leading to ankylosis and the relationship between inflammation and new tissue formation. None of these animal models, however, exactly mimics human SpA and the direct clinical relevance of the available models is sometimes heavily debated.

FUNDAMENTALS OF BONE FORMATION

To understand pathologic new bone formation in SpA, it is necessary to consider the basic mechanisms of skeletal development and turnover (**Fig. 2**). New bone formation leading to ankylosis is a process in which the new skeletal tissue is always formed in connection with existing bone but extends beyond its original border. For this feature the term, *osteoproliferation*, has been introduced,[9] but it may not well reflect the different cellular and molecular processes involved.[10] The processes involved in new bone formation in SpA are orchestrated by proliferation, differentiation, maturation, and migration of cells as well as cell death. Osteproliferation in SpA is a complex tissue remodeling process rather than simple proliferation of bone and shares similarities with joint remodeling in osteoarthritis.[11]

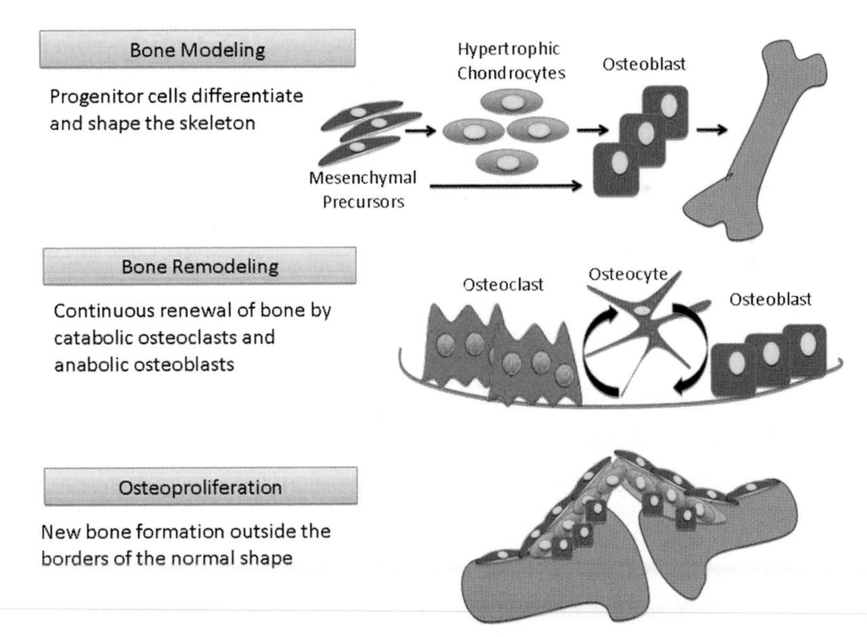

Fig. 2. Concepts of bone formation. Bone modeling is a developmental process that determines the shape and structure of the skeleton. In this well-orchestrated process, progenitors differentiate by endochondral or direct bone formation. Bone remodeling refers to the continuous renewal of the skeleton by bone resorbing osteoclasts (multinucleated cells) and bone-forming osteoblasts. The osteocytes are mechanosensitive cells and orchestrate the bone remodeling cycle. Bone modeling in SpA is a disease-associated process, in which new bone formation is occurring outside the original borders of the skeleton.

Bone remodeling in SpA should be distinguished from classical bone remodeling, which is the continuous renewal of the skeleton by the balanced activity of bone-forming osteoblasts and bone-resorbing osteoclasts, which is orchestrated by the mechanosensitive osteocytes.[12] The distinction between this physiologic process and pathologic bone formation becomes particularly clear in SpA: whereas new bone is excessively built up at the outer surface of the cortical bone, SpA patients paradoxically develop osteoporosis due to degradation of the trabecular bone of the vertebral bodies. These diverging remodeling types in the cortical and the trabecular bone of patients with SpA suggest that pathologic bone remodeling in SpA is fundamentally different from classical bone turnover.[13] Moreover, control of inflammation reverts the trabecular bone loss[13] but does not seem to affect the progression of ankylosis.[14–16]

Therefore, pathologic bone formation in SpA can be best understood from its parallels with bone development and growth, the so-called bone modeling (in contrast to remodeling) process.[17] Two different types of bone formation have been extensively described and cooperate to skeletal development and growth: (1) endochondral bone formation defines the skeletal elements through an intermediate cartilage stage, whereas (2) membranous bone formation results in direct new bone formation.[17] The former process builds up most of the skeletal elements, in particular in the appendicular skeleton, whereas the latter is important for the calvarial bones but also contributes to later stages of the development of long bones. In endochondral bone formation, skeletal progenitor cells first form cell condensations at the prospective sites (so-called anlagen) and thereby trigger a cascade of chondrogenic differentiation processes. Thus, mesenchymal progenitor cells first commit toward chondrocytes and start producing collagen type II and extracellular matrix proteoglycans, like aggrecan. Starting off as proliferating chondrocytes, they subsequently become prehypertrophic chondrocytes and finally terminally differentiated hypertrophic chondrocytes. These cells express vascular endothelial growth factor and matrix metalloproteinase (MMP) 13 and produce a different type of extracellular matrix, typically rich in type X collagen. The proangiogenic factors attract blood vessels and other progenitor cells, which allow breakdown of the calcified matrix and their replacement by bone based on the influx of osteoblast precursors. Typically, such ossification centers are found on both sides of the long bones and shape into the growth plates. As the skeletal element grows and develops its specific shape, a bony collar is formed at the borders of the bone through membranous bone formation.[17]

BONE FORMATION IN SPONDYLOARTHRITIS

The limited histology data available from SpA patients suggest that both endochondral and membranous bone formation seem to contribute to ankylosis.[18–22] Nevertheless, these processes appear less well orchestrated and structured than those during development and normal growth. Thus, so-called cartilage metaplasia, in which cartilage cells are found in a calcified matrix, was also identified in bone samples from patients with SpA.[18] Although formal proof is lacking, it seems likely that in SpA, joint-associated or spine-associated progenitor populations commit toward differentiation into either chondrocytes or osteoblasts. The multilineage potential of cell types, such as synovial, periosteal, and bone marrow cells, which are involved in SpA, has been demonstrated.[23–26] Nevertheless specific influx of already commited cells, such as fibrocytes[27] and pericytes,[28] as well as local endothelial-mesenchymal transition cannot be excluded as contributing mechanisms.[29]

MOLECULAR SIGNALING PATHWAYS IN BONE DEVELOPMENT

The developmental processes (described previously) are steered by several molecular pathways, including BMPs, Wnt proteins, hedgehog proteins, and fibroblast growth factors.[17] BMPs, Wnts, and hedgehogs have been studied in animal models of arthritis and in patient samples (discussed later) (**Fig. 3**).

BMPs were originally identified as protein factors isolated from bone matrix that can ectopically induce a full cascade of endochondral bone formation, when injected intramuscularly or subcutaneously in vivo.[30,31] These potent morphogens were subsequently demonstrated to play important roles not only in skeletal development but also in other organs systems and in early stages of development.[32] Increasing evidence suggests that BMPs have homeostatic or regulatory roles in different organ systems, including the skeleton (bone and cartilage), the kidney,[33] and the endocrine system postnatally.[34] BMPs are currently used in the clinic for the treatment of nonunion fractures and to obtain spinal ankylosis in patients with intervertebral disk degeneration.[35]

BMPs consist of a large family of ligands that can be divided into different subgroups. The numerous ligands and promiscuous receptor associations that are leading to the activation of distinct signaling cascades allow BMPs to have wide-ranging effects on distinct cell types.[36] The best-known downstream signaling event is activation of Smad proteins and activation of mitogen-activated protein kinases (MAPKs), such as p38 and ERK. In addition, regulatory mechanisms, including extracellular and intracellular antagonists, and complex association of coactivators and corepressors at the level of transcription are essential for the fine-tuning of this signaling system.[36] In skeletal development, BMPs play an essential role in the early phases of chondrogenesis by stimulating chondrogenic differentiation as well as in the late hypertrophic stages.[17] Most of these effects seem mediated by Smad signaling.

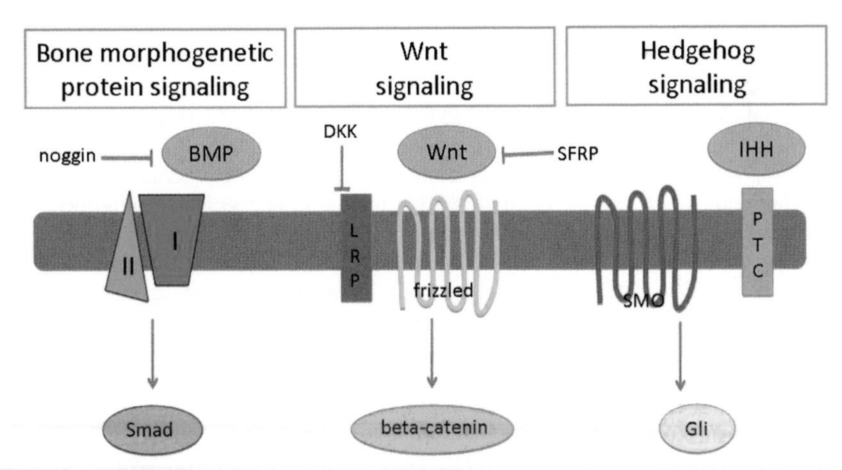

Fig. 3. Main signaling cascades studied in animal models of spondyloarthritis. BMPs activate type I and type II receptors leading to phosphorylation of intracellular Smad molecules. Wnts act through Frizzled receptors and lipoprotein-related protein (LRP) 5/6 receptors to stabilize β-catenin in the cytoplasm. When hedgehogs bind to the PTCH (PTC) receptor, SMO is activated and increases Gli proteins. Smads, β-catenin, and Glis transfer to the nucleus and influence gene transcription. Noggin, DKK1 (DKK), and secreted frizzled-related proteins (SFRPs) are BMP, LRP, and Wnt antagonists respectively, which have been studied in animal models. IHH, Indian hedgehog.

Wnt proteins were originally identified in cancer research and fruit fly development and much like BMPs direct early developmental processes as well as postnatal tissue homeostasis.[37,38] The Wnt family also mediates its effects by using complex ligand-receptor interactions as well as activation of different intracellular signaling cascades. Canonical Wnt signaling primarily involves β-catenin translocation to the nucleus.[38] Other downstream events include increased calcium signaling and direct effects on the cytoskeleton and cell polarity.[39] In skeletal development and biology, Wnts have stimulatory roles on bone formation and their expression seems regulated by the mechanosensing osteocytes.[39] Wnt stimulate new bone formation by direct effects on osteoblasts. Moreover, Wnt proteins tightly regulate articular cartilage homeostasis.[40–42]

Hedgehog proteins provide an essential feedback loop in bone development.[43] In combination with parathyroid hormone–related protein, Indian hedgehog defines the rate of chondrocyte proliferation and hypertrophy. Indian hedgehog binds to the Smoothened (SMO) and Patched (PTCH) receptor complex and leads to an activation of the Gli transcription factors.[44] Gli1 and Gli2 are considered transcriptional activators, whereas Gli3 acts as a transcriptional repressor.[44]

MOLECULAR SIGNALING PATHWAYS IN ANIMAL MODELS OF SPONDYLOARTHRITIS

The BMP pathway was the first cascade studied in animal models of SpA.[45] The spontaneous arthritis model in aging male DBA/1 mice develops after grouped caging of male mice and typically presents as oligoarthritis of the toes. This model is specifically characterized by a spurious phase of inflammation followed by extensive bone remodeling originating from the entheses.[46] The histomorphologic features of the model closely resemble the growth plate with consecutive phases of chondrocyte proliferation, condensation, differentiation, hypertrophy, and ultimately replacement by bone. Different BMPs are expressed during ankylosis in this mouse model of SpA and activation of the Smad signaling cascade is found in the early phases of the disease.[45] Noggin, a broad-spectrum endogenous BMP antagonist that interferes with ligand-receptor binding, was overexpressed in this model. The gene transfer resulted in inhibition of ankylosis both in preventive and therapeutic settings.[45] This inhibitory effect could be explained by interference of the antagonist with the Smad signaling cascade.

In a subsequent set of experiments, alternative BMP signaling cascades, in particular, activation of p38 MAPK, were studied.[47] Inhibition of p38 MAPK interfered with osteochondrogenic differentiation of progenitor cells in vitro but paradoxically showed opposite effects in vivo. Thus, inhibition of p38 MAPK in the spontaneous DBA/1 model using a chemical inhibitor stimulated rather than suppressed ankylosis.[47] This apparent paradox may be explained by the short half-life of the compound resulting in compensatory up-regulation and feedback systems in vivo.

The link between Wnt signaling and new bone formation in SpA has been established by a remarkable observation in the human tumor necrosis factor (TNF) transgenic mouse model of arthritis.[48,49] In this well-established model of joint destruction, the effect of blocking Dickkopf-1 (DKK1), a secreted Wnt antagonist, previously linked to bone loss, was studied. By blocking DKK1, the phenotype of the disease model shifted from joint destruction toward joint remodeling with formation of osteophytes in the peripheral joints and ankylosis of the sacroiliac joints.[48,49] This local phenomenon was accompanied by a systemic gain of bone, indicating that enhancing Wnt signaling in this model also affects bone remodeling in addition to bone modeling. DKK1 is a factor induced by TNF, which suggests that its up-regulation in arthritis makes it a master regulator of the overall phenotype of arthritis.[49,50] Blockade of DKK1 function is associated with activation of the canonical Wnt signaling pathway and increased levels and nuclear translocation of β-catenin. Currently, no data are available on the role of noncanonical Wnt signaling in joint remodeling.

Both BMPs and Wnts have multiple effects in different organ systems postnatally and blockade of these pathways may thus be associated with major toxicity. Hegehog signaling seems more restricted to developing bone and may theoretically have less general toxicity issues. A chemical compound that inhibits Hedghog signaling by directly interfering with SMO affects osteophyte development in the late stages of the serum transfer model of arthritis.[51] This model is typically destructive in its first phase, but on resolution of inflammation, rapid development of osteophytes is seen. This effect was specific for new bone formation because no effects were noticed on inflammation or systemic bone turnover.[51]

MARKERS OF NEW BONE FORMATION

The translation of animal model data to clonical useful data, in particular with regards to the prediction of structural damage, represents a challenge in SpA. As outlined previously, 2 different and contrasting features are found in the skeletons of patients with disease.[13] Inflammation leads to osteoporosis while at the same time, and in close proximity, new bone formation is progressing toward ankylosis. Therefore, any assessment of specific bone markers should be considered in this context, not only in cross-sectional analysis but also when the effect of a therapeutic intervention is evaluated in a longitudinal setting. This challenge affects not only the classical markers of bone and cartilage turnover, such as collagen breakdown and synthesis products, but also new markers associated with the pathways (discussed previously) that have recently been studied or proposed.

Some results have been reported based on classical bone and cartilage turnover analyses that typically highlight this complexity. Data obtained before the introduction of anti-TNF strategies indicated that patients with AS show enhanced levels of bone and cartilage degradation products (urinary pyridinium cross links) with normal ranges of bone formation markers (alkaline phosphatase and osteocalcin).[52] Other work showed increased cartilage turnover that correlated well with CRP levels and that could indicate either turnover of articular cartilage and intervertebral disks or, alternatively, reflect the ongoing process of endochondral bone formation.[53] Similar views can be derived from the analysis of type II collagen telopeptide, a marker of cartilage degradation.[54] Treatment with anti-TNF results in increased bone anabolism reflected by the levels of bone-specific alkaline phosphatase and decreased type I collagen telopeptide in parallel with changes in lumbar spine bone mineral density.[55] Tissue turnover reflected by MMP3 levels was earlier identified as a biomarker for radiographic progression in AS.[56]

Recently several studies have tried to translate the animal model data into human biomarkers. With regards to Wnt signaling, the initial study on DKK1 in mice included an analysis of DKK1 levels in AS patients, controls, and rheumatoid arthritis patients.[49] Based on a functional assay (binding to the LRP6 Wnt receptor), levels of DKK1 were consistently lower in AS patients. Within the GESPIC cohort, AS patients with low levels of DKK1 showed increased radiographic progression compared with those with higher levels.[57] These data were also based on the functional assay. Surprisingly, a classical sandwich ELISA using 2 anti-DKK1 antibodies demonstrated that patients with AS had significantly increased levels of DKK1.[58] Levels increased further on anti-TNF treatment but DKK1 itself was dysfunctional in a cell-based assay, explaining the discrepancy between both types of ELISA used.[58] Low sclerostin level, an osteocyte-specific Wnt antagonist,[57] was also strongly associated with radiographic progression in AS patients and correlated well with functional DKK levels.[57,59]

Consistent data on BMP serum levels are limited. A recent study suggested that patients with radiographic signs of ankylosis have higher serum levels of different BMPs compared with AS patients without signs of new bone formation and healthy controls.[60] Other studies, however, have not come forward with similar results.[61,62] This discrepancy phenomenon highlights one of the challenges in the field of biomarkers, in particular with regard to progression of ankylosis in SpA patients. Data sets are scattered and taken from diverse patient populations. There is a need to consistently replicate findings from one cohort in other independent cohorts much like what is common practice in the field of genetics.

LINKS BETWEEN INFLAMMATION AND NEW BONE FORMATION

The specific relationship between inflammation and new bone formation has been extensively debated over the past couple of years[9,10,63] because cohort studies failed to show a structural effect of TNF inhibitors (TNFi) over a 2-year period.[14–16] From these data, a long-term structural effect of TNFi can, however, not be completely excluded, although, if present, it may be mild. More data from early-stage disease are awaited, which may shed more light on the kinetics of interaction of inflammation and new bone formation in SpA. The negative data on the effect of TNFi on new bone formation in SpA contrast with the accumulating evidence that NSAID therapy shows substantial effects on new bone formation in SpA and retards structural progression.[64–66] First demonstrated in a landmark study with specific cyclooxygenase 2 inhibitor, celecoxib,[64] newer data demonstrate that this important feature is most likely a general effect of NSAIDs, provided that they are used continuously in SpA patients.[65,66]

Two different views on the relationship between inflammation and new bone formation in SpA have been developed. The first view supports a direct link between inflammation and new bone formation.[9] MRI studies have brought forward good evidence that active inflammatory lesions can evolve into remodeling lesions characterized by so-called fatty degeneration, which subsequently become sites of new bone formation.[67] According to this concept, active inflammation, including cytokines, such as TNF, may temporarily act as a brake on bone formation by up-regulating molecules, such as DKK1, that inhibit bone formation.[68] On resolution of inflammation and the decline of cytokines levels, new bone formation may become apparent. This view has a dual impact on the clinical concepts of disease treatment. First, this theory suggests that the use of TNFi, despite being highly effective to control inflammation, may automatically result in accelerated bone formation. Although increased bone formation is not seen in any of the cohort studies on TNFi until now, such effect may be masked by the anti-inflammatory effects of TNFi, which suppressed the development of the primary inflammatory lesions. Second, this concept suggests that an early and likely sustained intervention will have an impact on radiographic progression by preventing the development such primary lesions.[69]

The second view suggests that inflammation and new bone formation are linked but largely uncoupled processes.[10,70] Accordingly, inflammation and new bone formation should be considered complementary targets for the treatment of the disease. This view is supported by the observation that TNFi do not affect radiographic progression in either a positive or negative way[14–16] and by MRI data demonstrating that a large number of syndesmophytes appears at sites in which no preceding inflammation had been documented.[71] This hypothesis suggests that biomechanical factors, such as enthesial strain and microdamage, and infections may trigger both inflammation and bone modeling and that both of these processes together may determine the phenotype of SpA.

Exciting new data have recently emerged on the role of interleukin (IL)-23.[72,73] Polymorphisms in the IL-23 receptor gene have been associated with AS but also with related disorders, such as psoriatic arthritis.[74] In an elegant animal model study, Sherlock and colleagues[72] identified a T-cell population within the enthesis that is responsive to IL-23. Downstream events of the activation of this local cell population include triggering of different inflammatory cascades and pathways associated with new bone formation, such as Wnts and BMPs.[72] Although the data have been developed in a specific overexpression model in mice and are not corroborated in any translational setting, these observations provide a new concept in SpA. Increased IL-23 levels could be derived from the gut, thereby providing a molecular bridge for the long-standing relationship between gut and joint inflammation, from infection, including *Klebsiella pneumoniae*, a bacteria previously associated with AS but most likely also from entheseal damage and strain.[73]

HORIZONS AND CHALLENGES?

Understanding of the bone formation process in SpA is far from complete. Although concepts can be transposed from developmental biology toward disease pathology and have gained novel insights into some of the molecular pathways that trigger new bone formation in SpA, most of these insights need further work and confirmation in human disease and additional molecular specification in terms of the ligands, receptors, and pathways involved. The opposing views on the relationship between inflammation and new bone formation are likely to be merged into a common concept as further data accumulate. It seems likely that early intervention can result in a better outcome but the costs and toxicity may warrant this only for patients who are at risk for severe disability. Current markers and predictors, however, including genetics, are not yet ready for use in clinical practice and require large population confirmation and validation. Developing specific therapies against ankylosis remains a challenge with regard to effectiveness and also toxicity and long-term side effects. In this context, the importance of the effect of NSAIDs on ankylosis may not be underestimated. The eventual continued use of these drugs in patients with good disease control but a high risk for structural damage is a matter of debate. In summary, the past decade has faced enormous progress in understanding of structural damage in SpA. This progress cannot be uncoupled from the renewed interest in the field sparked by the development of the drugs like TNFi. Novel data also generate new avenues for research and there is confidence that future progress in research in the pathophysiology and clinics of SpA will improve understanding of this complex disease.

REFERENCES

1. Dougados M, Baeten D. Spondyloarthritis. Lancet 2011;377(9783):2127–37.
2. Machado P, Landewe R, Braun J, et al. Both structural damage and inflammation of the spine contribute to impairment of spinal mobility in patients with ankylosing spondylitis. Ann Rheum Dis 2010;69(8):1465–70.
3. Lories RJ, Baeten DL. Differences in pathophysiology between rheumatoid arthritis and ankylosing spondylitis. Clin Exp Rheumatol 2009;27(4 Suppl 55): S10–4.

4. Vleeming A, Volkers AC, Snijders CJ, et al. Relation between form and function in the sacroiliac joint. Part ii: biomechanical aspects. Spine (Phila Pa 1976) 1990;15(2):133–6.
5. Vleeming A, Stoeckart R, Volkers AC, et al. Relation between form and function in the sacroiliac joint. Part i: clinical anatomical aspects. Spine (Phila Pa 1976) 1990; 15(2):130–2.
6. Baraliakos X, Listing J, von der Recke A, et al. The natural course of radiographic progression in ankylosing spondylitis—evidence for major individual variations in a large proportion of patients. J Rheumatol 2009;36(5):997–1002.
7. Sieper J, Rudwaleit M, Baraliakos X, et al. The assessment of spondyloarthritis international society (asas) handbook: a guide to assess spondyloarthritis. Ann Rheum Dis 2009;68(Suppl 2):ii1–44.
8. Wanders AJ, Landewe RB, Spoorenberg A, et al. What is the most appropriate radiologic scoring method for ankylosing spondylitis? A comparison of the available methods based on the outcome measures in rheumatology clinical trials filter. Arthritis Rheum 2004;50(8):2622–32.
9. Sieper J, Appel H, Braun J, et al. Critical appraisal of assessment of structural damage in ankylosing spondylitis: implications for treatment outcomes. Arthritis Rheum 2008;58(3):649–56.
10. Lories RJ, Luyten FP, de Vlam K. Progress in spondylarthritis. Mechanisms of new bone formation in spondyloarthritis. Arthritis Res Ther 2009;11(2):221.
11. Lories RJ, Luyten FP. Bone morphogenetic protein signaling in joint homeostasis and disease. Cytokine Growth Factor Rev 2005;16(3):287–98.
12. Del Fattore A, Teti A, Rucci N. Bone cells and the mechanisms of bone remodelling. Front Biosci (Elite Ed) 2012;4:2302–21.
13. Carter S, Lories RJ. Osteoporosis: a paradox in ankylosing spondylitis. Curr Osteoporos Rep 2011;9(3):112–5.
14. van der Heijde D, Salonen D, Weissman BN, et al. Assessment of radiographic progression in the spines of patients with ankylosing spondylitis treated with adalimumab for up to 2 years. Arthritis Res Ther 2009;11(4):R127.
15. van der Heijde D, Landewe R, Baraliakos X, et al. Radiographic findings following two years of infliximab therapy in patients with ankylosing spondylitis. Arthritis Rheum 2008;58(10):3063–70.
16. van der Heijde D, Landewe R, Einstein S, et al. Radiographic progression of ankylosing spondylitis after up to two years of treatment with etanercept. Arthritis Rheum 2008;58(5):1324–31.
17. Lefebvre V, Bhattaram P. Vertebrate skeletogenesis. Curr Top Dev Biol 2010;90: 291–317.
18. Francois RJ, Gardner DL, Degrave EJ, et al. Histopathologic evidence that sacroiliitis in ankylosing spondylitis is not merely enthesitis. Arthritis Rheum 2000; 43(9):2011–24.
19. Francois RJ. Some pathological features of ankylosing spondylitis as revealed by microradiography and tetracycline labelling. Clin Rheumatol 1982;1(1):23–9.
20. Appel H, Maier R, Loddenkemper C, et al. Immunohistochemical analysis of osteoblasts in zygapophyseal joints of patients with ankylosing spondylitis reveal repair mechanisms similar to osteoarthritis. J Rheumatol 2010;37(4):823–8.
21. Appel H, Kuhne M, Spiekermann S, et al. Immunohistologic analysis of zygapophyseal joints in patients with ankylosing spondylitis. Arthritis Rheum 2006;54(9): 2845–51.
22. Appel H, Loddenkemper C, Grozdanovic Z, et al. Correlation of histopathological findings and magnetic resonance imaging in the spine of patients with ankylosing spondylitis. Arthritis Res Ther 2006;8(5):R143.

23. De Bari C, Dell'Accio F, Tylzanowski P, et al. Multipotent mesenchymal stem cells from adult human synovial membrane. Arthritis Rheum 2001;44(8):1928–42.
24. De Bari C, Dell'Accio F, Luyten FP. Human periosteum-derived cells maintain phenotypic stability and chondrogenic potential throughout expansion regardless of donor age. Arthritis Rheum 2001;44(1):85–95.
25. Pittenger MF, Mackay AM, Beck SC, et al. Multilineage potential of adult human mesenchymal stem cells. Science 1999;284(5411):143–7.
26. Jones EA, English A, Henshaw K, et al. Enumeration and phenotypic characterization of synovial fluid multipotential mesenchymal progenitor cells in inflammatory and degenerative arthritis. Arthritis Rheum 2004;50(3):817–27.
27. Lories RJ, Luyten FP. Activated fibrocytes: circulating cells that populate the arthritic synovium? Rheumatology (Oxford) 2010;49(4):617–8.
28. Kurth TB, Dell'accio F, Crouch V, et al. Functional mesenchymal stem cell niches in adult mouse knee joint synovium in vivo. Arthritis Rheum 2011;63(5):1289–300.
29. Medici D, Shore EM, Lounev VY, et al. Conversion of vascular endothelial cells into multipotent stem-like cells. Nat Med 2010;16(12):1400–6.
30. Urist MR. Bone: formation by autoinduction. Science 1965;150(3698):893–9.
31. Wozney JM, Rosen V, Celeste AJ, et al. Novel regulators of bone formation: molecular clones and activities. Science 1988;242(4885):1528–34.
32. Hogan BL. Bone morphogenetic proteins: multifunctional regulators of vertebrate development. Genes Dev 1996;10(13):1580–94.
33. Nakamura J, Yanagita M. Bmp modulators in kidney disease. Discov Med 2012; 13(68):57–63.
34. Otsuka F. Multiple endocrine regulation by bone morphogenetic protein system. Endocr J 2010;57(1):3–14.
35. Axelrad TW, Einhorn TA. Bone morphogenetic proteins in orthopaedic surgery. Cytokine Growth Factor Rev 2009;20(5–6):481–8.
36. Miyazono K, Maeda S, Imamura T. Bmp receptor signaling: transcriptional targets, regulation of signals, and signaling cross-talk. Cytokine Growth Factor Rev 2005;16(3):251–63.
37. Nusse R, Varmus H. Three decades of wnts: a personal perspective on how a scientific field developed. EMBO J 2012;31(12):2670–84.
38. Clevers H, Nusse R. Wnt/beta-catenin signaling and disease. Cell 2012;149(6): 1192–205.
39. Amin N, Vincan E. The wnt signaling pathways and cell adhesion. Front Biosci 2012;17:784–804.
40. Luyten FP, Tylzanowski P, Lories RJ. Wnt signaling and osteoarthritis. Bone 2009; 44(4):522–7.
41. Lodewyckx L, Lories RJ. Wnt signaling in osteoarthritis and osteoporosis: what is the biological significance for the clinician? Curr Rheumatol Rep 2009;11(1):23–30.
42. Lories RJ, Peeters J, Bakker A, et al. Articular cartilage and biomechanical properties of the long bones in frzb-knockout mice. Arthritis Rheum 2007;56(12): 4095–103.
43. Mackie EJ, Tatarczuch L, Mirams M. The skeleton: a multi-functional complex organ: the growth plate chondrocyte and endochondral ossification. J Endocrinol 2011;211(2):109–21.
44. Hui CC, Angers S. Gli proteins in development and disease. Annu Rev Cell Dev Biol 2011;27:513–37.
45. Lories RJ, Derese I, Luyten FP. Modulation of bone morphogenetic protein signaling inhibits the onset and progression of ankylosing enthesitis. J Clin Invest 2005;115(6):1571–9.

46. Lories RJ, Matthys P, de Vlam K, et al. Ankylosing enthesitis, dactylitis, and onychoperiostitis in male dba/1 mice: a model of psoriatic arthritis. Ann Rheum Dis 2004;63(5):595–8.
47. Braem K, Luyten FP, Lories RJ. Blocking p38 signalling inhibits chondrogenesis in vitro but not ankylosis in a model of ankylosing spondylitis in vivo. Ann Rheum Dis 2012;71(5):722–8.
48. Uderhardt S, Diarra D, Katzenbeisser J, et al. Blockade of dickkopf (dkk)-1 induces fusion of sacroiliac joints. Ann Rheum Dis 2010;69(3):592–7.
49. Diarra D, Stolina M, Polzer K, et al. Dickkopf-1 is a master regulator of joint remodeling. Nat Med 2007;13(2):156–63.
50. Polzer K, Diarra D, Zwerina J, et al. Inflammation and destruction of the joints–the wnt pathway. Joint Bone Spine 2008;75(2):105–7.
51. Ruiz-Heiland G, Horn A, Zerr P, et al. Blockade of the hedgehog pathway inhibits osteophyte formation in arthritis. Ann Rheum Dis 2012;71(3):400–7.
52. Marhoffer W, Stracke H, Masoud I, et al. Evidence of impaired cartilage/bone turnover in patients with active ankylosing spondylitis. Ann Rheum Dis 1995;54(7):556–9.
53. Kim TH, Stone M, Payne U, et al. Cartilage biomarkers in ankylosing spondylitis: relationship to clinical variables and treatment response. Arthritis Rheum 2005;52(3):885–91.
54. Vosse D, Landewe R, Garnero P, et al. Association of markers of bone- and cartilage-degradation with radiological changes at baseline and after 2 years follow-up in patients with ankylosing spondylitis. Rheumatology (Oxford) 2008;47(8):1219–22.
55. Appel H, Janssen L, Listing J, et al. Serum levels of biomarkers of bone and cartilage destruction and new bone formation in different cohorts of patients with axial spondyloarthritis with and without tumor necrosis factor-alpha blocker treatment. Arthritis Res Ther 2008;10(5):R125.
56. Maksymowych WP, Landewe R, Conner-Spady B, et al. Serum matrix metalloproteinase 3 is an independent predictor of structural damage progression in patients with ankylosing spondylitis. Arthritis Rheum 2007;56(6):1846–53.
57. Heiland GR, Appel H, Poddubnyy D, et al. High level of functional dickkopf-1 predicts protection from syndesmophyte formation in patients with ankylosing spondylitis. Ann Rheum Dis 2012;71(4):572–4.
58. Daoussis D, Liossis SN, Solomou EE, et al. Evidence that dkk-1 is dysfunctional in ankylosing spondylitis. Arthritis Rheum 2010;62(1):150–8.
59. Appel H, Ruiz-Heiland G, Listing J, et al. Altered skeletal expression of sclerostin and its link to radiographic progression in ankylosing spondylitis. Arthritis Rheum 2009;60(11):3257–62.
60. Chen HA, Chen CH, Lin YJ, et al. Association of bone morphogenetic proteins with spinal fusion in ankylosing spondylitis. J Rheumatol 2010;37(10):2126–32.
61. Park MC, Park YB, Lee SK. Relationship of bone morphogenetic proteins to disease activity and radiographic damage in patients with ankylosing spondylitis. Scand J Rheumatol 2008;37(3):200–4.
62. Wendling D, Cedoz JP, Racadot E, et al. Serum il-17, bmp-7, and bone turnover markers in patients with ankylosing spondylitis. Joint Bone Spine 2007;74(3):304–5.
63. Maksymowych WP, Elewaut D, Schett G. Motion for debate: the development of ankylosis in ankylosing spondylitis is largely dependent on inflammation. Arthritis Rheum 2012;64(6):1713–9.

64. Wanders A, Heijde D, Landewe R, et al. Nonsteroidal antiinflammatory drugs reduce radiographic progression in patients with ankylosing spondylitis: a randomized clinical trial. Arthritis Rheum 2005;52(6):1756–65.
65. Kroon F, Landewe R, Dougados M, et al. Continuous NSAID use reverts the effects of inflammation on radiographic progression in patients with ankylosing spondylitis. Ann Rheum Dis 2012. [Epub ahead of print].
66. Poddubnyy D, Rudwaleit M, Haibel H, et al. Effect of non-steroidal anti-inflammatory drugs on radiographic spinal progression in patients with axial spondyloarthritis: results from the German Spondyloarthritis Inception Cohort. Ann Rheum Dis 2012. [Epub ahead of print].
67. Chiowchanwisawakit P, Lambert RG, Conner-Spady B, et al. Focal fat lesions at vertebral corners on magnetic resonance imaging predict the development of new syndesmophytes in ankylosing spondylitis. Arthritis Rheum 2011;63(8): 2215–25.
68. Maksymowych WP. Disease modification in ankylosing spondylitis. Nat Rev Rheumatol 2010;6(2):75–81.
69. Maksymowych WP, Morency N, Conner-Spady B, et al. Suppression of inflammation and effects on new bone formation in ankylosing spondylitis: evidence for a window of opportunity in disease modification. Ann Rheum Dis 2012. [Epub ahead of print].
70. Lories RJ, de Vlam K, Luyten FP. Are current available therapies disease-modifying in spondyloarthritis? Best Pract Res Clin Rheumatol 2010;24(5): 625–35.
71. van der Heijde D, Machado P, Braun J, et al. Mri inflammation at the vertebral unit only marginally predicts new syndesmophyte formation: a multilevel analysis in patients with ankylosing spondylitis. Ann Rheum Dis 2012;71(3):369–73.
72. Sherlock JP, Joyce-Shaikh B, Turner SP, et al. Il-23 induces spondyloarthropathy by acting on ror-gammat(+) cd3(+)cd4(-)cd8(-) entheseal resident t cells. Nat Med 2012;18(7):1069–76.
73. Lories RJ, McInnes IB. Primed for inflammation: enthesis-resident t cells. Nat Med 2012;18(7):1018–9.
74. Burton PR, Clayton DG, Cardon LR, et al. Association scan of 14,500 nonsynonymous snps in four diseases identifies autoimmunity variants. Nat Genet 2007; 39(11):1329–37.

Pathophysiology and Role of the Gastrointestinal System in Spondyloarthritides

Peggy Jacques, MD, PhD[1], Liesbet Van Praet, MD[1],
Philippe Carron, MD, Filip Van den Bosch, MD, PhD,
Dirk Elewaut, MD, PhD*

KEYWORDS

• Pathophysiology • Inflammatory bowel disease • Ankylosing spondylitis

KEY POINTS

- Inflammatory bowel disease (IBD) is a well-known extra-articular manifestation in spondyloarthritis (SpA); about 6.5% of patients with ankylosing spondylitis develop IBD during the course of the disease.
- The pathogenesis of both SpA and IBD is considered to be the result of a complex interplay between the host (genetic predisposition), the immune system and environmental factors, notably microorganisms, leading to a disturbed immune system and chronic inflammation.
- Over the past decade, the role of tumor necrosis factor inhibition (infliximab, etanercept, adalimumab, golimumab) in improving signs and symptoms and overall quality of life has been well documented in various forms of SpA. Future research will clarify the role of other potential targets.

INTRODUCTION

In spondyloarthritis (SpA), there is a prominent and intriguing link between joint and gut, which has been broadly studied over the past 30 years. Inflammatory bowel disease (IBD) is a well-known extra-articular manifestation in SpA; about 6.5% of patients with ankylosing spondylitis (AS) develop IBD during the course of the disease. Furthermore, up to 60% of patients with AS show microscopic gut inflammation without obvious gastrointestinal discomfort.[1]

On the other hand, articular involvement (axial and peripheral) often hits patients primarily diagnosed with IBD. The reported incidence of asymptomatic sacroiliitis varies from 11% to 52% according to the detection technique,[2,3] with up to 10% developing AS. Arthritis is typically pauciarticular, transient, migratory, asymmetrical, and mostly nondeforming.

Department of Rheumatology, Ghent University Hospital, Belgium
[1] These authors contributed equally to this article.
* Corresponding author. Laboratory for Molecular Immunology and Inflammation, Department of Rheumatology, Ghent University Hospital, De Pintelaan 185, 9000 Ghent, Belgium.
E-mail address: Dirk.elewaut@ugent.be

Rheum Dis Clin N Am 38 (2012) 569–582
http://dx.doi.org/10.1016/j.rdc.2012.08.012 rheumatic.theclinics.com

Extensive research has been performed to clarify the role of gut inflammation in the pathogenesis of SpA. Despite substantial progress, the exact mechanisms by which gut inflammation triggers joint inflammation remain unclear.

This article focuses on the overlap between SpA and IBD and discusses future strategies in the treatment of SpA.

MICROSCOPIC GUT INFLAMMATION

One of the first forms of evidence for a relationship between bowel inflammation and peripheral arthritis stems from the clinical observation that peripheral joint inflammation may appear in genetically predisposed patients after a bacterial gut infection, such as *Salmonella typhimurium*, *Yersinia enterocolitica*, *Shigella*, and *Campylobacter jejuni*. The risk of the development of a reactive arthritis is genetically influenced, for example, by human leukocyte antigen (HLA)-B27, although clearly additional genes significantly modulate this risk.

Mielants and colleagues[1] observed a very high frequency of microscopic gut inflammation in patients with different forms of SpA. Up to two-thirds of patients with SpA showed microscopic signs of gut inflammation without obvious signs of gastrointestinal discomfort. Two histologic types of microscopic gut inflammation can be distinguished: acute and chronic inflammation.[4] This classification refers to the observed morphologic characteristics and not to the disease duration. In the acute type of inflammation, the normal mucosal structure is preserved and changes are limited to an infiltration of the epithelium with neutrophils and eosinophils, crypt abscess formation, and an infiltration of the lamina propria with polymorphonuclear cells. Chronic inflammation is characterized by a disturbed mucosal architecture, with crypt distortion, villous blunting and fusion, increased mixed lamina propria cellularity, and the presence of basal lymphoid aggregates.

Equally high frequencies of acute and chronic microscopic gut inflammation were recently observed in the Gent Inflammatory Arthritis and spoNdylitis cohorT (GIANT), a prospective observational cohort of patients diagnosed with SpA and classified according to the Assessment of SpondyloArthritis International Society (ASAS) criteria. In this cohort, about 50% of the patients showed microscopic gut inflammation, with the acute type of inflammation being present in up to 20% and the chronic type in up to 30% of patients (**Fig. 1**).

Importantly, the chronic type of inflammation may be considered as an early stage of Crohn disease (CD) and, additionally, as a risk factor for developing CD over time.[1] About 20% of the patients with chronic gut inflammation on baseline ileocolonoscopy evolved into overt IBD in a 5-year period.[1]

The impact of nonsteroidal antiinflammatory drugs (NSAIDs) on bowel inflammation in SpA has always been a topic of discussion. Often, patients with IBD are advised to avoid the use of NSAIDs to prevent disease exacerbation. Nevertheless, the association between NSAIDs and IBD flares cannot be considered as proven because the data are inconsistent. Several retrospective studies have been performed to elucidate the role of NSAIDs in causing flares of IBD; some found no association, whereas others reported a flare-up of symptoms.[5–10]

However, 2 randomized, controlled, double-blind trials in patients with inactive IBD receiving a cyclooxygenase 2–selective inhibitor (celecoxib/etoricoxib) or placebo[11,12] showed no significant difference in the frequency of disease exacerbation.

Regarding microscopic gut inflammation, comparable prevalence rates were observed among patients with SpA receiving antiinflammatory drugs compared with patients not treated with NSAIDs.[13] Furthermore, in arthritic controls treated with

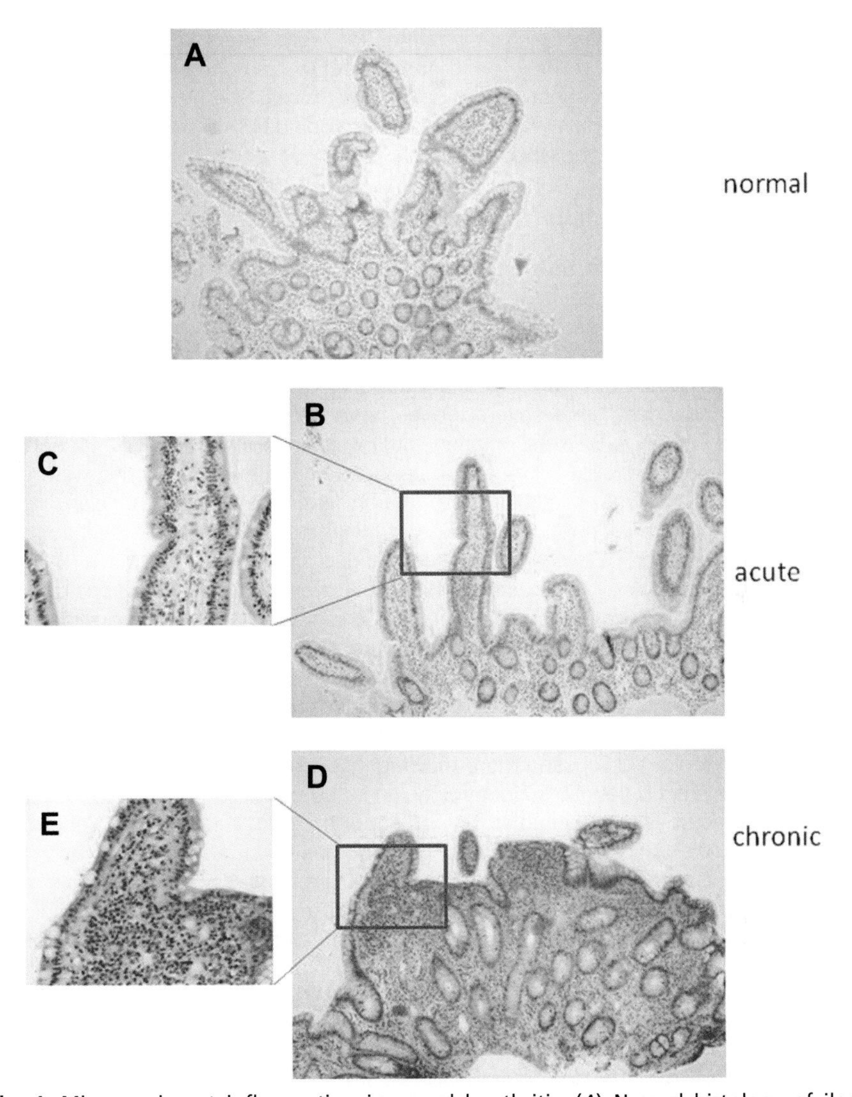

Fig. 1. Microscopic gut inflammation in spondyloarthritis. (*A*) Normal histology of ileal mucosa: straight crypts and slender villi; absence of inflammatory cell infiltrates (hematoxylin-eosin, original magnification ×10). (*B*) Focal active inflammation in mucosa with preserved architecture of villi and crypts (hematoxylin-eosin, original magnification ×10). (*C*) Higher magnification emphasizing an increased amount of granulocytes in villus and crypt epithelium with well-preserved epithelium (hematoxylin-eosin, original magnification ×40). (*D*) Chronic dense inflammatory cell infiltration of lamina propria with crypt and villus alterations (hematoxylin-eosin, original magnification ×10). (*E*) Higher magnification emphasizing active granulocytic infiltration of villus epithelium and chronic dense lymphoplasmacytic cellular infiltrate in the lamina propria (hematoxylin-eosin, original magnification ×40).

NSAIDs, no signs of microscopic gut inflammation were detected.[13] Similarly, in the authors' own GIANT cohort, they found normal, acute, and chronic gut involvement in 60%, 20%, and 20%, respectively, in patients with axial SpA not receiving NSAIDs versus 47.7%, 18.2%, and 34.1% in patients undergoing NSAID treatment (van praet and colleagues, 2012, unpublished data).

GENETICS AND ENVIRONMENT

The pathogenesis of both SpA and IBD is considered to be the result of a complex interplay between the host (genetic predisposition) and environmental factors, notably microorganisms, leading to a disturbed immune system and chronic inflammation.

Over the last couple of years, our understanding of the genetic basis of SpA has tremendously advanced, and several genes have been linked to SpA. Apart from the strong link with HLA-B27, association with genes involved in intracellular antigen processing (endoplasmic reticulum amino peptidase-1 [ERAP1] interacting with HLA-B27) and genes involved in cytokine production (especially those important in the regulation of the interleukin (IL)-17–IL-23 pathway) play a role in the susceptibility for AS.[14] Likewise, for IBD, multiple genetic markers are known.

In an Iceland genealogy database, a remarkable overlap in the genetic background between AS and IBD was revealed because there was an elevated cross-risk ratio between either of these diseases.[15] A 3-fold increased risk to develop IBD was identified in first-degree relatives of patients with AS; conversely, equal risk was found in relatives from patients with IBD being much more susceptible to develop AS. Hence, IBD and AS share a common genetic susceptibility, particularly in the IL-17–IL-23 pathway. This topic is discussed more thoroughly elsewhere in this issue.

Besides this shared genetic susceptibility, an inappropriate inflammatory response to intestinal microbes is assumed to play an important role. This role is supported by the detection of IBD-associated circulating antibodies to various microbial antigens, including anti-Saccharomyces cerevisiae antibodies, anti–Escherichiae coli outer membrane porin C, and perinuclear antineutrophil cytoplasmic antibodies.[16,17] In a study by De Vries and colleagues,[18] 55% of patients with AS without overt IBD showed at least one antibody associated with IBD.

Future research will have to address the role of these and other IBD-associated antimicrobial reactivities in SpA.

The Intestinal Microbiome and SpA-Associated Inflammation

Several hypotheses have been proposed to explain the close relationship between joint and gut inflammation in SpA. A first theory points at the potential role for intestinal bacteria in the origin of articular inflammation. Alterations in gut flora itself may be an important contributing factor, for example, caused by an abnormal number of microorganisms or by fluctuations in the composition of the microbial flora, which is generally referred to as the microbiome. In healthy individuals, immunologic tolerance to the gut microbiome is obtained, whereas this homeostatic balance is disrupted in patients with IBD, overall resulting in dysbiosis.[19] The composition of the intestinal flora in patients with IBD is altered compared with healthy individuals, resulting in a general loss in diversity,[20] a reduction in protective *Firmicutes* and *Bacteroidetes,* and a relative increase in *Enterobacteriaceae*, such as *E coli,* although their absolute numbers remained unaltered.[21] Whether these alterations are at the origin of inflammation or a result of defective immune balances remains incompletely resolved. Up until now, the causative species remain unidentified.[22–24]

On the other hand, the gut mucosal immune system is the first defense against invasion of pathogens, and the intestinal flora also directly influences the immune response. A dysfunctional interaction between gut bacteria and the mucosal immune system could result in immunologic intolerance. The intestinal epithelium plays a pivotal role in the primary defense against pathogens. One important cell type within the epithelium is Paneth cells. These intestinal secretory cells located at the bottom of the bowel crypts have the ability to secrete antimicrobial products, including lysozyme and defensins. Besides Paneth cells, goblet cells also secrete defensins.[25] Defensins are reduced in ileal Crohn disease in contrast with colonic Crohn or ulcerative colitis.[26,27] In ileal biopsy samples from patients with AS and chronic inflammation or recent-onset Crohn disease, a marked upregulation in Paneth cell antimicrobial peptides was observed.[28] Dysfunction of Paneth cells occurring during the early stages of intestinal inflammation may be a signature for development of bowel inflammation.[28]

The most compelling evidence for the pathogenic role of bacteria in the pathogenesis of gut and joint inflammation in SpA is derived from animal models. Germfree raised mice fail to develop a normal immune system and display reduced intestinal lymphoid tissue.[29,30] Furthermore, HLA-B27 transgenic rats reared in a germfree environment do not develop arthritis or colitis, whereas the restoration of intestinal flora leads to the development of colitis within weeks.[31]

The contribution of HLA B27 to the interrelationship of gut and joint inflammation remains unclear. Rosenbaum and colleagues[32] hypothesized that HLA-B27 positivity predisposes the individual to develop AS by modifying the composition of the endogenous flora and alter the immune response to infectious agents. Hence, there are various ways how HLA-B27 may be implicated. It encodes for a protein that presents antigens to induce immune responses but could also present arthritogenic peptides.[33] Furthermore, it regulates positive and negative selection of T cells in the thymus and can form dimers that are recognized by natural killer (NK) cells,[34] which might also promote inflammation and contribute to AS pathogenesis.

The most persuasive connection between the microbiome and SpA is the appreciation that certain bacterial species, such as *Chlamydia*, *Salmonella*, *Shigella*, *Yersinia*, and *Campylobacter*, can trigger reactive arthritis.

Cellular Targets in Gut and Joint Inflammation

The main cellular targets for these intracellular pathogens that are associated with SpA are macrophages.[35] Therefore, one of the most attractive hypotheses remains that trafficking of mononuclear cells from the intestine to the joints could be a critical factor in the development of gut and joint inflammation.[36] As such, macrophages could contribute to disease pathogenesis by the uptake of bacterial components in the intestine, followed by the presentation to T cells and migration to the joint. In support of this hypothesis, a particular subset of macrophages, expressing the scavenger receptor CD163, was enriched in the colon of patients with SpA and Crohn disease, even in noninflamed regions,[37] while this specific subset was also selectively increased in SpA synovium.[38] Global disease activity correlated well with the number of $CD163^+$ macrophages and polymorphonuclear cells in the synovium.[39] These cells are also an important source of proinflammatory cytokines, such as TNF.

However, the target cell responding to proinflammatory cytokine production may well be another cell type. This idea is supported by strong experimental evidence for the role of the stromal cells in gut and joint inflammation revealed in the $TNF^{\Delta ARE}$ mouse model. Chronic and dysregulated TNF production, caused by the deletion of the adenylate/uridylate (AU)-rich elements in the regulatory sequences of the murine

TNF genome, provokes simultaneous development of a Crohnlike inflammatory bowel disease and articular inflammation.[40] The articular inflammation shows substantial resemblance to the SpA concept because it involves peripheral synovitis, enthesitis, and sacroiliitis.[41] Signaling through TNF receptor I (TNFRI) seemed to be a prerequisite for the development of both gut inflammation and arthritis.[40] Yet, only recently is was demonstrated that selective TNFR1 expression within the stromal compartment, synovial fibroblasts and intestinal myofibroblasts, provided a sufficient target for TNF in the development of both gut and joint inflammation.[41] In addition, TNF production in intestinal epithelial cells was sufficient to cause murine Crohnlike ileitis; however, when TNFRI expression was limited to intestinal epithelial cells, deregulated TNF production was not sufficient to cause chronic inflammation.[42] In conclusion, epithelial-derived TNF can trigger the activation of the stroma, namely, the intestinal myofibroblasts residing in the deeper bowel wall layers.[41] Further research is required to unravel the precise effector pathways by which stromal cells can induce bowel inflammation and arthritic disease.

However, whether SpA is a disease driven by innate versus adaptive immunity is still unclear. In patients with SpA, the synovium is also infiltrated by T and B lymphocytes[43]; these T cells have an altered functional behavior with a decreased T_H1/T_H2 ratio.[44,45]

Therefore, aberrant trafficking of lymphocytes between the gut and the joint may be another mechanism for the combined intestinal and articular inflammation in SpA. Naive lymphocytes continuously recirculate in between different lymphoid organs until they encounter a specific antigen. Following an antigen encounter, homing of matured lymphocyte is mediated by a distinct set of adhesion molecules, such as integrins and selectins, and by chemokine receptors.[46] Homing to the intestine is mediated by 2 members of the β7 integrin subfamily: α4β7 and αEβ7.[46] The expression of the α4β7 integrin on memory T cells allows their binding to mucosal addressin cell adhesion molecule-1 (MadCAM-1), which is selectively expressed by mucosal endothelial cells, whereas the αEβ7 integrin, constitutively expressed by mucosal intraepithelial T cells, binds to E-cadherin, which is expressed on gut epithelial cells.[47] The interaction of the α4β7 integrin and MAdCAM-1 is thought to contribute to the chronic bowel inflammation.[48–50] A hallmark of Crohn disease (and other inflammatory conditions) is the recruitment and inappropriate retention of leukocytes, particularly T cells at the site of inflammation. Patients suffering from Crohn disease showed a reduced expression of αEβ7 on intraepithelial lymphocytes in the ileum even in noninflamed mucosa.[51] Also, mucosal lymphocytes isolated from inflamed bowel from patients with IBD were able to bind in vitro to inflamed synovial vessels.[36,52] In addition, it was shown that activated T cells carrying the α4β7 and αEβ7 integrins were enriched in inflamed synovial tissue in patients with early SpA.[53] However, the expression of the αEβ7 integrin could be modulated by the chronic inflammatory environment itself and local TGF-β production.[54,55]

As mentioned earlier, targeting of molecules involved in leukocyte trafficking or retention may provide promising new treatment options in IBD. Natalizumab, a recombinant humanized monoclonal antibody directed at the integrin subunit a4, systemically blocks the integrins α4β7 and α4β1 and was the first approved treatment in the class of selective adhesion molecule inhibitors for Crohn disease.[56] However, serious safety concerns (eg, increased incidence of the fatal infectious disease progressive multifocal leukoencephalopathy by decreasing immunosurveillance in the central nervous system) resulted in the temporarily withdrawal of the product. A more selective antibody, vedolizumab, directed against the α4β7 integrin also showed good clinical efficacy in Crohn disease[48] and ulcerative colitis.[57]

More recently, the contribution of the IL-23/IL-17 axis to SpA became widely appreciated. This finding is strongly supported by the fact that IL-23 receptor polymorphisms could confer protection against AS and associated conditions, such as psoriasis and IBD.[58,59] The IL-23/IL-17 axis is also strongly activated in the colon of HLA-B27 transgenic rats, concurrent with intestinal inflammation.[60] HLA-B27 misfolding and the subsequent unfolded protein response strongly increases the production of IL-23.[60]

Serum concentrations of IL-23 are elevated in patients with AS.[61,62] It remains, however, unclear how IL-23 is responsible for inflammation at different sites in SpA. IL-23 upregulation was also reported in microscopic gut inflammation (in the terminal ileum) in patients with AS in comparison with healthy controls.[61] However, this was not associated with a clear T_H17 polarization.

Recently, it was shown that a resident double-negative T-cell population within the entheseal region in collagen-antibody–induced arthritis mice is also highly responsive to IL-23, and these cells are able to produce proinflammatory cytokines, such as IL-6, IL-17, and IL-22, in response to IL-23 receptor engagement.[63]

Interestingly, innate immune cells are also capable of IL-17 production. It was recently reported by histologic analysis of zygapophyseal joints of patients with AS that $CD15^+$ neutrophils and myeloperoxidase-positive myeloid cells, but not classical T cells, are the major cellular sources of IL-17 in the inflamed bone marrow.[64] A specific subset of NK cells (NK-22 cells) that are located in the mucosa-associated lymphoid tissue secrete IL-22 in response to acute exposure to IL-23. Expression of the IL-22 receptor is restricted to mesenchymal cells. Therefore, IL-22 production by immune cells is thought to regulate inflammation and provide protection particularly at mucosal sites by controlling stromal responses.[65] Whether this pathway is also operational in the inflamed SpA joint remains elusive.

REGULATORY FEEDBACK OF GUT AND JOINT INFLAMMATION

Several studies have highlighted a variety of adaptive immune responses mediated by naturally occurring counter regulatory cells, such as T-regulatory (T_{REG}) cells and NK T (NKT) cells.[66,67] Nevertheless, these adaptive immune responses seem insufficient to combat inflammation in these inflammatory conditions.

Among these regulatory subsets, forkhead box P3 $Foxp3^+CD4^+$ T_{REG} cells have emerged as the most important cell type. These cells are able to suppress the proliferation and cytokine production of effector T cells mainly through direct cell-cell interactions.[67,68] Active Crohn disease is associated with a contraction of the peripheral blood T_{REG}-cell pool compared with healthy individuals and an only moderate expansion of these cells in intestinal lesions.[69,70] Therapy with anti-TNF antibodies (infliximab or adalimumab) enhances the number and suppressive function of peripheral blood $Foxp3^+$ T_{REG} cells, which is shown by reduced proliferation of effector T cells in patients with IBD.[71] Similarly, a good clinical response of patients with Crohn disease to infliximab was associated with a clear increase in peripheral blood T_{REG} cells and TGF-β levels when compared with nonresponders.[72]

Data on the frequency and role of T_{REG} cells in SpA are scarce. It was suggested that $Foxp3^+$ T_{REG} cells are actively recruited to the inflamed joints because these cells accumulated within the joints when compared with levels in peripheral blood during relapses.[73,74] A higher frequency of Foxp3+ T_{REG} cells was reported in patients with axial and peripheral SpA compared with those with definite AS and rheumatoid arthritis (RA). According to the investigators, this might contribute to the spontaneous resolution of peripheral SpA as compared with the more persistent joint inflammation in RA.[74]

In patients with AS with chronic intestinal inflammation, the activity of T_{REG} cells within the terminal ileum was demonstrated by high expression of IL-2, IL-10, TGF-β,

Table 1
Pipeline therapeutic options for IBD and AS

Agent	Mode of Action	IBD[80]	AS
Adalimumab	Neutralization of TNFα activity		
Infliximab	Neutralization of TNFα activity		
Certolizumab pegol	Neutralization of TNFα activity		81
Golimumab	Neutralization of TNFα activity		
Etanercept	Neutralization of TNFα activity		
Tocilizumab	Blockade of IL-6R		82
Tofacitinib	JAK3 inhibitor		
Natalizumab	Blockade of α4β1 and α4β7		
Vedolizumab	Blockade of α4β7 integrin		
PF547659	Blockade of human mucosal addressin cell adhesion molecule-1 (MAdCAM)		
Ustekinumab	Blockade of IL-12/23		83
Briakinumab	Blockade of IL-12/23		
Basiliximab	Blockade of IL-2R		
Daclizumab	Blockade of IL-2R		
Fontolizumab	Blockade of IFN-γ		
Sargramostim	GM-CSF		
Abatacept	Inhibitor of costimulation of T cells		84,85
Visilizumab	Anti-CD3 antibody		
Ocrelizumab	Anti-CD20 antibody		
Rituximab	Anti-CD20 antibody		86
Traficet	Chemokine receptor CCR9 antagonist		
Alicaforsen	Antisense oligonucleotide against ICAM-1 messenger RNA		
Secukinumab	Blockade of IL-17A		87
Vidofludimus	Inhibitor of IL-17A and IL-17F		

Positive outcome.

Potentially effective/ongoing trials.

Negative outcome.

No studies (clinicaltrials.gov July 17, 2012).

Abbreviations: GM-CSF, granulocyte-macrophage colony-stimulating factor; ICAM-1, intercellular adhesion molecule 1; IFN, interferon; JAK3, Janus kinase 3.

Foxp3, and signal transducer and activator of transcription (STAT5).[75] In addition, a significantly increased frequency of IL-10–producing $CD4^{+}CD25^{high}$ T_{REG} cells was detected both in lamina propria from ileal biopsy samples and in peripheral blood from these patients compared with healthy individuals.[75]

Another subset of regulatory T lymphocytes is NKT cells, which express an invariant T-cell receptor, the so-called invariant NKT (iNKT) cells. iNKT cells recognize endogenous or exogenous glycolipid antigens presented by the nonclassic major histocompatibility complex (MHC) molecule CD1d. The cells operate as sensors of microbial infections through recognition of microbial-derived glycolipid ligands. In $TNF^{\Delta ARE}$ mice, a model for spondyloarthritis, iNKT cells provide a naturally occurring feedback mechanism to dampen both intestinal and articular inflammation.[76] These cells operate through enhanced crosstalk with inflammatory dendritic cells, which express significantly higher levels of the nonclassic MHC molecule CD1d under chronic exposure of TNF. CD1d presents exogenous or endogenous glycolipid antigens to iNKT cells and induces the production of T_H1, T_H2, and T_H17 cells. Under chronic TNF exposure, iNKT cell activation does not require exogenous administration of glycolipid antigens, suggesting an enhanced presentation of endogenous ligands. Importantly, a similar increase in CD1d levels in patients with SpA was apparent.[76] However, the functional role of human iNKT cells requires further investigation.

THERAPEUTIC IMPLICATIONS OF BOWEL INFLAMMATION IN SPA

Over the past decade, the role of TNF inhibition (infliximab, etanercept, adalimumab, golimumab) in improving signs and symptoms and overall quality of life has been well documented in various forms of SpA. It also became clear tht the monoclonal antibodies neutralizing TNF are considerably more efficacious than etanercept in modulating extra-articular manifestations of SpA, even though a comparable efficacy is noted for both axial and peripheral joint manifestations.[77,78] This has been incorporated in the ASAS therapeutic recommendations for the management of AS.[79] Nevertheless, there is an urgent need for a new mode of action drugs that could be of benefit in patients that have an unsatisfactory clinical response or have severe side effects on TNF blocking agents. The common genetic susceptibility between AS and IBD and the relation between gut and joint in general in SpA is reflected in at least a partial therapeutic overlap between both diseases. **Table 1** shows the therapeutic (pipeline) options that are currently available or in clinical development for IBD, which may also become appropriate targets in SpA. There are, therefore, great expectations that a better understanding of the relation between gut and joint inflammation in SpA will broaden our therapeutic options in the near future in SpA.

REFERENCES

1. Mielants H, Veys EM, Cuvelier C, et al. The evolution of spondylarthropathies in relation to gut histology. II. Histological aspects. J Rheumatol 1995;22:2273–8.
2. Peeters H, Vander Cruyssen B, Laukens D, et al. Radiological sacroiliitis, a hallmark of spondylitis, is linked with CARD15 gene polymorphisms in patients with Crohn's disease. Ann Rheum Dis 2004;63:1131–4.
3. Davis P, Thomson ABR, Lentle BC. Quantitative sacroiliac scintigraphy in patients with Crohn's disease. Arthritis Rheum 1978;21:234–7.
4. Cuvelier C, Barbatis C, Mielants H, et al. Histopathology of intestinal inflammation related to reactive arthritis. Gut 1987;28:394–401.

5. Felder JB, Korelitz BI, Rajapakse R, et al. Effects of nonsteroidal antiinflammatory drugs on inflammatory bowel disease: a case-control study. Am J Gastroenterol 2000;95:1949–54.
6. Mahadevan U, Loftus EV Jr, Tremaine WJ, et al. Safety of selective cyclooxygenase-2 inhibitors in inflammatory bowel disease. Am J Gastroenterol 2002;97:910–4.
7. Matuk R, Crawford J, Abreu MT, et al. The spectrum of gastrointestinal toxicity and effect on disease activity of selective cyclooxygenase-2 inhibitors in patients with inflammatory bowel disease. Inflamm Bowel Dis 2004;10:352–6.
8. Takeuchi K, Smale S, Premchand P, et al. Prevalence and mechanism of nonsteroidal anti-inflammatory drug-induced clinical relapse in patients with inflammatory bowel disease. Clin Gastroenterol Hepatol 2006;4:196–202.
9. Reinisch W, Miehsler W, Dejaco C, et al. An open-label trial of the selective cyclooxygenase-2 inhibitor, rofecoxib, in inflammatory bowel disease-associated peripheral arthritis and arthralgia. Aliment Pharmacol Ther 2003;17:1371–80.
10. Biancone L, Tosti C, Geremia A, et al. Rofecoxib and early relapse of inflammatory bowel disease: an open-label trial. Aliment Pharmacol Ther 2004;19: 755–64.
11. Sandborn WJ, Stenson WF, Brynskov J, et al. Safety of celecoxib in patients with ulcerative colitis in remission: a randomized, placebo-controlled, pilot study. Clin Gastroenterol Hepatol 2006;4:203–11.
12. El Miedany Y, Youssef S, Ahmed I, et al. The gastrointestinal safety and effect on disease activity of etoricoxib, a selective cox-2 inhibitor in inflammatory bowel diseases. Am J Gastroenterol 2006;101:311–7.
13. Mielants H, Veys E. Ankylosing spondylitis and reactive arthritis : pathogenic aspects and therapeutic consequences. Ghent: Ghent University; 1988.
14. Reveille JD. Genetics of spondyloarthritis-beyond the MHC. Nat Rev Rheumatol 2012;8:296–304.
15. Thjodleifsson B, Geirsson AJ, Bjornsson S, et al. A common genetic background for inflammatory bowel disease and ankylosing spondylitis: a genealogic study in Iceland. Arthritis Rheum 2007;56:2633–9.
16. Rutgeerts P, Vermeire S. Serological diagnosis of inflammatory bowel disease. Lancet 2000;356(9248):2117–8.
17. Hoffman IEA, Demetter P, Peeters M, et al. Anti-saccharomyces cerevisiae IgA antibodies are raised in ankylosing spondylitis and undifferentiated spondyloarthropathy. Ann Rheum Dis 2003;62:455–9.
18. de Vries M, van der Horst-Bruinsma I, van Hoogstraten I, et al. pANCA, ASCA, and OmpC antibodies in patients with ankylosing spondylitis without inflammatory bowel disease. J Rheumatol 2010;37:2340–4.
19. Sartor RB. Mechanisms of disease: pathogenesis of Crohn's disease and ulcerative colitis. Nat Clin Pract Gastroenterol Hepatol 2006;3:390–407.
20. Ott SJ, Musfeldt M, Wenderoth DF, et al. Reduction in diversity of the colonic mucosa associated bacterial microflora in patients with active inflammatory bowel disease. Gut 2004;53:685–93.
21. Frank DN, St Amand AL, Feldman RA, et al. Molecular-phylogenetic characterization of microbial community imbalances in human inflammatory bowel diseases. Proc Natl Acad Sci U S A 2007;104:13780–5.
22. Friswell M, Campbell B, Rhodes J. The role of bacteria in the pathogenesis of inflammatory bowel disease. Gut Liver 2010;4:295–306.
23. Tannock GW. The bowel microbiota and inflammatory bowel diseases. Int J Inflam 2010;2010:954051.

24. Kang S, Denman SE, Morrison M, et al. Dysbiosis of fecal microbiota in Crohn's disease patients as revealed by a custom phylogenetic microarray. Inflamm Bowel Dis 2010;16:2034–42.
25. Frye M, Bargon J, Lembcke B, et al. Differential expression of human alpha- and beta-defensins mRNA in gastrointestinal epithelia. Eur J Clin Invest 2000;30:695–701.
26. Wehkamp J, Chu H, Shen B, et al. Paneth cell antimicrobial peptides: topographical distribution and quantification in human gastrointestinal tissues. FEBS Lett 2006;580:5344–50.
27. Wehkamp J, Salzman NH, Porter E, et al. Reduced Paneth cell alpha-defensins in ileal Crohn's disease. Proc Natl Acad Sci U S A 2005;102:18129–34.
28. Ciccia F, Bombardieri M, Rizzo A, et al. Over-expression of Paneth cell-derived anti-microbial peptides in the gut of patients with ankylosing spondylitis and subclinical intestinal inflammation. Rheumatology 2010;49:2076–83.
29. Cebra JJ, Periwal SB, Lee G, et al. Development and maintenance of the gut-associated lymphoid tissue (GALT): the roles of enteric bacteria and viruses. Dev Immunol 1998;6:13–8.
30. Glaister JR. Factors affecting the lymphoid cells in the small intestinal epithelium of the mouse. Int Arch Allergy Appl Immunol 1973;45:719–30.
31. Taurog JD, Richardson JA, Croft JT, et al. The germfree state prevents development of gut and joint inflammatory disease in HLA-B27 transgenic rats. J Exp Med 1994;180:2359–64.
32. Rosenbaum JT, Davey MP. Hypothesis: time for a gut check: HLA B27 predisposes to ankylosing spondylitis by altering the microbiome. Arthritis Rheum 2011;63(11):3195–8.
33. Benjamin R, Parham P. Guilt by association: HLA-B27 and ankylosing spondylitis. Immunol Today 1990;11:137–42.
34. Kollnberger S, Bird L, Sun MY, et al. Cell-surface expression and immune receptor recognition of HLA-B27 homodimers. Arthritis Rheum 2002;46:2972–82.
35. Granfors K. Do bacterial antigens cause reactive arthritis? Rheum Dis Clin North Am 1992;18:37–48.
36. Salmi M, Andrew DP, Butcher EC, et al. Dual binding capacity of mucosal immunoblasts to mucosal and synovial endothelium in humans: dissection of the molecular mechanisms. J Exp Med 1995;181:137–49.
37. Demetter P, De Vos M, Van Huysse JA, et al. Colon mucosa of patients both with spondyloarthritis and Crohn's disease is enriched with macrophages expressing the scavenger receptor CD163. Ann Rheum Dis 2005;64:321–4.
38. Baeten D, Demetter P, Cuvelier CA, et al. Macrophages expressing the scavenger receptor CD163: a link between immune alterations of the gut and synovial inflammation in spondyloarthropathy. J Pathol 2002;196:343–50.
39. Baeten D, Kruithof E, De Rycke L, et al. Infiltration of the synovial membrane with macrophage subsets and polymorphonuclear cells reflects global disease activity in spondyloarthropathy. Arthritis Res Ther 2005;7:R359–69.
40. Kontoyiannis D, Pasparakis M, Pizarro TT, et al. Impaired on/off regulation of TNF biosynthesis in mice lacking TNF AU-rich elements: implications for joint and gut-associated immunopathologies. Immunity 1999;10:387–98.
41. Armaka M, Apostolaki M, Jacques P, et al. Mesenchymal cell targeting by TNF as a common pathogenic principle in chronic inflammatory joint and intestinal diseases. J Exp Med 2008;205:331–7.
42. Roulis M, Armaka M, Manoloukos M, et al. Intestinal epithelial cells as producers but not targets of chronic TNF suffice to cause murine Crohn-like pathology. Proc Natl Acad Sci U S A 2011;108:5396–401.

43. Baeten D, Demetter P, Cuvelier C, et al. Comparative study of the synovial histology in rheumatoid arthritis, spondyloarthropathy, and osteoarthritis: influence of disease duration and activity. Ann Rheum Dis 2000;59:945–53.
44. Baeten D, Van Damme N, Van den Bosch F, et al. Impaired Th1 cytokine production in spondyloarthropathy is restored by anti-TNFalpha. Ann Rheum Dis 2001; 60:750–5.
45. Canete JD, Martinez SE, Farres J, et al. Differential Th1/Th2 cytokine patterns in chronic arthritis: interferon gamma is highly expressed in synovium of rheumatoid arthritis compared with seronegative spondyloarthropathies. Ann Rheum Dis 2000;59:263–8.
46. Johansson-Lindbom B, Agace WW. Generation of gut-homing T cells and their localization to the small intestinal mucosa. Immunol Rev 2007;215:226–42.
47. Cepek KL, Shaw SK, Parker CM, et al. Adhesion between epithelial cells and T lymphocytes mediated by E-cadherin and the alpha E beta 7 integrin. Nature 1994;372:190–3.
48. Feagan BG, Greenberg GR, Wild G, et al. Treatment of active Crohn's disease with MLN0002, a humanized antibody to the alpha4beta7 integrin. Clin Gastroenterol Hepatol 2008;6:1370–7.
49. Feagan BG, Greenberg GR, Wild G, et al. Treatment of ulcerative colitis with a humanized antibody to the alpha4beta7 integrin. N Engl J Med 2005;352: 2499–507.
50. Picarella D, Hurlbut P, Rottman J, et al. Monoclonal antibodies specific for beta 7 integrin and mucosal addressin cell adhesion molecule-1 (MAdCAM-1) reduce inflammation in the colon of scid mice reconstituted with CD45RBhigh CD4+ T cells. J Immunol 1997;158:2099–106.
51. Elewaut D, Van Damme N, De Keyser F, et al. Altered expression of alpha E beta 7 integrin on intra-epithelial and lamina propria lymphocytes in patients with Crohn's disease. Acta Gastroenterol Belg 1998;61:288–94.
52. Salmi M, Jalkanen S. Human leukocyte subpopulations from inflamed gut bind to joint vasculature using distinct sets of adhesion molecules. J Immunol 2001;166: 4650–7.
53. Elewaut D, De Keyser F, Van Den Bosch F, et al. Enrichment of T cells carrying beta7 integrins in inflamed synovial tissue from patients with early spondyloarthropathy, compared to rheumatoid arthritis. J Rheumatol 1998;25:1932–7.
54. Austrup F, Rebstock S, Kilshaw PJ, et al. Transforming growth factor-beta 1-induced expression of the mucosa-related integrin alpha E on lymphocytes is not associated with mucosa-specific homing. Eur J Immunol 1995;25:1487–91.
55. Brew R, West DC, Burthem J, et al. Expression of the human mucosal lymphocyte antigen, HML-1, by T cells activated with mitogen or specific antigen in vitro. Scand J Immunol 1995;41:553–62.
56. MacDonald JK, McDonald JW. Natalizumab for induction of remission in Crohn's disease. Cochrane Database Syst Rev 2007;(1):CD006097.
57. Parikh A, Leach T, Wyant T, et al. Vedolizumab for the treatment of active ulcerative colitis: a randomized controlled phase 2 dose-ranging study. Inflamm Bowel Dis 2012;18:1470–9.
58. Capon F, Di Meglio P, Szaub J, et al. Sequence variants in the genes for the interleukin-23 receptor (IL23R) and its ligand (IL12B) confer protection against psoriasis. Hum Genet 2007;122:201–6.
59. Duerr RH, Taylor KD, Brant SR, et al. A genome-wide association study identifies IL23R as an inflammatory bowel disease gene. Science 2006;314: 1461–3.

60. DeLay ML, Turner MJ, Klenk EI, et al. HLA-B27 misfolding and the unfolded protein response augment interleukin-23 production and are associated with Th17 activation in transgenic rats. Arthritis Rheum 2009;60:2633–43.
61. Ciccia F, Bombardieri M, Principato A, et al. Overexpression of interleukin-23, but not interleukin-17, as an immunologic signature of subclinical intestinal inflammation in ankylosing spondylitis. Arthritis Rheum 2009;60:955–65.
62. Melis L, Vandooren B, Kruithof E, et al. Systemic levels of IL-23 are strongly associated with disease activity in rheumatoid arthritis but not spondyloarthritis. Ann Rheum Dis 2010;69(3):618–23.
63. Sherlock JP, Joyce-Shaikh B, Turner SP, et al. IL-23 induces spondyloarthropathy by acting on ROR-γt+ CD3+CD4−CD8− entheseal resident T cells. Nat Med 2012;18:1069–76.
64. Appel H, Maier R, Wu P, et al. Analysis of IL-17+ cells in facet joints of patients with spondyloarthritis suggests that the innate immune pathway might be of greater relevance than the Th17-mediated adaptive immune response. Arthritis Res Ther 2011;13:R95.
65. Cella M, Fuchs A, Vermi W, et al. A human natural killer cell subset provides an innate source of IL-22 for mucosal immunity. Nature 2009;457:722–5.
66. Wu L, Van Kaer L. Natural killer T cells and autoimmune disease. Curr Mol Med 2009;9:4–14.
67. Wing K, Sakaguchi S. Regulatory T cells exert checks and balances on self tolerance and autoimmunity. Nat Immunol 2010;11:7–13.
68. von Boehmer H. Mechanisms of suppression by suppressor T cells. Nat Immunol 2005;6:338–44.
69. Maul J, Loddenkemper C, Mundt P, et al. Peripheral and intestinal regulatory CD4+ CD25(high) T cells in inflammatory bowel disease. Gastroenterology 2005;128:1868–78.
70. Saruta M, Yu QT, Fleshner PR, et al. Characterization of FOXP3+CD4+ regulatory T cells in Crohn's disease. Clin Immunol 2007;125:281–90.
71. Boschetti G, Nancey S, Sardi F, et al. Therapy with anti-TNFalpha antibody enhances number and function of Foxp3(+) regulatory T cells in inflammatory bowel diseases. Inflamm Bowel Dis 2011;17:160–70.
72. Di Sabatino A, Biancheri P, Piconese S, et al. Peripheral regulatory T cells and serum transforming growth factor-beta: relationship with clinical response to infliximab in Crohn's disease. Inflamm Bowel Dis 2010;16:1891–7.
73. Cao D, van Vollenhoven R, Klareskog L, et al. CD25brightCD4+ regulatory T cells are enriched in inflamed joints of patients with chronic rheumatic disease. Arthritis Res Ther 2004;6:R335–46.
74. Appel H, Wu P, Scheer R, et al. Synovial and peripheral blood CD4+FoxP3+ T cells in spondyloarthritis. J Rheumatol 2011;38:2445–51.
75. Ciccia F, Accardo-Palumbo A, Giardina A, et al. Expansion of intestinal CD4+CD25(high) Treg cells in patients with ankylosing spondylitis: a putative role for interleukin-10 in preventing intestinal Th17 response. Arthritis Rheum 2010;62:3625–34.
76. Jacques P, Venken K, Van Beneden K, et al. Invariant natural killer T cells are natural regulators of murine spondylarthritis. Arthritis Rheum 2010;62:988–99.
77. Van Praet L, Van den Bosch F, Mielants H, et al. Mucosal inflammation in spondylarthritides: past, present, and future. Curr Rheumatol Rep 2011;13:409–15.
78. Elewaut D, Matucci-Cerinic M. Treatment of ankylosing spondylitis and extra-articular manifestations in everyday rheumatology practice. Rheumatology 2009;48:1029–35.

79. Braun J, van den Berg R, Baraliakos X, et al. 2010 update of the ASAS/EULAR recommendations for the management of ankylosing spondylitis. Ann Rheum Dis 2011;70:896–904.
80. Danese S. New therapies for inflammatory bowel disease: from the bench to the bedside. Gut 2012;61:918–32.
81. Certolizumab pegol in subjects with active axial spondyloarthritis. 2012. Available at: ClinicalTrials.gov[online].
82. Sieper J, Porter-Brown B, Thompson L, et al. Tocilizumab (TCZ) is not effective for the treatment of ankylosing spondylitis (AS): results of a phase 2, international, multicentre, randomised, double-blind, placebo-controlled trial. Ann Rheum Dis 2012;71(Suppl 3):110.
83. Ustekinumab for the Treatment of Patients with Active Ankylosing Spondylitis (TOPAS). 2012. Available at: ClinicalTrials.gov[online].
84. Song IH, Heldmann F, Rudwaleit M, et al. Treatment of active ankylosing spondylitis with abatacept: an open-label, 24-week pilot study. Ann Rheum Dis 2011;70:1108–10.
85. Lekpa FK, Farrenq V, Canoui-Poitrine F, et al. Lack of efficacy of abatacept in axial spondylarthropathies refractory to tumor-necrosis-factor inhibition. Joint Bone Spine 2012;79:47–50.
86. Song IH, Heldmann F, Rudwaleit M, et al. Different response to rituximab in tumor necrosis factor blocker-naive patients with active ankylosing spondylitis and in patients in whom tumor necrosis factor blockers have failed: a twenty-four-week clinical trial. Arthritis Rheum 2010;62:1290–7.
87. Baraliakos X, Braun J, Laurent DD, et al. Interleukin-17A blockade with secukinumab reduces spinal inflammation in patients with ankylosing spondylitis as early as week 6, as detected by magnetic resonance imaging. Arthritis Rheum 2011;63:2486D.

Therapy for Spondyloarthritis

The Role of Extra-articular Manifestations (Eye, Skin)

Philippe Carron, MD, Liesbet Van Praet, MD,
Peggy Jacques, MD, PhD, Dirk Elewaut, MD, PhD,
Filip Van den Bosch, MD, PhD*

KEYWORDS

• Therapy • Spondyloarthritis • Extra-articular manifestations • Psoriasis • Uveitis

KEY POINTS

- IBD, psoriasis and uveitis are typical spondyloarthritis concept-related extra-articular manifestations.
- Although frequently prescribed, limited evidence-based data on the efficacy of conventional DMARDS such as sulphasalazine, methotrexate and cyclosporin on extra-articular manifestations are available.
- Besides the well-established beneficial effects on rheumatological manifestations, biologics targeting TNF-alpha also have an impact on the extra-articular manifestations with a potential more profound efficacy of monoclonal antibodies versus soluble receptor constructs.

INTRODUCTION

Spondyloarthritis (SpA) can be considered one of the prototypes (besides rheumatoid arthritis) of an inflammatory rheumatic disease. The locomotor system is, of course, prominently involved with arthritis, enthesitis, dactylitis, sacroiliitis, and/or axial disease; but besides the rheumatologic component, other body systems are frequently affected. The authors' consider extra-articular manifestations all the medical conditions and symptoms that are not directly related to the locomotor system. SpA is now classified according to its predominant presenting symptom, which can be axial (encompassing forms with clear-cut radiographic involvement previously named ankylosing spondylitis [AS] as well as nonradiographic forms) or peripheral (arthritis associated with inflammatory bowel disease, some forms of psoriatic arthritis, and reactive

Department of Rheumatology, Ghent University Hospital, De Pintelaan 185, Ghent 9000, Belgium
* Corresponding author.
E-mail address: filip.vandenbosch@ugent.be

Rheum Dis Clin N Am 38 (2012) 583–600
http://dx.doi.org/10.1016/j.rdc.2012.08.017 **rheumatic.theclinics.com**

arthritis). In SpA, extra-articular manifestations can be divided in 2 groups: those related to the SpA concept, such as involvement of the skin, eye, gut, or urogenital system, and those more reflecting chronic, longstanding inflammation, which involve the heart, lung, kidney, and nerves.[1] The concept-related manifestations are relatively frequent (20%–60%), can occur at any moment of the disease evolution (sometimes as the first manifestation), and can sometimes be related to axial or peripheral joint inflammation.[2] Many studies have found higher incidences of extra-articular manifestations to be a consequence of uncontrolled systemic inflammation.[3] Besides inflammatory bowel diseases, such as Crohn disease and ulcerative colitis, which is dealt by Jacques P and colleagues, with in a separate article in this issue, the major concept-related extra-articular manifestations are located in the eye (acute anterior uveitis) and the skin (psoriasis). This review focuses on the possible implications of these nonrheumatologic manifestations with regard to the treatment of SpA.

ACUTE ANTERIOR UVEITIS

Acute anterior uveitis (AAU) is the most common form of uveitis, with an annual incidence rate of about 8 cases per 100 000 population.[4] Although anterior uveitis is usually the most easily managed form of uveitis, recurrences may result in severe visual loss. The disease primarily affects only the anterior chamber of the eye. A typical attack has a sudden onset and is unilateral (but in subsequent attacks the other eye may be involved); local redness, pain, photophobia, and reduced vision are the cardinal symptoms. An attack usually lasts up to 6 to 12 weeks. In most cases, local treatment is sufficient; however, relapses are frequent. Prolonged, uncontrolled anterior uveitis can extend into the posterior part of the eye with the formation of synechiae and secondary glaucoma. From an ophthalmologic point of view, it can be a significant cause of vision loss.[5,6] AAU is a prominent manifestation of spondyloarthritides with a strong link with human leukocyte antigens (HLA) B27, occurring in 30% to 40% of patients with AS. About 50% of patients with AAU as an initial presentation have or will develop a form of SpA. Power and colleagues[7] found that patients who are HLA-B27 positive have a more severe clinical course with a significantly higher rate of recurrent inflammatory attacks and, hence, a higher incidence of ocular complications, supporting the need for more aggressive therapeutic strategies. Banares and colleagues[8] also described a relationship between anterior uveitis and bowel inflammation (in 60% of patients with AS-related uveitis), with a close relation between the recurrence of uveitis and the presence of chronic intestinal inflammation.

PSORIASIS

Psoriasis is a chronic, autoimmune, inflammatory skin disorder affecting about 2% of the Caucasian population.[9] In Europe, it is estimated to affect 5.1 million people. The most common form of psoriasis is plaque psoriasis, which occurs in approximately 80% of all patients with psoriasis. Some patients with psoriasis develop a specific form of inflammatory arthritis termed *psoriatic arthritis* (PsA), which is characterized by chronic inflammation of the joints, entheses, and spine. Although previously considered to be a relatively mild form of arthritis, there has been growing appreciation that PsA can be destructive and deforming with an indolent and progressive course.[10–12] The exact prevalence of PsA in patients with psoriasis is unknown. Reported prevalences vary depending on the population studied and the method of assessment, but the true estimate is likely around 30%.[13,14] The skin and nail lesions in SpA are largely identical to isolated skin disease (mostly plaque psoriasis); but the lesions are sometimes localized on more atypical localizations, such as the palms of hands and feet (palmoplantar pustulosis). There are no data supporting a parallelism between the activity of psoriasis and the locomotor inflammation.

TREATMENT: GENERAL PRINCIPLES

The individual treatment of patients with SpA is extremely challenging because of the heterogeneous character of the diseases that are part of this family of interrelated conditions. Not only is there a different therapeutic approach depending on whether the main presenting rheumatologic manifestation is back pain, arthritis, enthesitis, or dactylitis but also the presence and the extent of extra-articular manifestations significantly influences the therapeutic decisions in an individual patient. Recently, the 2010 update of the Assessment of Spondyloarthritis International Society/European League Against Rheumatism (ASAS/EULAR) recommendations for the management of AS was published.[15] As with other guidelines, they introduced the concept of overarching principles, stating that AS is a potentially severe disease with diverse manifestations, usually requiring multidisciplinary treatment coordinated by the rheumatologist, with the primary goal of maximization of long-term health-related quality of life through the control of symptoms and inflammation, prevention of progressive structural damage, and the preservation/normalization of function and social participation. It is explicitly stated that the treatment should be tailored according to the current manifestations of the disease (axial, peripheral, entheseal, and extra-articular symptoms and signs) as well as the level of current symptoms, clinical findings, and prognostic indicators.

The optimal management requires a combination of nonpharmacologic treatment modalities, such as patient education and regular exercise, and pharmacologic therapy. Nonsteroidal antiinflammatory drugs (NSAIDs) are recommended as the first-line drug treatment for patients with pain and stiffness. Corticosteroid injections can be directed to the local site of musculoskeletal inflammation, but the use of systemic glucocorticoids for axial disease is not supported by evidence. Likewise, there is no evidence for the efficacy of disease-modifying antirheumatic drugs (DMARDs), including sulfasalazine and methotrexate, for the treatment of axial disease, but sulfasalazine may be considered in patients with peripheral arthritis. Although again not supported by evidence, most rheumatologists will also try methotrexate in predominant peripheral spondyloarthritis. Finally, anti–tumor necrosis factor (TNF) therapy should be given to patients with persistently high disease activity despite conventional treatments. With regard to axial and articular/entheseal disease manifestations, there is no evidence for a significant difference in efficacy of the various available TNF inhibitors (infliximab, etanercept, adalimumab, golimumab). However, a specific recommendation is reserved for extra-articular manifestations and comorbidities; these frequently observed conditions, such as psoriasis, uveitis, and inflammatory bowel disease, should be managed in collaboration with the respective specialists. In these cases, a differential efficacy of the available conventional and biologic treatment modalities may play an important role. In this article, the authors review the relevance of extra-articular manifestations for therapeutic decisions, with a specific focus on the eye and the skin.

EFFICACY OF SPA TREATMENTS ON PSORIASIS

Conventional Treatments

Traditional systemic treatment of psoriasis with methotrexate, retinoids, and cyclosporine has been in use for more than 20 years and still represents the first-line systemic treatment in Europe for patients with psoriasis who cannot be controlled with topical agents or phototherapy. Because of the important psoriasis burden on patient life, there is evidence of an increasing use of systemic agents in psoriasis over the past 10 years when compared with previous years.[16] There is a high level of heterogeneity regarding the practical daily life use of conventional systemic treatments in psoriasis. Despite the fact that only a few prospective, randomized, placebo-controlled studies of the conventional systemic agents exist, recommendations have been generated to guide physicians on the best use of traditional agents in psoriasis.[17] The authors present here an overview of the efficacy of the most commonly used treatments of SpA or PsA on psoriasis.

Nonsteroidal antiinflammatory drugs

Evidently, NSAIDs do not play a role in the treatment of skin or nail psoriasis. Drugs, such as indomethacin and ibuprofen, have occasionally been reported to exacerbate psoriasis, although additional well-controlled studies are still needed.[18,19] Because psoriasis is a very complex disease and its activity is often unpredictable, clinical studies of adverse drug effects on psoriasis have been difficult to conduct.

Sulfasalazine

Evidence for the efficacy of sulfasalazine on skin psoriasis is scarce, as it was only evaluated in a small prospective, randomized, double-blind, placebo-controlled study.[20] Twenty-three patients received active treatment (ranging from 1.5–4.0 g of daily sulfasalazine), and 6 patients discontinued because of the side effects. In the remaining 17 patients, 7 had marked (60%–89%) change and another 7 had moderate (30%–59%) improvement. The placebo arm (n = 27) had only one subject who showed moderate improvement, whereas the rest of the group had only minimal improvement or worsening of psoriasis.

Methotrexate

Dermatologists were among the first to embrace methotrexate as an antiinflammatory/immune-modulating agent, with Edmunson and Guy[21] reporting its efficacy in the treatment of psoriasis in 1958. One of the earliest studies with methotrexate, in 50 patients, reported more than 50% improvement in psoriasis in 82% of patients.[22] It has since been claimed that greater than 90% clearance could be achieved in 30% to 50% of patients treated aggressively with methotrexate.[23] There are no randomized placebo-controlled trials evaluating methotrexate in patients with plaque psoriasis. Three well-designed active-comparator studies that evaluated the efficacy of methotrexate were performed in the last decade.[24–26] Heydendael and colleagues[24] compared methotrexate with cyclosporine in moderate to severe chronic plaque psoriasis; in this trial, at 16 weeks of treatment, there was no significant advantage of one drug over the other with a psoriasis area and severity (PASI) 75 response in 60% versus 71% for methotrexate and cyclosporine, respectively. Saurat and colleagues[26] performed a double-blind placebo-controlled study of methotrexate, designed to compare the safety and efficacy of adalimumab, methotrexate, and placebo in 250 patients. After 16 weeks of treatment, PASI 75 improvement was 19% for placebo, 36% for methotrexate, and 80% for adalimumab. For those patients in the methotrexate arm of the study, methotrexate was initiated at a low weekly dosage of 7.5 mg for 2 weeks, followed by 10 mg weekly for 2 weeks, and then 15 mg for 4 weeks. Thereafter, an increase in the dosage of methotrexate was permitted depending on the response and the presence or absence of toxicity. After 8 weeks, if patients in the methotrexate arm had achieved a PASI 50 response, no further increase in the methotrexate dosage was allowed. Methotrexate seems as effective as maintenance therapy in plaque psoriasis.

Cyclosporine

Cyclosporine is a highly effective and rapidly acting systemic agent belonging to the family of immunosuppressant drugs known as calcineurin inhibitors. The original observation that cyclosporine is an effective therapy for psoriasis was the consequence of an investigation for the treatment of arthritis. Four patients in the study group had PsA; in these patients, the high doses of cyclosporine in use at that time cleared the patients of psoriasis within 2 weeks of therapy initiation. Indeed, it was this and subsequent observations in the 1980s that provided added evidence that psoriasis is a T-cell-mediated dermatosis.[27–29] The only placebo-controlled analysis of cyclosporine enrolled 85 adult patients with moderate to severe psoriasis into 3 dosing arms (3.0, 5.0, and 7.5 mg/kg daily); a fourth group received placebo.[30] Efficacy was measured after 8 weeks and quantified the patients becoming "clear or almost clear." The analysis by intention to treat showed that cyclosporine improved psoriasis in a dose-dependent manner, with clear or almost clear results achieved by 36% in the cyclosporine 3.0 mg/kg daily group, 65% in the 5.0 mg/kg daily group, 80% in the 7.5 mg/kg daily group, and 0% in the placebo group. These results were statistically significant. Multiple other studies added to the evidence that cyclosporine given at a dosage of 3 mg/kg daily for 12 to 16 weeks leads to rapid and dramatic improvement in psoriasis with a PASI 75 response in 50% to 70% of patients and even a PASI 90 response in 30% to 50% of cases.[31–34] Because of concerns of organ (renal) toxicity, cyclosporine is used mainly in short-term (12 weeks) intermittent courses.

Leflunomide

Leflunomide has demonstrated some usefulness in treating cutaneous psoriasis. One published prospective, multicenter, randomized, double-blind, placebo-controlled study showed mild efficacy for the treatment of psoriasis.[35] In this study, 182 adult patients with psoriasis and PsA were randomized to either placebo or leflunomide given as 20 mg daily for 6 consecutive months. Patients had a baseline body surface area of psoriasis involvement that was greater than 3% and were allowed low-dose systemic corticosteroids (about 15% of the leflunomide-treated group). After 24 weeks of treatment, 17% of the leflunomide-treated patients achieved a PASI 75 versus 8% receiving placebo ($P = .048$).

Although larger, prospective, well-powered, placebo-controlled studies would be useful to provide further evidence-based information on conventional treatments in psoriasis, it can be concluded from the current available literature that methotrexate is effective and well tolerated in appropriately selected patients who are adequately monitored for potential toxicities. Cyclosporine suffers from dose-related nephrotoxicity and hypertension that impede its use as a long-term agent for most patients. Given this restriction, cyclosporine is an effective drug for rapid clearing in most patients, serving as an excellent bridging agent that can be used safely for periods of 2 to 12 months. Sulfasalazine and leflunomide have poor evidence substantiating their use as monotherapy in plaque psoriasis.[36]

Biologics

As mentioned, conventional systemic therapies for psoriasis are not effective in all patients and they may be associated with toxicities that can limit their long-term use. In recent years, biologic therapies have offered new, exciting treatment options with improved safety and efficacy for the treatment of psoriasis. The biologic therapies used in psoriasis are defined by their mode of action and can be classified into 3 categories: T-cell modulating agents (alefacept, efalizumab), agents that block TNF-alpha, and inhibitors of interleukin (IL)12/23 (ustekinumab). In clinical trials, the toxicity of biologicals has usually been mild to moderate, although severe side effects have been described. The use of a biological may be considered when patients cannot tolerate or are unresponsive to conventional systemic therapy.

T-cell modulating therapy

In 2003, alefacept and efalizumab were the first biologic agents to be approved by the Food and Drug Administration for the treatment of psoriasis. In the European Union, only efalizumab was approved for the treatment of moderate to severe plaque psoriasis. Efalizumab is a monoclonal antibody binding to the human CD11a subunit in leukocyte function antigen-1 (LFA-1), thereby blocking the binding of LFA-1 to intracellular adhesion molecule-1; this causes loss of activation, adhesion, and migration of T cells. In 2009, efalizumab was withdrawn from the market because of 3 cases of progressive multifocal leukoencephalopathy described in patients on long-term (>3 years) therapy. Alefacept, a recombinant dimeric fusion protein, is made up of the terminal portion of leukocyte function antigen-3 (LFA-3), blocking the signal between LFA-3 on antigen-presenting cells and the CD2 molecule on T cells. As a consequence, the activation and proliferation of T lymphocytes is inhibited. Using a weekly dosage of 15 mg administered intramuscularly, PASI 75 scores at week 12 were found to range between 21% and 35%.[37] In a PsA study, alefacept in combination with methotrexate was shown to improve arthritis significantly, with 54% ACR 20 responders compared with 23% in the methotrexate-alone group ($P<.001$).[38] However, in November 2011, Astellas Pharma voluntarily withdrew alefacept from the market for business reasons.

TNF-blocking agents

The potential importance of TNF in the pathophysiology of psoriasis is underscored by the observation that there are elevated levels of this cytokine in both the affected skin and serum of patients with psoriasis. These elevated levels have a significant correlation with psoriasis severity as measured by the PASI score, and a reduction to normal levels is observed after successful treatment with TNF-blocking agents. Currently, the 4 anti-TNF agents available for the treatment of signs and symptoms of AS are also indicated for PsA,[39–42] with a fifth agent, certolizumab, for which preliminary results of a phase III study were recently reported.[43] Of these agents, 3 (infliximab, adalimumab, and etanercept) were formally evaluated in phase III psoriasis studies,[44–46] leading to their indication for the treatment of moderate to severe psoriasis. Results of the skin responses (PASI 75) in the pivotal phase III studies on psoriasis and PsA (secondary end point) as well as the American College of Rheumatology (ACR) 20 response in PsA are summarized for the 5 different anti-TNF agents in **Table 1**.

Table 1
Efficacy of anti-TNF agents on psoriasis (PASI 75 response)

	Psoriasis Trials		PsA Trials		
TNF-blocker	**Dose**	**PASI 75 (%)**	**Dose**	**PASI 75 (%)**	**ACR 20 (%)**
Etanercept	25 mg biw	34 (wk 12)	25 mg biw	26 (wk 12)	73
	50 mg biw	49 (wk 12)	—	—	—
Infliximab	5 mg/kg	80 (wk 10)	5 mg/kg	64 (wk 14)	58
Adalimumab	40 mg q2w	71 (wk 16)	40 mg q2w	49 (wk 12)	58
Golimumab	—	—	50 mg q4w	40 (wk 14)	51
Certolizumab	—	—	200 mg q2w	47 (wk 12)	58

Despite the fact that there are no head-to-head comparisons for any of the TNF-blockers, remarkable similarities are observed in the percentage of patients that experience at least a PASI 75 response when exposed to a monoclonal antibody targeting TNF. With the etanercept dosage classically used in rheumatology (50 mg SC [subcutaneously] weekly), a lower percentage of PASI 75 responders were observed both in the pivotal psoriasis and PsA trials. For all anti-TNF agents, the percentage of patients with at least a 75% improvement of the PASI score continues to improve with longer treatment (with a plateau usually being reached at week 24). Infliximab (chimeric) and adalimumab (fully human) are 2 monoclonal antibodies that bind specifically to soluble and membrane-bound TNF. They are currently approved for the treatment of psoriasis. Infliximab is administered intravenously at a dosage of 5 mg/kg at weeks 0, 2, and 6 and then every 8 weeks.[44] Patients are less likely to develop antibodies against infliximab if they are continuously treated rather than on an as-needed basis; also, clinical responses are better maintained with continuous compared with intermittent therapy.[47] Infliximab is remarkable for the rapidity of clinical response. However, loss of efficacy may occur over time. Some dermatologists prescribe low-dose methotrexate concurrently with the goal of decreasing the formation of antibodies against infliximab and, hence, maintaining clinical efficacy over time. The dosing regimen for adalimumab in psoriasis is slightly different from the conventional dosage used in rheumatologic indications and consists of 80 mg given subcutaneously the first week, followed by 40 mg given the next week, and then every 2 weeks thereafter.[45] Rebound does not typically occur when adalimumab is discontinued; however, skin clearance is better maintained with continuous use. Etanercept is a recombinant human TNF-alpha receptor (p75) protein fused with the Fc portion of immunoglobulin G1 (IgG1). The dosing of etanercept differs in psoriasis compared with its other indications. The approved regimen is 50 mg given subcutaneously twice weekly for the first 12 weeks followed by 50 mg weekly thereafter.[46] Dosing is continuous. Some patients showed a loss of clinical response after 12 weeks when the dose was reduced from 50 mg twice weekly to 50 mg once weekly. Contrary to rheumatoid and PsA whereby TNF inhibitors, including etanercept, are often used in combination with methotrexate, all clinical studies in psoriasis have been performed with etanercept as a monotherapy. Continuous and interrupted etanercept therapy was effective, with greater improvements observed in the continuous arm at week 24. Most patients regained their response after the reinitiation of etanercept.[48]

Ustekinumab

IL-12 and IL-23 have important roles in the pathophysiology of psoriasis. Ustekinumab is a human monoclonal antibody with high affinity for the p40 subunit of IL-12 and IL-23. The drug is indicated for the treatment of psoriasis. Two large, double-blind, placebo-controlled, phase III studies (Phoenix 1 and 2) in patients with moderate to severe psoriasis were conducted in parallel in the United States and Europe.[49,50] The primary outcome in both studies was PASI 75 at week 12. Combining the results of both studies (including almost 2000 patients with psoriasis), a PASI 75 response at week 12 was observed in 66.7% of the ustekinumab 45-mg group (administered subcutaneously at week 0 and 4), 75.7% of the ustekinumab 90-mg dosage group, and only 3.7% of the placebo group ($P<.0001$ for both ustekinumab groups vs placebo). Ustekinumab is currently the only drug for which a randomized, active-controlled, parallel, 3-arm study (ACCEPT [Active Comparator (CNTO1275/Enbrel) Psoriasis Trial] trial) was performed; ustekinumab 45 and 90 mg, respectively, was compared with etanercept 50 mg twice weekly.[51] PASI 75 at week 12 was achieved by 56.8% of patients in the etanercept group compared with 67.5% (P =.012) and 73.8% (P<.001) in the ustekinumab 45- and 90-mg group, respectively.

Based on a successful phase II, double-blind, randomized, placebo-controlled study of ustekinumab in patients with active PsA (42.1% of patients in the active treatment group experienced an ACR 20 response at week 12 compared with only 14.3% in the placebo-dosed cohort),[52] a large phase III study was designed for which preliminary results were recently reported at the EULAR 2012 meeting.[53] Patients with active PsA (n = 615) were randomized to ustekinumab 45 mg, 90 mg, or placebo at weeks 0, 4, and every 12 weeks thereafter. A significantly greater proportion of ustekinumab patients (42.4% and 49.5% for ustekinumab 45 and 90 mg, respectively) had ACR 20 response at week 24 compared with placebo (22.8%; P<.001). Enthesitis and dactylitis also improved significantly in the active treated group. Currently, the drug is also under investigation for the treatment of AS (Ustekinumab for the Treatment of Patients with Active Ankylosing Spondylitis, which is a 28-week, prospective, open-label, proof-of-concept study; ClinicalTrials.gov identifier: NCT01330901). Ustekinumab also induced a clinical response in patients with moderate to severe Crohn disease.[54]

EFFICACY OF SPA TREATMENTS ON OPHTHALMOLOGIC MANIFESTATIONS

Conventional Treatments

Patients with occasional flares of AAU usually respond well to local topical treatment with corticosteroids and cycloplegic agents, and systemic corticosteroids or immunosuppressive drugs are usually not necessary. However, there seems to be ophthalmologic consensus that in patients with 3 or more flares during a 1-year period or with recurrence of inflammation close to cessation of the topical therapy, further systemic treatment is indicated. Because of the low prevalence of uveitis, new systemic treatments have historically been integrated into practice as a result of their success in controlling other autoimmune inflammatory disorders and subsequent anecdotal evidence based on small case series published by uveitis specialists. Larger retrospective cohort studies and a few small clinical trials have added further evidence.

NSAIDs

NSAIDs are the cornerstone of pharmacologic treatment in patients with predominant axial involvement in SpA. Although most data on the use of NSAIDS, particularly aspirin, in ocular inflammation deal with postoperative inflammation prophylaxis, NSAIDs were also used (before the emergence of corticosteroids) in the treatment of uveitis.[55–58] In a retrospective analysis, Fiorelli and colleagues[59] report on the use of prophylactic oral NSAIDs in the prevention of recurrences of uveitis in patients with recurrent anterior uveitis: 59 patients with recurrent uveitis and a follow-up period of at least 1 year before and after beginning oral NSAID therapy (celecoxib: n = 30, diflunisal: n = 29) were included. The average number of relapses before systemic NSAID therapy was 2.84 per person-year follow-up; this declined to 0.53 while on NSAID therapy (P<.001). All patients remained in remission for an average of 18.22 months. The difference between the relapse rate while on celecoxib versus diflunisal therapy was not statistically significant; however, patients on celecoxib remained in remission longer than those on diflunisal (21.0 vs 15.34 months; P<.001). The selective cyclooxygenase-2 inhibitor celecoxib was much better tolerated when compared with the nonselective NSAID diflunisal. Although data from a randomized controlled trial would be required to further evaluate the efficacy of NSAIDs for the treatment of recurrent AAU, the data indicate that systemic NSAID therapy provides an intermediate step between corticosteroid therapy and long-term immunosuppressive agents.

Sulfasalazine

A possible effect of sulfasalazine in the prevention of recurrent attacks of SpA-associated uveitis was first suggested by Dougados and colleagues[60] in a retrospective study on 22 patients. When flares of AAU are frequent, 2 studies showed that sulfasalazine could diminish the number of recurrences. In an open, prospective study the number of uveitis flares diminished from 3.4 in the pretreatment year to 0.9 (P = .007): in 5 patients there were no flares during the year of treatment; only 1 patients (undifferentiated SpA) was considered a nonresponder.[61] In another study, 22 patients with AS were included if they had experienced at least 2 recurrent acute attacks of uveitis in the last year in combination with chronic intestinal inflammation determined by biopsy.[62] Patients were randomized to receive either sulfasalazine (n = 10) or no treatment (n = 12). Ileocolonoscopic evaluation with bowel biopsy was performed before treatment on all patients and in 8 patients on sulfasalazine and 9 patients in the control group at the end of the study. The duration of the study was 36 months in all patients. A statistically significant difference in favor of sulfasalazine was observed between the 2 groups regarding the number of recurrences (P = .016). In patients on sulfasalazine, new episodes of uveitis were also less severe. A higher incidence of chronic intestinal inflammation was observed at the end of the study in the control group (3 out of 8 for sulfasalazine vs 7 out of 9 for control), although this difference did not reach statistical significance.

Methotrexate

Severe uveitis that is determined to be chronic and noninfectious often requires the introduction of a corticosteroid-sparing immunomodulatory treatment to control inflammation and avoid undesirable complications associated with chronic use of high-dose corticosteroids.[63] Several immunomodulatory therapy classes are currently used to treat uveitis, including antimetabolites, calcineurin inhibitors, alkylating agents, and biologic drugs. In a retrospective cohort study on different forms of noninfectious ocular inflammatory disease, complete suppression of inflammation sustained for more than 28 days was achieved within 6 months after adding methotrexate in 55.6% of patients with anterior uveitis; corticosteroid-sparing success was achieved in 46.1% of patients.[64] A recent survey among uveitis specialists looked at practice patterns regarding the prescription of corticoid-sparing therapy.[65] Azathioprine was not prescribed because of a lack of effectiveness, whereas the main concern for cyclosporine and cyclophosphamide was safety/tolerability. In this survey, methotrexate was the most commonly used initial treatment of anterior, intermediate, and posterior/panuveitis (85%, 57%, and 37%) and the most preferred for anterior uveitis (55%).

Mycophenolate mofetil

In the survey mentioned earlier, mycophenolate mofetil (MMF), an immunosuppressive agent that was shown in a retrospective case series of 60 patients with noninfectious uveitis to be generally effective and well tolerated, was the most preferred systemic treatment option for intermediate and posterior/panuveitis. Control of intraocular inflammation was achieved in 43 out of 60 patients (72%) after 1 year of MMF treatment. The probability of discontinuing prednisolone was 40% after 5 years of therapy. Recurrences of uveitis occurred in 6 out of 21 patients after MMF discontinuation.[66]

Biologics

The advent of biologic agents targeting TNF-alpha has provoked a revolution in the treatment of spondyloarthritis. At this moment, 4 different anti-TNF agents are indicated for the treatment of signs and symptoms of AS and PsA: etanercept, which is a dimeric soluble form of the TNF-receptor, and infliximab, adalimumab, and golimumab, which are all anti-TNF monoclonal antibodies. At this moment, and despite the fact that no head-to-head comparisons are available, it seems that the efficacy of the different compounds in phase III clinical trials is comparable regarding both axial and peripheral/entheseal rheumatologic symptoms.[67–70] Despite the fact that it was not the primary aim of these studies to evaluate the efficacy of these biologics with regard to extra-articular manifestations, a meta-analysis of the different published trials allowed for an estimation of the occurrence of inflammatory bowel disease[71] and uveitis.[72] Data from 4 placebo-controlled trials and 3 open-label studies with anti-TNF agents were analyzed, providing a global database of 717 patients: a history of anterior uveitis was reported in 236 (32,9%). Follow-up data on the incidence of uveitis were available for 397 patients. Both etanercept and infliximab significantly reduced the incidence of uveitis flares compared with placebo (placebo: 15.6 per 100 patient-years; infliximab: 3.4 per 100 patient-years; etanercept: 7.9 per 100 patient-years; *P* = .01 TNF-inhibitors vs placebo). This statistical significance was stronger for infliximab (*P* = .005) than for etanercept (*P* = .05); however, the differences between both TNF-inhibitors did not reach statistical significance (*P* = .08). The flare rate for etanercept was confirmed in a larger analysis of all etanercept AS clinical trials: In double-blind placebo-controlled trials, the uveitis rate with etanercept was 8.6 compared with 19.3 per 100 patient-years in the placebo group (*P* = .03). In the double-blind active comparator study, uveitis rates were similar for etanercept and sulfasalazine. In the long-term extension studies (1136.9 patient-years) a rate of 12.0 events per 100 patient-years was found.[73]

However, over the past years, several case reports were published, linking the first attack of uveitis to the treatment of rheumatic diseases with TNF blockers; this seemed to be a particular problem with etanercept.[74,75] Guignard and colleagues[76] reported results from a retrospective study of 46 patients with anti-TNF treated SpA that experienced at least 1 flare of uveitis (13 etanercept, 33 infliximab or adalimumab). The number of uveitis flares per 100 patient-years before and during anti-TNF treatment was 51.8 versus 21.4 with all anti-TNF drugs (*P* = .03), 54.6 versus 58.5 with etanercept (*P* = .92), and 50.6 versus 6.8 with anti-TNF antibodies (*P* = .001). These results allowed the calculation of the number needed to treat, which was 2 for anti-TNF antibodies versus 125 for the TNF soluble receptor, meaning that treating 2 patients with an anti-TNF monoclonal antibody avoids one uveitis flare in one patient over 1 year; in this study, etanercept was not efficacious. Moreover, 2 patients who never had uveitis before anti-TNF developed uveitis while taking etanercept, raising the question of a paradoxic effect of etanercept on ophthalmologic manifestations of SpA. Galor and colleagues[77] reported on the effectiveness of etanercept and infliximab regarding the actual treatment of refractory inflammatory eye diseases; patients treated with infliximab had a significant decrease in uveitis recurrences after starting therapy compared with those treated with etanercept (59% vs 0%; *P* = .004). Coates and colleagues[78] described new-onset uveitis in 5 patients with previously asymptomatic AS (4 etanercept, 1 infliximab). In these cases, the presentation of uveitis was atypical for AS because all patients had involvement of both eyes concurrently. Moreover, 4 out of the 5 patients were women, which is in contrast with the typical demographic profile of AS, which has a male predominance. Finally, the severity (3 patients sustained permanent damage to their sight) and poor response to treatment was unusual, requiring discontinuation of the anti-TNF agent; in one patient, there was a recurrence of the uveitis on rechallenge with etanercept. In summary, until today 42 cases of inflammatory eye disease thought to be associated with the use of etanercept have been reported in the literature: 33 uveitis, 8 scleritis, 1 orbital myositis, concerning

Table 2
Pipeline therapeutic options for psoriasis, uveitis, and AS

Agent	Mode of Action	Psoriasis[81]	Uveitis[82]	AS
Adalimumab	Neutralization of TNFα activity			
Infliximab	Neutralization of TNFα activity			
Certolizumab pegol	Neutralization of TNFα activity			83
Golimumab	Neutralization of TNFα activity			
Etanercept	Neutralization of TNFα activity			
Ustekinumab	Blockade of IL-12/23			84
Briakinumab	Blockade of IL-12/23			
Brodalumab	Blockade of IL-17RA			
Secukinumab	Blockade of IL-17A			85
LY2439821	Blockade of IL-17A			
Fezakinumab	Blockade of IL-22			
AEB071	Protein kinase C inhibitor			
BMS-582.949	Mitogen-activated protein kinase inhibitor (p38)			
Lestaurtinib	Tyrosine kinase inhibitor			
Tofacitinib	JAK3 inhibitor			
ASP-015K	JAK3 inhibitor			
Apremilast	Phosphodiesterase 4 inhibitor			86
SRT2104	Sirtuine enzyme 1 activator			
SCH527123	Antagonist of CXCR1 and CXCR2			
AbGn-168	Antibody inducing apoptosis of late-stage activated T cells			
BT-061	CD4 specific antibody			
CF101	A3AR agonist			
VB-201	Oxidized phospholipid small molecule			
ACT128800	Oral S1P receptor agonist			
RWJ-445.380	Cathepsin S inhibitor			
Voclosporin	Calcineurin inhibitor	87		
Anakinra	IL-1R-inhibitor			
Tocilizumab	Blockade of IL-6R			88
Daclizumab	Blockade of IL-2R			

(*continued on next page*)

Table 2
(continued)

Agent	Mode of Action	Psoriasis[81]	Uveitis[82]	AS
Basiliximab	Blockade of IL-2R			
Rituximab	Anti-CD20 antibody			89
Abatacept	Inhibitor of costimulation of T cells			90,91

Positive outcome.

Potentially effective/ongoing trials.

Negative outcome.

No studies (clinicaltrials.gov August 11, 2012).

Abbreviation: JAK 3, Janus kinase 3.

16 patients with rheumatoid arthritis, 10 with juvenile idiopathic arthritis, 14 with ankylosing spondylitis, and 2 with psoriatic SpA. Dechallenge was performed in 28 patients, leading to the resolution of symptoms. Rechallenge was done in 6 cases, with clear exacerbation.[79] In an attempt to clarify this question, Lim and colleagues[80] analyzed 2 drug event databases in the United States and found that etanercept is indeed associated with a higher incidence of uveitis than adalimumab and infliximab. The investigators concluded that etanercept is less effective for the treatment and prevention of flares of uveitis but does not seem to induce uveitis; and if uveitis occurs under an etanercept regimen, it seems logical to switch to another TNF blocker. Recently, 2 other TNF-alpha inhibitors for systemic use (certolizumab and golimumab) were introduced to the market, but no experience in the treatment of uveitis is available yet. For the treatment of anterior uveitis, a new topical TNF blocker for topical use is under development (exploratory study on topical ESBA150 in acute anterior uveitis; ClinicalTrials.gov identifier: NCT00823173). Although this approach promises to avoid systemic side effects, complications, and inconveniences during application, its effectiveness cannot be evaluated at present.

New Therapeutic Targets

Despite the established, well-documented improvements regarding signs, symptoms, and overall quality of life as a consequence of (predominantly TNF-targeting) biologics, there is still room for improvement and (especially in the diseases belonging to the SpA concept) a need for a new mode of action drugs. Further exploration of the common genetic susceptibility and the immune mechanisms underlying inflammation in the joints, axial skeleton, eye, skin, and gut of patients with SpA may provide valuable clues leading to new therapeutic breakthroughs. **Table 2** summarizes therapeutic (pipeline) options currently available or in clinical development for psoriasis and uveitis, which may also become appropriate treatment targets in SpA.

Therapeutic Strategy in Case of Extra-articular Manifestations

With the more widespread use of traditional systemic treatments and the advent of biologic therapies (antibodies, receptors) targeting TNF, it is clear that rheumatologists now have a powerful armamentarium for the treatment of patients with spondyloarthritides. As stated in the recently updated ASAS/EULAR recommendations for the

Table 3
Summary of the efficacy of conventional and biologic treatments on rheumatologic and extra-articular manifestations

	Joint	Spine	Gut	Eye	Skin
NSAID	+	++	Flare*	(+)	Flare*
Sulfasalazine	+	-	+	+	?
Methotrexate	+ (PsA)	-	?	+	+
Cyclosporine	+ (PsA)	-	-	+	++
Anti-TNF MoAb	+++	+++	+++ (IFX, ADA)	+++	+++ (IFX, ADA)
Etanercept	+++	+++	-	+	++
Ustekinumab	++ (PsA)	?	+	?	+++

Abbreviations: ADA, adalimumab; IFX, infliximab; MoAB, monoclonal antibody; -, no efficacy; +, moderate efficacy; ++, good efficacy; +++, very good efficacy; ?, unknown.
* no randomised controlled trials.

management of AS, there is no evidence for a significant effect of traditional DMARDs or a difference in efficacy of the various TNF inhibitors on the rheumatologic manifestations of SpA. However, the presence of SpA-related extra-articular manifestations (eye, skin, gut) may provide a basis for a more rational choice of these systemic and biologic treatments. Based on the literature summarized in this article, the authors provide a global overview of the efficacy of these therapies on the different SpA manifestations in **Table 3**.

It seems self-evident that the management of these complex disorders in a multidisciplinary setting together with the respective specialist (gastroenterology, dermatology, ophthalmology) would be beneficial for the individual patient. There is now emerging evidence, at least in psoriasis and PsA, that this approach indeed results in better care.[92]

Better knowledge of the critical pathogenetic pathways underlying rheumatologic as well as extra-articular manifestations has helped to create new treatment approaches that interfere with specific molecules induced in the body during the inflammatory process. The use of biologic agents targeting TNF-alpha has provided a real-life proof of concept of this paradigm.

REFERENCES

1. Mielants H, Van den Bosch F. Extra-articular manifestations. Clin Exp Rheumatol 2009;27(4 Suppl 55):S56–61.
2. Vander Cruyssen B, Ribbens C, Boonen A, et al. The epidemiology of ankylosing spondylitis and the commencement of anti-TNF therapy in daily rheumatology practice. Ann Rheum Dis 2007;66:354–9.
3. Elewaut D, Matucci-Cerinic M. Treatment of ankylosing spondylitis and extra-articular manifestations in everyday rheumatology practice. Rheumatology 2009;48:1029–35.
4. Rothova A, van Veenedaal WG, Linssen A, et al. Clinical features of acute anterior uveitis. Am J Ophthalmol 1987;103:137–45.
5. Nussenblatt RB. The natural history of uveitis. Int Ophthalmol 1990;14:303–8.
6. Rothova A, Suttorp-van Schulten MS, Frits Treffers W, et al. Causes and frequency of blindness in patients with intraocular inflammatory disease. Br J Ophthalmol 1996;80(4):332–6.

7. Power WJ, Rodriguez A, Pedroza-Seres M, et al. Outcomes in anterior uveitis associated with the HLA-B27 haplotype. Ophthalmology 1998;105:1646–51.
8. Banares A, Jover JA, Fernandez B, et al. Bowel inflammation in anterior uveitis and spondyloarthropathy. J Rheumatol 1995;22:1112–7.
9. Schon MP, Boehncke WH. Psoriasis. N Engl J Med 2005;352(18):1899–912.
10. Brockbank J, Gladman D. Diagnosis and management of psoriatic arthritis. Drugs 2002;62(17):2447–57.
11. Zachariae H. Prevalence of joint disease in patients with psoriasis: implications for therapy. Am J Clin Dermatol 2003;4(7):441–7.
12. Mease P, Goffe BS. Diagnosis and treatment of psoriatic arthritis. J Am Acad Dermatol 2005;52(1):1–19.
13. Zachariae H, Zachariae R, Blomqvist K, et al. Quality of life and prevalence of arthritis reported by 5,795 members of the Nordic Psoriasis Associations. Data from the Nordic Quality of Life Study. Acta Derm Venereol 2002;82(2):108–13.
14. Gladman DD, Antoni C, Mease P, et al. Psoriatic arthritis: epidemiology, clinical features, course, and outcome. Ann Rheum Dis 2005;64(Suppl 2):ii14–7.
15. Braun J, van den Berg R, Baraliakos X, et al. 2010 update of the ASAS/EULAR recommendations for the management of ankylosing spondylitis. Ann Rheum Dis 2011;70:896–904.
16. Strowd LC, Yentzer BA, Fleischer AB Jr, et al. Increasing use of more potent treatments for psoriasis. J Am Acad Dermatol 2009;60:478–81.
17. Menter A, Korman NJ, Elmets CA, et al. Guidelines of care for the management of psoriasis and psoriatic arthritis: section 4. Guidelines of care for the management and treatment of psoriasis with traditional systemic agents. J Am Acad Dermatol 2009;61(3):451–85.
18. Abel EA, DiCicco LM, Orenberg EK, et al. Drugs in exacerbation of psoriasis. J Am Acad Dermatol 1986;15:1007–22.
19. Ben-Chetrit E, Rubinow A. Exacerbation of psoriasis by ibuprofen. Cutis 1986;38:45.
20. Gupta AK, Ellis CN, Siegel MT, et al. Sulfasalazine improves psoriasis: a double-blind analysis. Arch Dermatol 1990;126:487–93.
21. Edmunson WF, Guy WB. Treatment of psoriasis with folic acid antagonists. AMA Arch Derm 1958;78:200–3.
22. Nyfors A, Brodthagen H. Methotrexate for psoriasis in weekly oral doses without any adjunctive therapy. Dermatologica 1970;140:345–55.
23. Jeffes EW III, Weinstein GD. Methotrexate and other chemotherapeutic agents used to treat psoriasis. Dermatol Clin 1995;13:875–90.
24. Heydendael VM, Spuls P, Opmeer BC, et al. Methotrexate versus cyclosporine in moderate-to-severe chronic plaque psoriasis. N Engl J Med 2003;349:658–65.
25. Flytstrom I, Stenberg B, Svensson A, et al. Methotrexate versus cyclosporin in psoriasis: effectiveness, quality of life and safety. A randomized controlled trial. Br J Dermatol 2008;158:116–21.
26. Saurat JH, Stingl G, Dubertret L, et al. Efficacy and safety results from the randomized controlled comparative study of adalimumab vs methotrexate vs placebo in patients with psoriasis (CHAMPION). Br J Dermatol 2008;158:558–66.
27. Griffiths CE, Powles AV, Leonard JN, et al. Clearance of psoriasis with low dose cyclosporine. Br Med J (Clin Res Ed) 1986;293:731–2.
28. Ellis CN, Gorsulowsky DC, Hamilton TA, et al. Cyclosporine improves psoriasis in a double-blind study. JAMA 1986;256:3110–6.

29. Van Joost T, Bos JD, Heule F, et al. Low-dose cyclosporine A in severe psoriasis. A double-blind study. Br J Dermatol 1988;118:183–90.
30. Ellis CN, Fradin MS, Messana JM, et al. Cyclosporine for plaque-type psoriasis: results of a multidose, double-blind trial. N Engl J Med 1991;324:277–84.
31. Berth-Jones J, Henderson CA, Munro CS, et al. Treatment of psoriasis with intermittent short course cyclosporin (Neoral): a multicenter study. Br J Dermatol 1997;136:527–30.
32. Faerber L, Braeutigam M, Weidinger G, et al. Cyclosporine in severe psoriasis: results of a meta-analysis in 579 patients. Am J Clin Dermatol 2001;2:41–7.
33. Ho VC, Griffiths CE, Albrecht G, et al. Intermittent short courses of cyclosporine (Neoral) for psoriasis unresponsive to topical therapy: a 1-year multicenter, randomized study; the PISCES Study Group. Br J Dermatol 1999;141:283–91.
34. Ho VC, Griffiths CE, Berth-Jones J, et al. Intermittent short courses of cyclosporine microemulsion for the long-term management of psoriasis: a 2-year cohort study. J Am Acad Dermatol 2001;44:643–51.
35. Kaltwasser J, Nash P, Gladman D, et al. Efficacy and safety of leflunomide in the treatment of psoriatic arthritis and psoriasis: a multinational, double-blind, randomized, placebo-controlled clinical trial. Arthritis Rheum 2004;50:1939–50.
36. Paul C, Gallini A, Maza A, et al. Evidence-based recommendations on conventional systemic treatments in psoriasis: systematic review and expert opinion of a panel of dermatologists. J Eur Acad Dermatol Venereol 2011;25(Suppl 2):2–11.
37. Lebwohl M, Christophers E, Langley R, et al, Alefacept Clinical Study Group. An international, randomized, double-blind, placebo-controlled phase 3 trial of intramuscular alefacept in patients with chronic plaque psoriasis. Arch Dermatol 2003;139:719–27.
38. Mease PJ, Gladman DD, Keystone EC. Alefacept with methotrexate for the treatment of psoriatic arthritis: results from a double-blind, placebo-controlled study. Arthritis Rheum 2006;54:1638–45.
39. Mease PJ, Goffe BS, VanderStoep A, et al. Etanercept in the treatment of psoriatic arthritis and psoriasis: a randomised trial. Lancet 2000;356:385–90.
40. Antoni C, Krueger GG, de Vlam K, et al, IMPACT 2 Investigators. Infliximab improves signs and symptoms of psoriatic arthritis: results of the IMPACT 2 trial. Ann Rheum Dis 2005;64:1150–7.
41. Mease PJ, Gladman DD, Ritchlin CT, et al, Adalimumab Effectiveness in Psoriatic Arthritis Trial Study Group. Adalimumab for the treatment of patients with moderately to severely active psoriatic arthritis: results of a double-blind, randomized, placebo-controlled trial. Arthritis Rheum 2005;52:3279–89.
42. Kavanaugh A, McInnes I, Mease P, et al. Golimumab, a new human tumor necrosis factor alpha antibody, administered every four weeks as a subcutaneous injection in psoriatic arthritis: twenty-four-week efficacy and safety results of a randomized, placebo-controlled study. Arthritis Rheum 2009;60:976–86.
43. Mease PJ, Fleischmann R, Deodhar A, et al. Effect of certolizumab pegol on signs and symptoms in patients with psoriatic arthritis: 24-week results of a phase 3 double-blind, randomized, placebo-controlled study (RAPID-PSA). Ann Rheum Dis 2012;71(Suppl 3):150.
44. Chaudhari U, Romano P, Mulcahy LD, et al. Efficacy and safety of infliximab monotherapy for plaque-type psoriasis: a randomised trial. Lancet 2001;357:1842–7.
45. Menter A, Tyring SK, Gordon K, et al. Adalimumab therapy for moderate to severe psoriasis: a randomized, controlled phase III trial. J Am Acad Dermatol 2008;58:106–15.

46. Leonardi CL, Powers JL, Matheson RT, et al, Etanercept Psoriasis Study Group. Etanercept as monotherapy in patients with psoriasis. N Engl J Med 2003;349: 2014–22.
47. Menter A, Feldman SR, Weinstein GD, et al. A randomized comparison of continuous vs intermittent infliximab maintenance regimens over 1 year in the treatment of moderate-to-severe plaque psoriasis. J Am Acad Dermatol 2007; 56(31):e1–15.
48. Moore A, Gordon KB, Kang S, et al. A randomized, open-label trial of continuous versus interrupted etanercept therapy in the treatment of psoriasis. J Am Acad Dermatol 2007;56:598–603.
49. Leonardi CL, Kimball AB, Papp KA, et al. Efficacy and safety of ustekinumab, a human interleukin-12/23 monoclonal antibody, in patients with psoriasis: 76-week results from a randomised, double- blind, placebo-controlled trial (PHOENIX 1). Lancet 2008;371:1665–74.
50. Papp KA, Langley RG, Lebwohl M, et al. Efficacy and safety of ustekinumab, a human interleukin-12/23 monoclonal antibody, in patients with psoriasis: 52-week results from a randomised, double-blind, placebo-controlled trial (PHOENIX 2). Lancet 2008;371:1675–84.
51. Griffiths CE, Strober BE, van de Kerkhof P, et al. Comparison of ustekinumab and etanercept for moderate-to-severe psoriasis. N Engl J Med 2010;362: 118–28.
52. Gottlieb AB, Menter A, Mendelsohn A, et al. Ustekinumab, a human interleukin 12/23 monoclonal antibody, for psoriatic arthritis: randomised, double-blind, placebo-controlled, crossover trial. Lancet 2009;373:633–40.
53. McInnes IB, Kavanaugh A, Gottlieb AB, et al, on behalf of the PSUMMIT I Study Group. Ustekinumab in patients with active psoriatic arthritis: results of the phase 3 multicenter, double-blind, placebo-controlled PSUMMIT I study. Ann Rheum Dis 2012;71(Suppl 3):107.
54. Sandborn WJ, Feagan BG, Fedorak RN, et al, Ustekinumab Crohn's Disease Study Group. A randomized trial of ustekinumab, a human interleukin-12:23 monoclonal antibody, in patients with moderate-to-severe Crohn's disease. Gastroenterology 2008;135:1130–41.
55. Perkins ES, MacFaul PA. Indomethacin in the treatment of uveitis: a double blind trial. Trans Ophthalmol Soc UK 1965;85:53–8.
56. March W, Coniglione TC. Ibuprofen in the treatment of uveitis. Ann Ophthalmol 1985;17:103–4.
57. Hunter PJ, Fowler PD, Wilkinson P. Treatment of anterior uveitis: comparison of oral oxyphenbutazone and topical steroids. Br J Ophthalmol 1973;57:892–6.
58. Olson NY, Lindsley CB, Godfrey WA. Non-steroidal anti-inflammatory drug therapy in chronic childhood iridocyclitis. Am J Dis Child 1988;142:1289–92.
59. Fiorelli VM, Bhat P, Foster CS. Nonsteroidal anti-inflammatory therapy and recurrent acute anterior uveitis. Ocul Immunol Inflamm 2010;18(2):116–20.
60. Dougados M, Berenbaum F, Maetzel A, et al. Prevention of acute anterior uveitis associated with spondylarthropathy induced by salazosulfapyridine. Rev Rhum Ed Fr 1993;60:81–3.
61. Munoz-Fernandez S, Hidalgo V, Fernandez-Melon J, et al. Sulfasalazine reduces the number of flares of acute anterior uveitis over a one-year period. J Rheumatol 2003;30:1277–9.
62. Benitez-del-Castillo JM, Garcia-Sanchez J, Iradier R, et al. Sulfasalazine in the prevention of anterior uveitis associated with ankylosing spondylitis. Eye 2000; 14:340–3.

63. Jabs DA, Rosenbaum JT, Foster CS, et al. Guidelines for the use of immunosuppressive drugs in patients with ocular inflammatory disorders: recommendations of an expert panel. Am J Ophthalmol 2000;130(4):492–513.
64. Gangaputra A, Newcomb CW, Liesegang TL, et al, Systemic Immunosuppressive Therapy for Eye Diseases Cohort Study. Methotrexate for ocular inflammatory diseases. Ophthalmology 2009;116:2188–98.
65. Esterberg E, Acharya NR. Corticosteroid-sparing therapy: practice patterns among uveitis specialists. J Ophthalmic Inflamm Infect 2012;2:21–8.
66. Doycheva D, Zierhut M, Blumenstock G, et al. Long-term results of therapy with mycophenolate mofetil in chronic non-infectious uveitis. Graefes Arch Clin Exp Ophthalmol 2011;249(8):1235–43.
67. Davis JC, van der Heijde D, Braun J, et al, Enbrel AS Study Group. Recombinant human tumor necrosis factor receptor (etanercept) for treating ankylosing spondylitis: a randomized, controlled trial. Arthritis Rheum 2003;48:3230–6.
68. van der Heijde D, Dijkmans B, Geusens P, et al, ASSERT study group. Efficacy and safety of infliximab in patients with ankylosing spondylitis: results of a randomized, placebo-controlled trial. Arthritis Rheum 2005;52:582–91.
69. van der Heijde D, Kivitz A, Schiff MH, et al, ATLAS Study Group. Efficacy and safety of adalimumab in patients with ankylosing spondylitis: results of a multicenter, randomized, double-blind, placebo-controlled trial. Arthritis Rheum 2006;54:2136–46.
70. Inman RD, Davis JC, van der Heijde D, et al. Efficacy and safety of golimumab in patients with ankylosing spondylitis; results of a randomized, double-blind, placebo-controlled, phase III trial. Arthritis Rheum 2008;58:3402–12.
71. Braun J, Baraliakos X, Listing J, et al. Differences in the incidence of flares or new onset of inflammatory bowel disease in patients with ankylosing spondylitis exposed to therapy with anti-tumor necrosis factor alpha agents. Arthritis Rheum 2007;57:639–47.
72. Braun J, Baraliakos X, Listing J, et al. Decreased incidence of anterior uveitis in patients with ankylosing spondylitis treated with the anti-tumor necrosis factor agents infliximab and etanercept. Arthritis Rheum 2005;52:2447–51.
73. Sieper J, Koenig A, Baumgartner S, et al. Analysis of uveitis rates across all etanercept ankylosing spondylitis clinical trials. Ann Rheum Dis 2010;69:226–9.
74. Reddy AR, Backhouse OC. Does etanercept induce uveitis? Br J Ophthalmol 2003;87:925.
75. Taban M, Dupps WJ, Mandell B, et al. Etanercept (Enbrel)-associated inflammatory eye disease: case report and review of the literature. Ocul Immunol Inflamm 2006;14:145–50.
76. Guignard S, Gossec L, Salliot C, et al. Efficacy of tumour necrosis factor blockers in reducing uveitis flares in patients with spondylarthropathy: a retrospective study. Ann Rheum Dis 2006;65:1631–4.
77. Galor A, Perez VL, Hammel JP, et al. Differential effectiveness of etanercept and infliximab in the treatment of ocular inflammation. Ophthalmology 2006;113(12):2317–23.
78. Coates LC, McGonagle DG, Bennett AN, et al. Uveitis and tumour necrosis factor blockade in ankylosing spondylitis. Ann Rheum Dis 2008;67:729–30.
79. Gaujoux-Viala C, Giampietro C, Gaujoux T, et al. Scleritis: a paradoxical effect of etanercept? Etanercept-associated inflammatory eye disease. J Rheumatol 2012;39(2):233–9.
80. Lim LL, Fraunfelder FW, Rosenbaum JT. Do tumor necrosis factor inhibitors cause uveitis? A registry-based study. Arthritis Rheum 2007;56:3248–52.

81. Ryan C, Abramson A, Patel M, et al. Current investigational drugs in psoriasis. Expert Opin Investig Drugs 2012;21:473–87.
82. Gomes Bittencourt M, Sepah YJ, Do DV, et al. New treatment options for noninfectious uveitis. Dev Ophthalmol 2012;51:134–61.
83. Certolizumab pegol in subjects with active axial spondyloarthritis. Available at: ClinicalTrials.gov [Identifier: NCT01087762]. Accessed August 11, 2012.
84. Ustekinumab for the Treatment of Patients With Active Ankylosing Spondylitis (TOPAS). Available at: ClinicalTrials.gov [Identifier: NCT01330901]. Accessed August 11, 2012.
85. Baraliakos X, Braun J, Laurent DD, et al. Interleukin-17A blockade with secukinumab reduces spinal inflammation in patients with ankylosing spondylitis as early as week 6, as detected by magnetic resonance imaging. Arthritis Rheum 2011; 63:2486D.
86. Study of apremilast to treat subjects with active ankylosing spondylitis (POSTURE). Available at: ClinicalTrials.gov [Identifier: NCT01583374]. Accessed August 11, 2012.
87. Papp K, Bissonnette R, Rosoph L, et al. Efficacy of ISA247 in plaque psoriasis: a randomised, multicentre, double-blind, placebo-controlled phase III study. Lancet 2008;371:1337–42.
88. Sieper J, Porter-Brown B, Thompson L, et al. Tocilizumab (TCZ) is not effective for the treatment of ankylosing spondylitis (AS): results of a phase 2, international, multicentre, randomised, double-blind, placebo-controlled trial. Ann Rheum Dis 2012;71(Suppl 3):110.
89. Song IH, Heldmann F, Rudwaleit M, et al. Different response to rituximab in tumor necrosis factor blocker-naive patients with active ankylosing spondylitis and in patients in whom tumor necrosis factor blockers have failed: a twenty-four-week clinical trial. Arthritis Rheum 2010;62:1290–7.
90. Lekpa FK, Farrenq V, Canouï-Poitrine F, et al. Lack of efficacy of abatacept in axial spondyloarthropathies refractory to tumor-necrosis-factor inhibition. Joint Bone Spine 2012;79:47–50.
91. Song IH, Heldmann F, Rudwaleit M, et al. Treatment of active ankylosing spondylitis with abatacept: an open-label, 24-week pilot study. Ann Rheum Dis 2011;70: 1108–10.
92. Velez NF, Wei-Passanese EX, Husni ME, et al. Management of psoriasis and psoriatic arthritis in a combined dermatology and rheumatology clinic. Arch Dermatol Res 2012;304:7–13.

Therapeutic Controversies in Spondyloarthritis

Nonsteroidal Anti-Inflammatory Drugs

Denis Poddubnyy, MD[a,*], Désirée van der Heijde, MD[b]

KEYWORDS

- Spondyloarthritis • Ankylosing spondylitis • ASAS
- Nonsteroidal anti-inflammatory drugs • Therapy

KEY POINTS

- Nonsteroidal anti-inflammatory drugs (NSAIDs) represent a first-line therapy in axial spondyloarthritis, including ankylosing spondylitis.
- NSAIDs are highly effective in reduction of spondyloarthritis symptoms, including pain and stiffness.
- NSAIDs also reduce activity of systemic inflammation and might have a (small) impact on the activity of local inflammatory lesions in the sacroiliac joints and the spine.
- NSAIDs are able to reduce progression of structural damage in the spine if administered continuously, especially in patients who already have signs of structural damage (syndesmophytes) and elevated C-reactive protein and/or erythrocyte sedimentation rate.
- Cardiovascular, gastrointestinal, renal, and hepatic risks should be taken into account if an NSAID is administered, especially if a long-term and continuous treatment is anticipated.

INTRODUCTION

Nonsteroidal anti-inflammatory drugs (NSAIDs) are considered a first-line therapy in patients with axial spondyloarthritis (axSpA), including ankylosing spondylitis (AS).[1] Beyond NSAIDs, only tumor necrosis factor α (TNF-α) blockers are currently available and effective for treating axial signs and symptoms of patients with active axSpA.[1,2] In contrast to rheumatoid arthritis, for example, disease-modifying antirheumatic drugs and corticosteroids play only a minor role in the management of axSpA, and only in the case of peripheral joint involvement.[3,4] In the joint ASAS (Assessment of SpondyloArthritis international Society) and EULAR (European League Against Rheumatism) recommendations for the management of axSpA, continuous treatment with NSAIDs

Disclosures: Denis Poddubnyy has received consultancy and speaking fees from Merck; Désirée van der Heijde has received consultancy fees from Merck and Pfizer.
[a] Rheumatology, Medical Department I, Campus Benjamin Franklin, Charité Universitätsmedizin Berlin, Hindenburgdamm 30, Berlin 12203, Germany; [b] Department of Rheumatology, Leiden University Medical Center, PO Box 9600, 2300 RC Leiden, The Netherlands
* Corresponding author.
E-mail address: denis.poddubnyy@charite.de

Rheum Dis Clin N Am 38 (2012) 601–611
http://dx.doi.org/10.1016/j.rdc.2012.08.005 **rheumatic.theclinics.com**

is preferred for patients with persistently active symptomatic disease.[1] Continuous treatment with NSAIDs, however, raises safety issues. In a survey on the application of the ASAS/EULAR recommendations, 38% of European rheumatologists mentioned safety concerns as the main barrier for not using NSAIDs more consistently in patients with AS.[5]

This article discusses the current role of NSAIDs in axSpA treatment, including the risks and benefits of NSAID use and current trends for more individualized treatment strategies.

CLINICAL EFFICACY OF NSAIDS

So far, clinical trials with NSAIDs have only been performed in patients with established AS. However, based mainly on clinical experience, NSAIDs can be expected also to be highly effective in patients with nonradiographic axSpA (nr-axSpA), or those with axSpA who did not develop (yet) radiographic sacroiliitis. Thus, patients with nr-axSpA should be treated with NSAIDs similarly to those with AS.[6] Furthermore, NSAIDs also play an important role in the management of patients with predominant peripheral spondyloarthritis,[1,7] who show only a limited response to conventional disease-modifying antirheumatic drugs.[1]

High clinical efficacy of NSAIDs for treating axial signs and symptoms of active axSpA/AS was shown (against placebo and an active comparator) in several clinical trials with nonselective cyclooxygenase (COX) inhibitors and selective COX-2 antagonists.[8–11] All NSAIDs, independently from their COX selectivity, are nearly equally effective in their therapeutic doses for reducing pain and stiffness in axSpA/AS. Nonetheless, great individual variation exists in response to and tolerability of NSAIDs. In general, trying at least one NSAID, but frequently several others, is worthwhile in case one is found to be ineffective. This sampling is also frequently performed in clinical practice: more than 20% of 1080 patients with AS who participated in a survey on NSAID use in Germany reported that they used at least 2 different NSAIDs (5% used $\geq$3 NSAIDs) within the past year.[12]

Good or very good improvement of AS symptoms is usually reported by 60% to 80% of patients treated with NSAIDs.[7,8,11] In contrast, this level of response is only reported by approximately 15% of patients with chronic low back pain from noninflammatory causes.[7] Furthermore, a good response to NSAID treatment is also used as a diagnostic approach to differentiate chronic back pain of inflammatory origin from other causes.[7] Moreover, good pain control is necessary to perform physiotherapy effectively. Many clinical trials showed that reduction of pain and stiffness during NSAID therapy was associated with improvement of functional status in patients with AS measured using the Bath Ankylosing Spondylitis Functional Index.[8,11,13] Up to 35% of active patients with AS treated with a full dose of an NSAID can fulfill even the ASAS criteria for partial remission.[8,14] In a survey performed in Germany, almost 20% of the patients with AS reported complete pain control with NSAIDs, and another 60% of the patients reported a reduction in pain level from one-quarter to one-half.[12]

In most cases, NSAIDs reduce pain and stiffness rapidly, and a full effect can normally be observed after 48 to 72 hours. In some cases, a longer treatment period (up to 2 weeks) is necessary to achieve the complete anti-inflammatory and analgesic effect of an NSAID.[8] However, if a response is not experienced within 2 weeks, it is unlikely to occur with continued treatment.

To judge the therapeutic effect of an NSAID in a patient with axSpA/AS, a full therapeutic (inflammatory) dose is usually required. The dose and the intake frequency could be, however, adjusted based on the patient's symptom intensity. In some patients with AS, a moderate dose might be sufficient for long-term treatment, whereas in others the highest tolerated dose might be necessary to achieve an optimal effect. On the group level, a higher efficacy could be demonstrated in patients treated with a higher dose of celecoxib (400 vs 200 mg/d),[11] etoricoxib (120 vs 90 mg/d),[8] or meloxicam (22.5 vs 15 mg/d)[9] compared with a lower dose.

Recently, the ASAS developed a recommendation for collecting, analyzing, and reporting NSAID intake in clinical trials and/or epidemiologic studies in axSpA.[15] An index of NSAID intake was proposed, taking both dose and duration into account (**Box 1**). This index includes an NSAID equivalent score, which represents a standardized dose of an NSAID taken. Daily diclofenac dose of 150 mg (maximal recommended dose for treatment of arthritis) was accepted by consensus as a reference value, with the equivalent score of 100.[15] Equivalent doses of other widely used NSAIDs are presented in **Table 1**. Daily doses of NSAIDs presented in table can be considered as full therapeutic doses for treatment of axSpA/AS.

INFLUENCE OF NSAIDS ON LOCAL AND SYSTEMIC INFLAMMATION IN axSpA

The high clinical efficacy of NSAIDs in axSpA indicates that their anti-inflammatory properties are more relevant for reducing pain and stiffness in this disease than their analgesic capacity only. However, the data indicating effective control of systemic and local inflammation with NSAIDs are limited.

C-reactive protein (CRP) is a sensitive marker of systemic inflammation, and an elevated level of CRP could be found in approximately 50% of the patients with axSpA.[16] Elevated serum CRP level was found recently to be an independent predictor of radiographic sacroiliitis progression (including progression from nr-axSpA to AS)[17] and of progression of structural damage in the spine.[18] NSAIDs are able to decrease CRP serum level significantly already after 12 weeks of treatment, as shown in 2 recent studies in AS.[10,11]

Even more clinically appealing might be a reduction of local inflammation in the sacroiliac joints and spine. However, until now no solid data showed whether NSAIDs influence active inflammation in the axial skeleton as detected on MRI. **Fig. 1** represents a case of near-complete resolution of active sacroiliitis after 2 weeks of treatment with a full dose of an NSAID for active axSpA. In the study by Jarrett and colleagues,[19] 22 patients who were eligible for the biologic therapy (ie, who did not respond to previous therapy with NSAIDs) were treated with 90 mg of etoricoxib for 6 weeks. Not surprisingly, this group of patients also showed no substantial improvement on MRI; only 13 of 60 active inflammatory lesions in the axial skeleton improved, whereas 5 lesions worsened or appeared during treatment.

Box 1
Formula for calculating the ASAS index of NSAID intake

$$\text{Index of NSAID intake} = \text{NSAID equivalent score} \times \frac{\text{Days of intake during period of interest} \times \text{Days per week}}{\text{Period of interest in days}}$$

Example: patient took diclofenac, 75 mg every day over the last 4 weeks that was also a period of interest. Index of NSAID intake = 50 (equivalent score for 75 mg of diclofenac every day) × 28 (4 weeks of intake) × 7/7 (the NSAID was taken daily)/28 (period of interest) = 50.

Data from Dougados M, Simon P, Braun J, et al. ASAS recommendations for collecting, analysing and reporting NSAID intake in clinical trials/epidemiological studies in axial spondyloarthritis. Ann Rheum Dis 2011;70(2):249–51.

Table 1
Daily doses of NSAIDs equivalent to diclofenac 150 mg/d (NSAID equivalent score = 100)

NSAID	Dose Therapeutically Equivalent to 150 mg of Diclofenac (Full Therapeutic Dose) in AS (mg)
Aceclofenac[a]	200
Celecoxib	400
Etodolac	600
Etoricoxib[a]	90
Flurbiprofen	200
Ibuprofen	2400
Indomethacin	150
Ketoprofen	200
Meloxicam	15
Naproxen	1000
Nimesulide[b]	200
Phenylbutazone[c]	400
Piroxicam	20
Tenoxicam[a]	20

[a] Currently not available in the United States.
[b] Not available in the United States, limited available in the European Union for short-term (up to 2 weeks) treatment of acute pain and primary dysmenorrhoea.
[c] Not available in the United States, limited available in the European Union for short-term (up to 1 week) treatment.
Data from Dougados M, Simon P, Braun J, et al. ASAS recommendations for collecting, analysing and reporting NSAID intake in clinical trials/epidemiologic studies in axial spondyloarthritis. Ann Rheum Dis 2011;70(2):249–51.

Important data concerning the influence of NSAIDs on active inflammation were obtained in the recent infliximab as first line therapy in patients with early active axial spondyloarthritis trial (INFAST). In this study, patients with very early axSpA (symptom duration not longer than 3 years) were randomized to either naproxen plus infliximab or naproxen alone. Combination therapy with a TNF-α blocker and an NSAID was clearly superior to an NSAID alone; partial remission after 28 weeks of treatment was achieved in 62% of the patients in the combination arm, but was also observed in

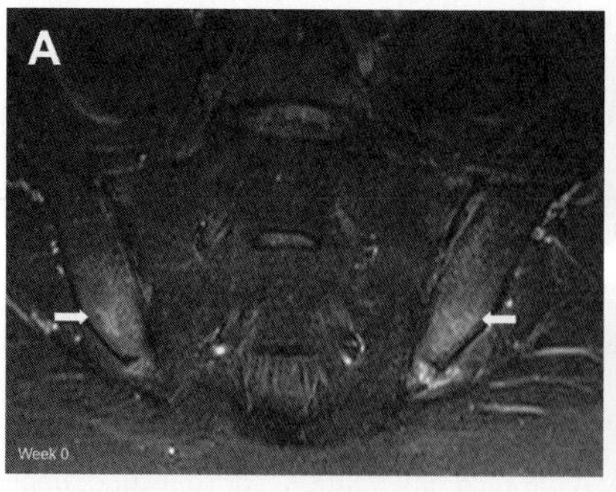

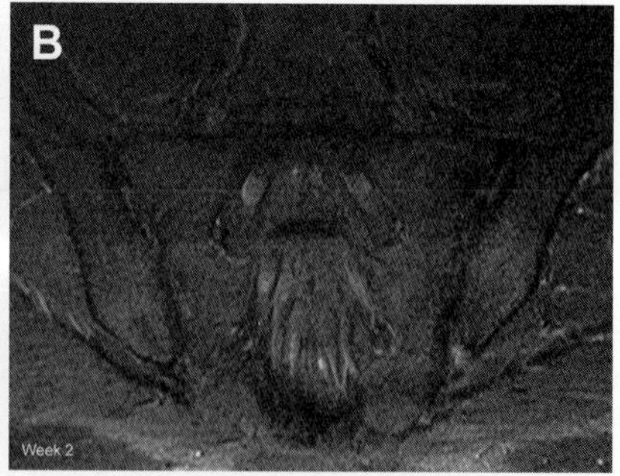

Fig. 1. MRI of sacroiliac joints in STIR sequence before (*A*) and 2 weeks after (*B*) treatment with a full dose of an NSAID. Near-complete resolution of active inflammation (*arrows*) is seen after 2 weeks.

a substantial proportion of patients (35%) in the naproxen alone arm. Complete absence of active inflammatory lesions in the sacroiliac joints was observed at week 28 in 5.9% of the patients treated with naproxen (compared with 27.6% in the naproxen plus infliximab group), whereas no patients in this arm (18.1% in the combined arm) were free of inflammation in both spine and sacroiliac joints.[14] However, because this study had no placebo arm, whether the resolution of the inflammation in the sacroiliac joints was a result of the naproxen use or the natural course of the disease is unclear.

These data indicate clearly that, although NSAIDs might have some influence on active inflammation in the axial skeleton, inflammation (in axial skeleton or systemic) might persist even when there is absence or good control of symptoms. Whether this asymptomatic inflammation, indicated by elevated serum CRP or osteitis on MRI, has clinical relevance is currently unclear. Current treatment recommendations rely mainly on symptoms,[1,2] and therefore no treatment modification is generally recommended for patients who respond well to NSAIDs but still have some signs of systemic or local inflammation.

INFLUENCE OF NSAIDS ON RADIOGRAPHIC SPINAL PROGRESSION IN AXSPA/AS

The high efficacy of NSAIDs in reducing clinical symptoms, and to some extent reducing signs of systemic inflammation (CRP), raises the question whether NSAIDs are only symptomatically effective or whether they might have an additional effect on the long-term outcome of axSpA/AS.

Radiographic spinal progression, which is mostly related to the process of new bone formation, or the development of syndesmophytes leading to the bony ankylosis of the spine (**Fig. 2**), seems to be an important determinant of long-term outcome in axSpA. Currently available data indicate a clear (although nonlinear) association

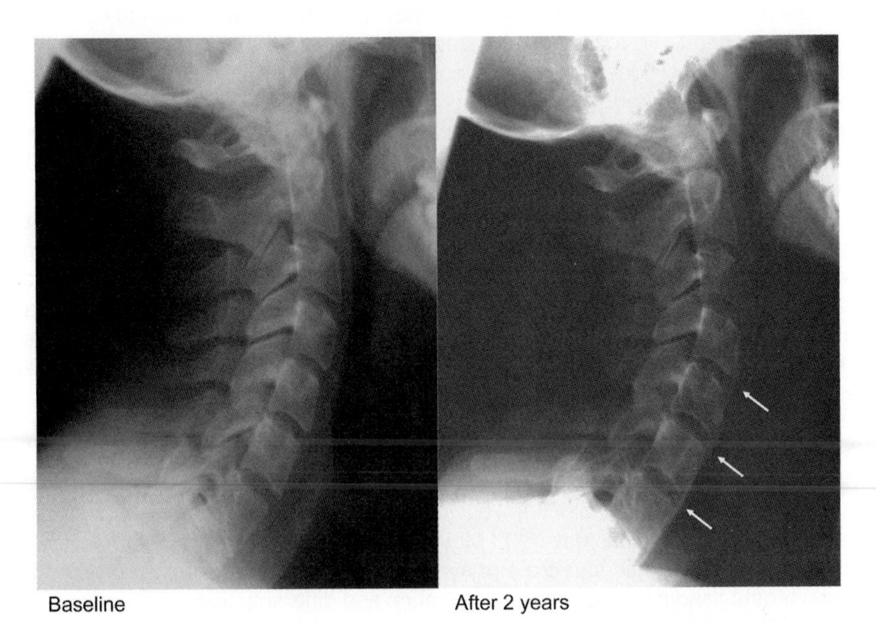

Fig. 2. Radiographs of the cervical spine in a lateral view of a patient with AS performed 2 years apart, showing a very quick radiographic progression with development of several new bridging syndesmophytes (*arrows*) over 2 years.

between radiographic damage in the spine and impaired spinal mobility[20,21] and reduction of physical function.[21,22] Therefore, retardation of radiographic spinal progression represents a logical treatment target in axSpA.

Years ago, Boersma[23] showed that continuous use of phenylbutazone was associated with retardation of spinal ossification in AS. In a more recent study by Wanders and colleagues,[24] continuous (daily) use of NSAIDs (all starting with celecoxib but changing to other NSAIDs in cases of clinical inefficacy or intolerance) was also associated with an inhibition of radiographic progression in the spine over 2 years compared with on-demand use. The most recent data from the German Spondyloarthritis Inception Cohort supports these findings. High NSAID intake (NSAID intake index $\geq$50) over 2 years was associated with lower radiographic spinal progression compared with low NSAID intake (NSAID intake index $<$50) in patients with AS. In nr-axSpA, no significant differences in radiographic progression were seen between patients with high and low NSAID intake, which was most likely related to the low level of spinal damage in general in this group.

Retardation of radiographic spinal progression during NSAID therapy was nearly exclusively seen in patients with risk factors for this progression (presence of syndesmophytes at baseline and elevated CRP). Radiographic spinal progression rate as assessed by a mean worsening of the modified Stoke Ankylosing Spondylitis Spinal Score (mSASSS)[25] over 2 years was 4.36 $\pm$ 4.53 in patients with low NSAID intake versus 0.14 $\pm$ 1.80 in those with high intake (P = .02).[26] The recent post hoc analysis[27] of the data from the study by Wanders and colleagues confirmed these findings. An inhibitory effect of continuous NSAID use was observed in patients with elevated acute-phase reactants (CRP or erythrocyte sedimentation rate [ESR]) only. For instance, in the subgroup of patients with elevated time-averaged CRP, the mean mSASSS progression over 2 years was 1.7 $\pm$ 2.8 in those with on-demand NSAID intake versus 0.2 $\pm$ 1.6 in those with continuous NSAID intake (P = .003), whereas in the subgroup with normal CRP, no difference in a mean mSASSS change was seen (0.8 $\pm$ 1.1 vs 0.9 $\pm$ 1.8, respectively, for the on-demand and continuous arms; P = .62). Similarly, a difference between on-demand and continuous arms in terms of percentages of patients who showed radiographic spinal progression (defined as an mSASSS worsening by at least 2 units over 2 years) was seen exclusively in the subgroups with elevated acute-phase reactants (CRP or ESR); in the patients with elevated CRP, the percentages of progressors were 38% versus 13%, respectively (P = .011).[27]

Defining the patient type that would benefit from continuous treatment at most is necessary for the development of individualized treatment strategies for axSpA. However, clinical indications for NSAID therapy defined by the level of pain and stiffness currently have clear priority over radiographic indications. Practically, this means that the need for NSAID treatment should be justified based on symptom levels, whereas risk factors for radiographic progression (such as syndesmophytes or elevated acute-phase reactants) play a secondary role. The mechanism of NSAID inhibition of radiographic spinal progression in AS is not fully understood. However, this effect clearly cannot be attributable only to the anti-inflammatory properties of NSAIDs, because the most potent anti-inflammatory drugs currently available for the treatment of AS (TNF-α blockers) have failed to slow radiographic spinal progression over 2 years in clinical trials.[28–30] Most likely, NSAIDs inhibit new bone formation in the spine (morphologic substrate of syndesmophytes and ankylosis) through preventing prostaglandin E2–dependent replication and differentiation of osteoblasts[31,32] and inhibiting prostaglandin-dependent angiogenesis, which is required for osteogenesis.[33] Because retardation of new bone formation is related to COX-2 inhibition, no substantial differences are expected between various NSAIDs, because in therapeutic concentrations, all NSAIDs, independent of their COX selectivity, inhibit COX-2 to nearly the same extent.[34]

Given the good anti-inflammatory capacity of TNF blockers in AS but their failure to stop new bone formation, a trial combining a TNF blocker and an NSAID would be of interest to determine whether this combination could inhibit new bone formation, in addition to suppressing inflammation and improving signs and symptoms. This clinical question is also important to answer because it will determine whether patients at risk for radiographic progression should be advised to continue the use of NSAIDs when they are no longer necessary for symptom modification.

SAFETY OF NSAIDS AND RISK/BENEFIT ESTIMATION OF NSAID THERAPY IN SPA

Serious safety concerns are always raised when long-term NSAID treatment is discussed. Several safety aspects are related to NSAID treatment, such as gastrointestinal, cardiovascular, renal, hepatic, and allergic reactions. The most common and clinically relevant are the first 2, which are discussed further.

Gastrointestinal toxicity is a well-known adverse effect during NSAID treatment, which is related mainly to inhibition of prostaglandin synthesis in the gastric mucosa. The most important aspect of the gastrointestinal toxicity is gastroduodenal ulceration and development of ulcer complications, such as gastrointestinal bleeding, perforation, and gastric outlet obstruction. Three large trials comparing COX-2–selective with nonselective NSAIDs showed a rate of serious gastrointestinal events (symptomatic gastroduodenal ulcers and ulcer complications) of 0.67 to 1.85 per 100 patient-years for COX-2–selective inhibitors and 0.97 to 3.21 per 100 patient years for nonselective NSAIDs.[35–37] At the same time, the rate of complications only (without symptomatic ulcers) was approximately 1 or less per 100 patient years for both COX-2–selective and nonselective NSAIDs.[35–37]

The risk of gastrointestinal adverse events is strongly dependent on the presence of risk factors, and therefore it can be recommended that patients be stratified according to gastrointestinal risk before NSAIDs are administered, and overall risk be reevaluated in case of a risk profile change. The following risk factors should be taken into account: previous gastrointestinal events, especially if complicated; age; concomitant use of anticoagulants, corticosteroids, and other NSAIDs, including low-dose aspirin and high-dose NSAID therapy; chronic debilitating disorders, especially cardiovascular disease; and *Helicobacter pylori* infection (a potential advantage exists to testing for *H pylori* infection and eradicating the infection if positive in patients requiring long-term NSAID therapy, especially those with a history of ulcers).[38]

The American College of Gastroenterology recently recommended the following patient stratification system according to risk of NSAID gastrointestinal toxicity[38]:

1. High risk
   a. History of a previously complicated ulcer, especially recent
   b. Multiple (>2) risk factors
2. Moderate risk
   a. Age >65 years
   b. High-dose NSAID therapy
   c. A previous history of uncomplicated ulcer
   d. Concurrent use of aspirin (including low-dose), corticosteroids, or anticoagulants
3. Low risk
   a. No risk factors

Prevention of NSAID gastrointestinal toxicity includes use of gastroprotectors (proton pump inhibitors or misoprostol), use of selective COX-2 inhibitors instead of nonselective ones, and eradication of *H pylori* infection.[38,39] To define an appropriate method of prevention, cardiovascular risk should be also taken into account.

Current evidence suggests that both selective COX-2 inhibitors (coxibs) and nonselective NSAIDs, with the possible exception of full-dose naproxen, increase cardiovascular risk. This effect was clearly shown in a meta-analysis of randomized trials by Kearney and colleagues[40] and confirmed later in a large population-based study from Denmark[41] and the most recent meta-analysis by Trelle and colleagues.[42] Furthermore, no difference seems to exist between coxibs (at least for those that are currently marketed, celecoxib and etoricoxib) and nonselective NSAIDs in their influence on cardiovascular risk.[43,44]

Obviously, the individual cardiovascular risk depends on numerous well-known traditional cardiovascular risk factors, such as smoking, diabetes, age, previous cardiovascular events, and NSAID dose used. Large clinical trials showed that rates of cardiovascular events were especially low in younger patients and those with low baseline cardiovascular risk (less than 1 event per 100 patient years).[44,45] This finding is especially relevant for the current discussion, because SpA is a disease of young people starting normally in the third decade of life.

As suggested by the American College of Gastroenterology, nonselective NSAIDs can be administered safely in patients with low cardiovascular risk (who do not take low-dose aspirin) and low gastrointestinal risk. A selective COX-2 inhibitor or a combination of a nonselective NSAID with a gastroprotector should be used in patients with moderate gastrointestinal risk, and an alternative therapy or, if not possible, the combination of a coxib and a gastroprotector should be considered in patients with high gastrointestinal risk.[38]

In patients with high cardiovascular risk (defined as a need for low-dose aspirin intake) and low or moderate gastrointestinal risk, the combination of naproxen with gastroprotective agents is recommended. If both cardiovascular and gastrointestinal risks are high, NSAIDs should be generally avoided and an alternative therapy should be considered.[38]

Most of the data concerning NSAID safety originate from clinical trials including patients with rheumatoid arthritis or osteoarthritis. Nonetheless, in the 3 available long-term NSAID trials in patients with AS ($\geq$1 year), no toxicity signals different from those discussed earlier were reported and the incidences of adverse events or discontinuations from adverse events did not differ significantly within treatment groups or between treatment and placebo groups.[8,9,24]

In the recent observational study from Norway, frequent use of NSAIDs in AS was clearly associated with decreased overall mortality.[46] These data require confirmation, but it could be speculated that anti-inflammatory effects of NSAIDs, reflected by the decrease in the serum CRP level, might counterbalance the increase of the cardiovascular risk in AS related to systemic inflammation and the NSAID treatment itself.[47]

Thus, taking into account the relative young age and the low comorbidity in patients with AS, serious adverse events can be expected to occur in approximately 1% or fewer per year if patients are treated with a full dose of an NSAID. An NSAID should be selected according to its expected benefit in a given patient and according to the patient's risk profile to help achieve a favorable benefit/risk ratio.[47]

SUMMARY

NSAIDs are highly effective in reducing symptoms of axSpA, including AS, and therefore considered a first-line therapy in this disease. NSAIDs might have an impact on radiographic spinal progression in AS if administered continuously. The greatest effect on radiographic progression is expected in patients with syndesmophytes who have an elevated CRP. However, the primary goal of treatment in patients with AS should be to eliminate symptoms, whereas retardation of radiographic progression represents a secondary goal of treatment, although relevant for the long-term outcome. Careful assessment of the cardiovascular, gastrointestinal, renal, and hepatic risk profile is required before administering an NSAID, especially if a long-term and continuous treatment is expected. Regular reassessment of the risks in patients treated with continuous NSAIDs is recommended.

REFERENCES

1. Braun J, van den Berg R, Baraliakos X, et al. 2010 update of the ASAS/EULAR recommendations for the management of ankylosing spondylitis. Ann Rheum Dis 2011;70(6):896–904.
2. van der Heijde D, Sieper J, Maksymowych WP, et al. 2010 update of the international ASAS recommendations for the use of anti-TNF agents in patients with axial spondyloarthritis. Ann Rheum Dis 2011;70(6):905–8.
3. Haibel H, Rudwaleit M, Braun J, et al. Six months open label trial of leflunomide in active ankylosing spondylitis. Ann Rheum Dis 2005;64(1):124–6.
4. Haibel H, Brandt HC, Song IH, et al. No efficacy of subcutaneous methotrexate in active ankylosing spondylitis: a 16-week open-label trial. Ann Rheum Dis 2007;66(3):419–21.
5. Gossec L, Dougados M, Phillips C, et al. Dissemination and evaluation of the ASAS/EULAR recommendations for the management of ankylosing spondylitis: results of a study among 1507 rheumatologists. Ann Rheum Dis 2008;67(6):782–8.
6. Braun A, Saracbasi E, Grifka J, et al. Identifying patients with axial spondyloarthritis in primary care: how useful are items indicative of inflammatory back pain? Ann Rheum Dis 2011;70(10):1782–7.
7. Amor B, Dougados M, Listrat V, et al. Are classification criteria for spondylarthropathy useful as diagnostic criteria? Rev Rhum Engl Ed 1995;62(1):10–5.
8. van der Heijde D, Baraf HS, Ramos-Remus C, et al. Evaluation of the efficacy of etoricoxib in ankylosing spondylitis: results of a fifty-two-week, randomized, controlled study. Arthritis Rheum 2005;52(4):1205–15.
9. Dougados M, Gueguen A, Nakache JP, et al. Ankylosing spondylitis: what is the optimum duration of a clinical study? A one year versus a 6 weeks non-steroidal anti-inflammatory drug trial. Rheumatology (Oxford) 1999;38(3):235–44.
10. Barkhuizen A, Steinfeld S, Robbins J, et al. Celecoxib is efficacious and well tolerated in treating signs and symptoms of ankylosing spondylitis. J Rheumatol 2006;33(9):1805–12.
11. Sieper J, Klopsch T, Richter M, et al. Comparison of two different dosages of celecoxib with diclofenac for the treatment of active ankylosing spondylitis: results of a 12-week randomised, double-blind, controlled study. Ann Rheum Dis 2008;67(3):323–9.
12. Zochling J, Bohl-Buhler MH, Baraliakos X, et al. Nonsteroidal anti-inflammatory drug use in ankylosing spondylitis–a population-based survey. Clin Rheumatol 2006;25(6):794–800.
13. Gossec L, van der Heijde D, Melian A, et al. Efficacy of cyclo-oxygenase-2 inhibition by etoricoxib and naproxen on the axial manifestations of ankylosing spondylitis in the presence of peripheral arthritis. Ann Rheum Dis 2005;64(11):1563–7.

14. Sieper J, Lenaerts J, Wollenhaupt J, et al. Double-blind, placebo-controlled, 28-week trial of efficacy and safety of infliximab plus naproxen vs naproxen alone in patients with early, active axial spondyloarthritis treated with a submaximal dose of NSAIDs: preliminary results of INFAST Part I. Ann Rheum Dis 2012; 71(Suppl 3):247.
15. Dougados M, Simon P, Braun J, et al. ASAS recommendations for collecting, analysing and reporting NSAID intake in clinical trials/epidemiological studies in axial spondyloarthritis. Ann Rheum Dis 2011;70(2):249–51.
16. Poddubnyy DA, Rudwaleit M, Listing J, et al. Comparison of a high sensitivity and standard C reactive protein measurement in patients with ankylosing spondylitis and non-radiographic axial spondyloarthritis. Ann Rheum Dis 2010;69(7):1338–41.
17. Poddubnyy D, Rudwaleit M, Haibel H, et al. Rates and predictors of radiographic sacroiliitis progression over 2 years in patients with axial spondyloarthritis. Ann Rheum Dis 2011;70(8):1369–74.
18. Poddubnyy D, Haibel H, Listing J, et al. Baseline radiographic damage, elevated acute-phase reactant levels, and cigarette smoking status predict spinal radiographic progression in early axial spondylarthritis. Arthritis Rheum 2012;64(5):1388–98.
19. Jarrett SJ, Sivera F, Cawkwell LS, et al. MRI and clinical findings in patients with ankylosing spondylitis eligible for anti-tumour necrosis factor therapy after a short course of etoricoxib. Ann Rheum Dis 2009;68(9):1466–9.
20. Wanders A, Landewe R, Dougados M, et al. Association between radiographic damage of the spine and spinal mobility for individual patients with ankylosing spondylitis: can assessment of spinal mobility be a proxy for radiographic evaluation? Ann Rheum Dis 2005;64(7):988–94.
21. Machado P, Landewe R, Braun J, et al. Both structural damage and inflammation of the spine contribute to impairment of spinal mobility in patients with ankylosing spondylitis. Ann Rheum Dis 2010;69(8):1465–70.
22. Landewe R, Dougados M, Mielants H, et al. Physical function in ankylosing spondylitis is independently determined by both disease activity and radiographic damage of the spine. Ann Rheum Dis 2009;68(6):863–7.
23. Boersma JW. Retardation of ossification of the lumbar vertebral column in ankylosing spondylitis by means of phenylbutazone. Scand J Rheumatol 1976;5(1):60–4.
24. Wanders A, Heijde D, Landewe R, et al. Nonsteroidal antiinflammatory drugs reduce radiographic progression in patients with ankylosing spondylitis: a randomized clinical trial. Arthritis Rheum 2005;52(6):1756–65.
25. Creemers MC, Franssen MJ, van't Hof MA, et al. Assessment of outcome in ankylosing spondylitis: an extended radiographic scoring system. Ann Rheum Dis 2005;64(1):127–9.
26. Poddubnyy D, Rudwaleit M, Haibel H, et al. Effect of non-steroidal anti-inflammatory drugs on radiographic spinal progression in patients with axial spondyloarthritis: results from the German spondyloarthritis inception cohort. Ann Rheum Dis 2012;71(10):1616–22.
27. Kroon F, Landewe R, Dougados M, et al. Continuous NSAID use reverts the effects of inflammation on radiographic progression in patients with ankylosing spondylitis. Ann Rheum Dis 2012;71(10):1623–9.
28. van der Heijde D, Landewe R, Einstein S, et al. Radiographic progression of ankylosing spondylitis after up to two years of treatment with etanercept. Arthritis Rheum 2008;58(5):1324–31.
29. van der Heijde D, Landewe R, Baraliakos X, et al. Radiographic findings following two years of infliximab therapy in patients with ankylosing spondylitis. Arthritis Rheum 2008;58(10):3063–70.

30. van der Heijde D, Salonen D, Weissman BN, et al. Assessment of radiographic progression in the spines of patients with ankylosing spondylitis treated with adalimumab for up to 2 years. Arthritis Res Ther 2009;11(4):R127.
31. Blackwell KA, Raisz LG, Pilbeam CC. Prostaglandins in bone: bad cop, good cop? Trends Endocrinol Metab 2010;21(5):294–301.
32. Zhang X, Schwarz EM, Young DA, et al. Cyclooxygenase-2 regulates mesenchymal cell differentiation into the osteoblast lineage and is critically involved in bone repair. J Clin Invest 2002;109(11):1405–15.
33. Raisz LG. Prostaglandins and bone: physiology and pathophysiology. Osteoarthritis and cartilage / OARS. Osteoarthritis Cartilage 1999;7(4):419–21.
34. Vane SJ. Differential inhibition of cyclooxygenase isoforms: an explanation of the action of NSAIDs. J Clin Rheumatol 1998;4(Suppl 5):s3–10.
35. Silverstein FE, Faich G, Goldstein JL, et al. Gastrointestinal toxicity with celecoxib vs nonsteroidal anti-inflammatory drugs for osteoarthritis and rheumatoid arthritis: the CLASS study: a randomized controlled trial. Celecoxib long-term arthritis safety study. JAMA 2000;284(10):1247–55.
36. Laine L, Curtis SP, Cryer B, et al. Assessment of upper gastrointestinal safety of etoricoxib and diclofenac in patients with osteoarthritis and rheumatoid arthritis in the Multinational Etoricoxib and Diclofenac Arthritis Long-term (MEDAL) programme: a randomised comparison. Lancet 2007;369(9560):465–73.
37. Schnitzer TJ, Burmester GR, Mysler E, et al. Comparison of lumiracoxib with naproxen and ibuprofen in the Therapeutic Arthritis Research and Gastrointestinal Event Trial (TARGET), reduction in ulcer complications: randomised controlled trial. Lancet 2004;364(9435):665–74.
38. Lanza FL, Chan FK, Quigley EM. Guidelines for prevention of NSAID-related ulcer complications. Am J Gastroenterol 2009;104(3):728–38.
39. Lanas A, Hunt R. Prevention of anti-inflammatory drug-induced gastrointestinal damage: benefits and risks of therapeutic strategies. Ann Med 2006;38(6):415–28.
40. Kearney PM, Baigent C, Godwin J, et al. Do selective cyclo-oxygenase-2 inhibitors and traditional non-steroidal anti-inflammatory drugs increase the risk of atherothrombosis? Meta-analysis of randomised trials. BMJ 2006;332(7553):1302–8.
41. Fosbol EL, Gislason GH, Jacobsen S, et al. Risk of myocardial infarction and death associated with the use of nonsteroidal anti-inflammatory drugs (NSAIDs) among healthy individuals: a nationwide cohort study. Clin Pharmacol Ther 2009; 85(2):190–7.
42. Trelle S, Reichenbach S, Wandel S, et al. Cardiovascular safety of non-steroidal anti-inflammatory drugs: network meta-analysis. BMJ 2011;342:c7086.
43. White WB, Faich G, Borer JS, et al. Cardiovascular thrombotic events in arthritis trials of the cyclooxygenase-2 inhibitor celecoxib. Am J Cardiol 2003;92(4):411–8.
44. Cannon CP, Curtis SP, FitzGerald GA, et al. Cardiovascular outcomes with etoricoxib and diclofenac in patients with osteoarthritis and rheumatoid arthritis in the Multinational Etoricoxib and Diclofenac Arthritis Long-term (MEDAL) programme: a randomised comparison. Lancet 2006;368(9549):1771–81.
45. Solomon SD, McMurray JJ, Pfeffer MA, et al. Cardiovascular risk associated with celecoxib in a clinical trial for colorectal adenoma prevention. N Engl J Med 2005; 352(11):1071–80.
46. Bakland G, Gran JT, Nossent JC. Increased mortality in ankylosing spondylitis is related to disease activity. Ann Rheum Dis 2011;70(11):1921–5.
47. Song IH, Poddubnyy DA, Rudwaleit M, et al. Benefits and risks of ankylosing spondylitis treatment with nonsteroidal antiinflammatory drugs. Arthritis Rheum 2008;58(4):929–38.

Therapeutic Controversies

Tumor Necrosis Factor α Inhibitors in Ankylosing Spondylitis

I.H. Song, MD, PhD[a], W.P. Maksymowych, FRCP(C)[b,*]

KEYWORDS

- TNF-α inhibitor • Ankylosing spondylitis • Efficacy • Immunogenicity
- Extraarticular manifestations • Uveitis • Magnetic resonance imaging
- Radiographic progression

KEY POINTS

- Four TNF blockers are available for the treatment of ankylosing spondylitis (AS), including infliximab, etanercept (ETN), adalimumab, and golimumab.
- For the treatment of active AS, only nonsteroidal anti-inflammatory drugs (NSAIDs) and the tumor necrosis factor α (TNF-α) inhibitors (in this article, termed *TNF blockers*) are recommended if patients primarily present with axial manifestations.
- Approximately 40% to 50% of AS patients treated with TNF blockers show a marked improvement of their disease activity, as measured by the Assessments in Spondyloarthritis International Society (ASAS) 40 percent response criterion.

INTRODUCTION

For the treatment of active AS, only NSAIDs and the TNF blockers are recommended if patients primarily present with axial manifestations.[1] Approximately 40% to 50% of AS patients treated with TNF blockers show a marked improvement of their disease activity, as measured by the BASDAI.[2–5]

This review aims at discussing the role of TNF blockers in the treatment of AS/axial spondyloarthritis (SpA) with a special focus on limitations and controversies. Although

Disclosures: I.H.S.: consulting fees or other remuneration from Pfizer Pharmaceuticals, Merck Sharp Dohme/Schering Plough, and Abbott Immunology Pharmaceuticals. W.P.M.: consultant and/or speaker fees and/or grants Abbott, Amgen, Bristol Myers Squibb, Eli-Lilly, Janssen, Merck, Pfizer, and Union chimique belge (UCB).

[a] Rheumatology, Charité Medical University, Campus Benjamin Franklin, Berlin, Germany; [b] Department of Medicine, University of Alberta, 562 Heritage Medical Research Building, Edmonton, Alberta T6G 2S2, Canada

* Corresponding author.

E-mail address: walter.maksymowych@ualberta.ca

Rheum Dis Clin N Am 38 (2012) 613–633
http://dx.doi.org/10.1016/j.rdc.2012.08.004 rheumatic.theclinics.com

the introduction of TNF blockers has revolutionized treatment of AS, treating physicians are aware of certain limitations. When looking for answers to controversial questions about TNF blockers in AS, experience shows that part of the answer is derived from treatment with RA, because in RA there is longer experience with TNF blockers. RA and AS are substantially different diseases, however, which share the common feature that TNF-α plays a major role in disease. This review outlines and discusses 8 major controversies that focus on treatment efficacy, treatment strategies involving the use of TNF blockers in real-world practice, and safety aspects specific to their use in SpA.

CONTROVERSY 1: ARE THERE SPECIFIC INDICATIONS FOR USING SPECIFIC TNF BLOCKERS BECAUSE OF DIFFERENCES IN EFFICACY? WHAT IS THE EVIDENCE FOR DIFFERENCES IN TREATMENT EFFICACY FOR EXTRA-ARTICULAR MANIFESTATIONS OF SPA?

As described previously, the efficacy of TNF blockers in AS for treating axial disease is similar.[2–5] It is also known, however, that patients with AS suffer from peripheral arthritis[6] and a substantial proportion of patients from extraarticular manifestations, such as enthesitis, psoriasis, inflammatory bowel disease (IBD), or acute anterior uveitis (AAU).[7–9]

Acute Anterior Uveitis

AAU represents one of the most common extraarticular manifestations, affecting approximately 30% to 50% of AS patients.[8] In cases of failure of topical glucocorticosteroids, TNF blockers are considered an effective treatment option. The question, however, is whether there is evidence that one TNF blocker is more efficacious than another.

A few case series described new onset or flares of AAU in patients on TNF blocker treatment, which was ETN in many cases.[10–14] Consistent with these case reports, 3 retrospective case series reported a lack of impact of ETN on AAU.[15–17] Guignard and colleagues[15] reported data from French patients with SpA, showing differences in the efficacy of TNF blockers in reducing AAU flares. Of 46 patients with AAU, 33 patients were treated with anti-TNF monoclonal antibodies (infliximab [IFX] [n = 25] or adalimumab [ADA] [n = 8]) and 13 patients received ETN. Subgroup analysis showed that the incidence of AAU remained unchanged with ETN treatment (54.6 vs 58.5 per 100 patient years), whereas there was a statistically significant reduction during treatment with IFX (47.4 vs 9.0 per 100 patient-years) or ADA (60.5 vs 0 per 100 patient years).

Cobo-Ibanez and colleagues[16] reported approximately 150 patients with SpA on TNF blocker therapy of whom 19 (12.7%) had AAU before starting treatment (15 had AS, 2 had undifferentiated SpA, and 2 had psoriasis). Of these 19 patients, 10 received ETN and 9 received IFX, and 1 patient was switched from ETN to IFX because of recurrent uveitis flares. The incidence of AAU in IFX-treated patients was 61.7 and 2.6 per 100 patient-years before and after treatment, respectively. In the ETN group, however, an increase of AAU flares from 34.3 before treatment to 60 per 100 patient-years after starting therapy was observed.

A 12-week open-label study with ADA demonstrated reduced rates of AAU in patients with AS (n =1250).[18] A significant reduction in AAU rates was found when treatment before and during ADA was compared (15 vs 7.4 per 100 patient-years) in the whole group of patients and flare rates were reduced by 50%. Subgroup analysis showed consistent findings in several subgroups, including patients with a history of AAU or patients with symptomatic AAU at baseline. The strength of this study was the large sample size and prospective study design but no comparator was used and study duration was limited to 12 weeks.

Braun and colleagues[19] compared AAU flare data from different AS clinical trials that included 4 placebo-controlled studies with TNF blockers (2 with ETN and 2 with IFX) and 3 open-label studies. Further information about the course of AAU was provided for 397 of 717 initially identified patients, of whom 90 were exposed to IFX and 297 to ETN for a total of 146 and 430 patient years, respectively. Although the frequency of AAU in the placebo group was 15.6 per 100 patient-years, for patients treated with TNF blockers a mean of only 6.8 AAU flares per 100 patient-years was found. In this study, a nonsignificant lower frequency of AAU flares was observed in patients treated with IFX compared with patients treated with ETN (3.4 per 100 patient-years vs 7.9 per 100 patient-years, respectively).

Finally, Sieper and colleagues[20] assessed the frequency of AAU in an analysis of different clinical trials of ETN in patients with AS (3 open label, 1 active controlled [sulfasalazine as comparator], and 4 placebo controlled). A significant difference was found in AAU event rates per 100 patient years in favor of ETN versus placebo: 8.6 versus 19.3. Compared with sulfasalazine, similar AAU event rates were found for ETN: 10.7 for ETN versus 14.7 for sulfasalazine.

Fig. 1 summarizes some of the data about AAU event rates per 100 patient years from several trials.

In conclusion, there seems little doubt that ETN does not increase the AAU event rate, as originally suggested by retrospective data. Whether ETN is efficacious in reducing AAU event rates is difficult to establish with certainty because exposure to placebo was short term (12–24 weeks) in clinical trials and the AAU event rate varied widely in placebo patients between clinical trials. Consequently, estimation of AAU event rate in placebo patients by summing data from different trials and presenting event rate per 100 patient years may not reflect an appropriate event rate. Overall, the data suggest that either IFX or ADA is a better choice in the minority of patients with frequent attacks of AAU.

Inflammatory Bowel Disease and Psoriasis

Several studies have demonstrated that IFX substantially improves gastrointestinal signs and symptoms of Crohn disease (CD) and ulcerative colitis as well as associated axial and peripheral joint inflammation.[21,22] The same is true for ADA, which was approved in 2007 for treatment of CD.[23] Conversely, treatment of patients with IBD and associated SpA with ETN showed that signs and symptoms of IBD worsened after 12 weeks of treatment even though articular symptoms had improved.[24] This is not surprising because ETN is not indicated for the treatment of CD.[25,26] For ETN there are even some case reports that CD persists or even flares during ETN therapy.[24,27] IFX and ADA are, therefore, preferred anti-TNF agents compared with ETN in the setting of IBD.

The 3 TNF blockers, IFX, ETN and ADA, are approved and indicated for treatment of psoriasis[23,25,28] and no head-to head comparisons are available. The weight of evidence does not support a preferred TNF blocker agent.

Enthesitis

Enthesitis is a characteristic finding in SpA patients and is considered an ASAS core outcome domain for the evaluation of AS.[29] The frequency of enthesitis differs in AS/SpA, ranging between approximately 40% and 50% in different cohorts.[9,30–32] For the assessment of enthesitis by clinical examination different indices have been developed, such as the Mander index,[33] the Stoke Enthesitis Index,[34] the University of

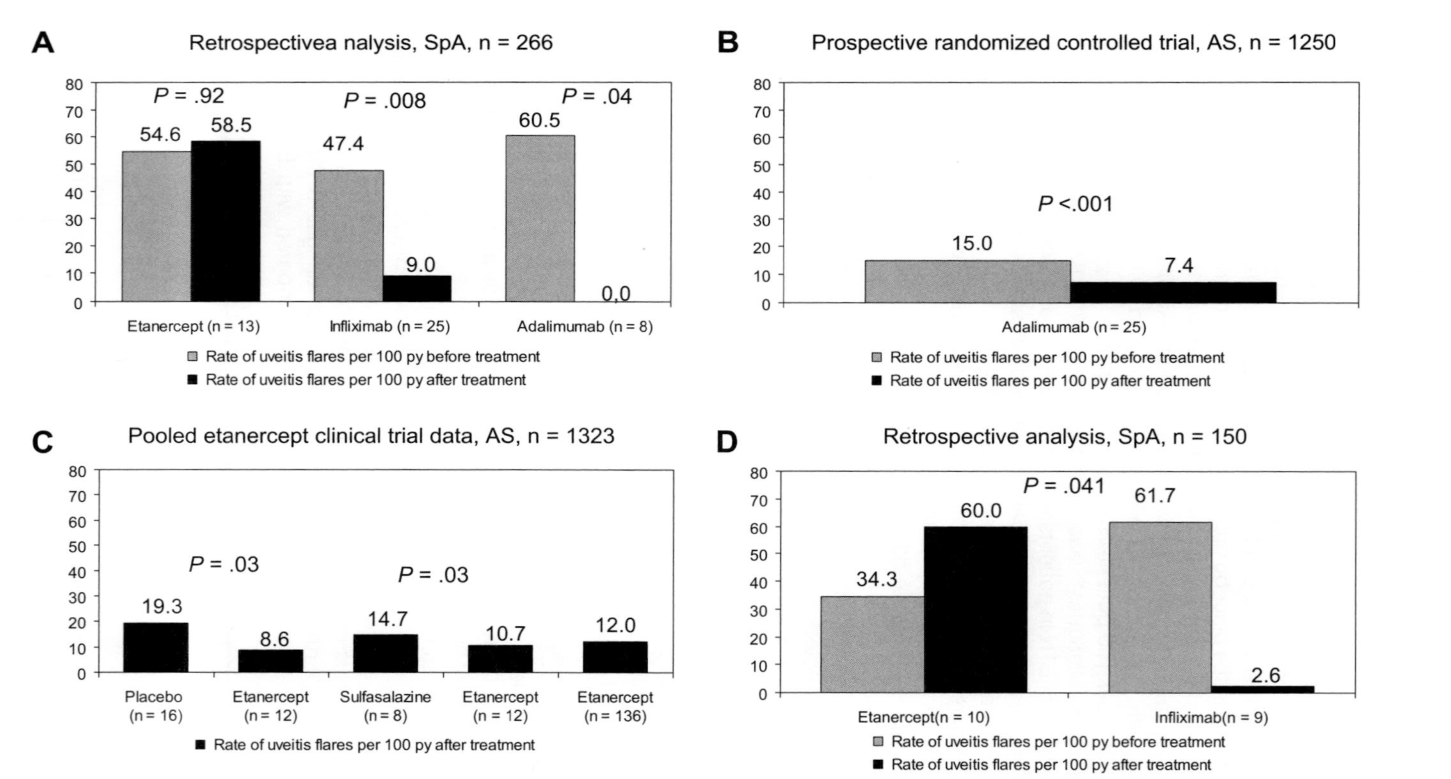

Fig. 1. Illustration of rates of AAU flares per 100 patient-years during treatment with different TNF-α–blocking agents in different studies. py, patient years; uveitis, acute anterior uveitis. (*Data from* (*A*) Guignard S, Gossec L, Salliot C, et al. Efficacy of tumour necrosis factor blockers in reducing uveitis flares in patients with spondylarthropathy: a retrospective study. Ann Rheum Dis 2006; 65(12):1631–4; (*B*) Rudwaleit M, Rodevand E, Holck P, et al. Adalimumab effectively reduces the rate of anterior uveitis flares in patients with active ankylosing spondylitis: results of a prospective open-label study. Ann Rheum Dis 2009; 68(5):696–701; (*C*) Sieper J, Koenig A, Baumgartner S, et al. Analysis of uveitis rates across all etanercept ankylosing spondylitis clinical trials. Ann Rheum Dis 2010; 69(1):226–9; (*D*) Cobo-Ibanez T, del Carmen Ordonez M, Munoz-Fernandez S, et al. Do TNF-blockers reduce or induce uveitis? Rheumatology (Oxford) 2008; 47(5):731–2)

San Francisco index,[35] the Maastricht Ankylosing Spondylitis Enthesitis Score (MASES),[36] the Berlin enthesitis score,[37] and the Spondyloarthritis Research Consortium of Canada (SPARCC) score.[38] None of these clinical indices has been fully validated. Most placebo-controlled trials of TNF blockers have not shown a consistent impact of treatment on enthesitis scores with the exception of ADA in the Adalimumab trial evaluating long-term efficacy and safety for ankylosing spondylitis (ATLAS) trial.[3] IFX did not significantly decrease enthesitis scores measured by either the Mander index in the ankylosing spondylitis study for the evaluation of recombinant infliximab therapy (ASSERT) study or the Berlin enthesitis score in the German study. Several different indices were assessed in the GO-RAISE trial of golimumab in AS, including the MASES, Berlin, and San Francisco scores, with a significant effect observed only using the San Francisco score. There was also no effect of ADA on the MASES in a placebo-controlled trial of patients with nonradiographic axial SpA (ABILITY I).[39] In contrast to the lack of effect on clinical enthesitis, there is evidence that enthesitis evident on MRI improves after TNF blocker treatment as shown in the HEEL study, in which patients with SpA and MRI-proved heel enthesitis were successfully treated with ETN,[40] or a trial in which whole-body MRI was able to show that enthesitis at various sites is significantly reduced by ETN in patients with early axial SpA (ESTHER trial).[41]

The discrepancy in the impact of TNF blocker therapy on clinical and MRI features of enthesitis may reflect the complete lack of correlation between clinical and MRI features[42] and the importance of training and a standardized approach to the clinical assessment of enthesitis. The available data do not support the case for preferential use of any specific TNF- blocker in patients with active enthesitis.

CONTROVERSY 2: IS IT POSSIBLE TO REDUCE THE DOSE OF A TNF BLOCKER (EG, BY INCREASING DOSING INTERVALS) OR EVEN STOP TREATMENT WITH A TNF BLOCKER SO THAT DRUG-FREE REMISSION BECOMES POSSIBLE?

A few clinical trials have dealt with the question of whether patients can remain in a low disease activity state or remission with a reduced dose of a TNF blocker or even after discontinuation of active treatment with a TNF blocker.

In a Spanish study, dose reduction of ETN was performed according to the treating rheumatologist and patient preference in patients with well-controlled disease activity defined as a BASDAI less than 4 and normal C-reactive protein (CRP) values; dose reduction was possible in 16 of 51 (32%) patients with different dose reduction schemes.[43]

Another retrospective study from South Korea assessed 109 AS patients in a real-life setting in whom dosing intervals for ETN were increased from 4.7 days at 3 months to 12.1 days at 21 months. BASDAI values declined from 8.5 to 0.6 after 21 months, which was accompanied by a decrease in CRP.[44] A dose reduction of ETN from 50 mg once weekly to a maintenance dose of 25 mg once weekly has been investigated in another Korean study, including 27 AS patients.[45]

A recent analysis of a retrospective French study assessed dose changes in clinical practice in 189 AS patients where the mean follow-up was 45.5 months.[46] In these patients, a state of low disease activity/remission was achieved in 65 patients (35%). The adjustment of TNF blocker dose was observed approximately 50 times and resulted in keeping the state of low disease activity in the majority of patients. For IFX, the mean dose intervals ranged between 7 and 15 weeks (mean interval for IFX increased from 8.3 weeks at 6 months to 9.7 weeks at 36 months). The most frequently performed dose modification for ADA was increasing the dose interval from 2 to

3 weeks (mean intervals for ADA application was 3.1 weeks at 6 months and 3.5 weeks at 24 months). For ETN, the most frequently observed dose modification was the use of 25 mg once weekly or 50 mg every 10 to 14 days (mean intervals for ETN 25 mg/50 mg application were 6.6 days/12.3 days at 6 months and 8.0 days/10.0 days at 36 months). Among patients reaching remission, no dose increase was necessary until the end of follow-up for 13 of 26 patients on IFX, 4 of 17 patients on ETN, and 2 of 5 patients on ADA. The cumulative probability of continuation of the TNF blocker after dose adjustment was approximately 80% at 12 months, approximately 70% at 24 months, and approximately 60% at 36 months.

The studies where TNF blockers were completely discontinued in patients who reached a state of inactive disease or remission showed flare rates of approximately 100% in patients with AS after several years of therapy with IFX[47] or ETN,[48] 83% in patients with nonradiographic axial SpA after 1 year of ADA,[49] and 60% of patients with axial SpA with a symptom duration of less than 3 years after 16 weeks of IFX.[50]

The latest trial providing data on drug-free remission are from the 2-year data of the ESTHER trial, which assessed ETN versus sulfasalazine in early axial SpA.[51] All patients had to have an MRI showing active inflammatory lesions on MRI at baseline. After 1 year of treatment, only those patients who were in ASAS remission and free of active inflammation on MRI were followed without active treatment for 1 more year. Although 33% of ETN patients retained this strict remission criterion (MRI and clinical remission) at year 1, only 8% of ETN-treated patients stayed in drug-free remission at year 2.

A reservation with the evaluation of studies that assessed flare rates is that different definitions for low disease activity or remission as well as flare were used. In longstanding disease in AS, it may be difficult for patients to attain a BASFI of less than or equal to 20 of 100, which is necessary for the ASAS remission criteria.[52] It has been proposed that remission may be more appropriately defined by using the Ankylosing Spondylitis Disease Activity Score definition for low disease activity state (score <1.3).[53]

The opposite question is whether some AS patients would benefit from a dose increase. For golimumab, 100 mg subcutaneously every 4 weeks was not superior to 50 mg subcutaneously every 4 weeks.[5] For ETN, a recent study evaluated whether 50 mg subcutaneously twice weekly is more efficacious than 50 mg subcutaneously once weekly[54] in a randomized placebo-controlled setting. At week 12, ASAS 20 and ASAS 40 response rates were not statistically different between the 2 treatment groups (31% vs 30% and 23% vs 18%, respectively).

To summarize, there are data that dose reduction may be possible in some patients. Treatment discontinuation may be possible in a small minority (10%) of patients with early axial SpA although the vast majority of patients clinically show a relapse, requiring resumption of TNF blocker treatment.

CONTROVERSY 3: ANTICHIMERIC ANTIBODIES—ARE THEY OF CLINICAL SIGNIFICANCE IN PATIENTS RECEIVING TNF BLOCKERS?

In RA, it has been shown that antibodies against TNF blockers may develop, which is associated with reduced efficacy of TNF blockers.[55]

In AS, a few smaller studies have investigated the development of antibodies to TNF blockers. For example, one study assessed 60 AS patients, of whom 20 patients per treatment group were treated with IFX, ETN, and ADA and then followed prospectively for 12 months. Antibodies against IFX, ETN, and ADA were found in 20%, 0%, and 30%, respectively.[56]

Another small study that assessed 8 AS patients treated with IFX for 24 weeks found that 2 patients developed antibodies to IFX and low trough IFX levels and this was associated with a lack of clinical response and infusion reactions.[57] In contrast, Krzysiek and colleagues[58] did not find any association of anti-IFX antibodies or trough IFX concentration and response to treatment. A similar study with a higher number of AS patients (n = 35) and a slightly longer follow-up (6 months) assessed the relationship between antibody formation against ADA and efficacy and side effects. Of 11 patients (31%) who developed antibodies to ADA with low or undetectable ADA levels, 9 were clinical nonresponders and 1 suffered from an allergic reaction.

When the same group of researchers evaluated antibody formation against ETN, in a group of 53 AS patients, serum drug levels increased to 2.7 mg/L after 3 months to 3.0 mg/L after 6 months with no difference between responders and nonresponders and no antibodies to ETN were identified.[59] This has also been noted in other rheumatic diseases,[60] so failure of clinical response in AS patients cannot be due to anti-ETN antibodies.

In the most recent study from a Spanish group, Plasencia and colleagues[61] conducted a 4-year retrospective study of 94 patients with axial SpA (50 with AS, 12 with undifferentiated SpA, 22 with psoriatic arthritis [PsA], and 10 with IBD]). All patients were treated with IFX (5 mg/kg). Antibodies to IFX were found in approximately 25% of patients, mostly after the sixth infusion, and patients with antibodies presented with higher disease activity at follow-up, shorter drug survival (4.3 years vs 8.2 years), and more adverse events. Anti-IFX antibodies developed less frequently in patients taking concomitant methotrexate (MTX) (11% vs 35%) and patients taking MTX had higher IFX serum concentrations. A limitation of this study is that data were not stratified according to diagnosis and it is unclear whether treatment with MTX had any beneficial clinical effects. In addition, it is unclear to what degree the development of anti-IFX antibodies was an independent factor contributing to lack of treatment response because no regression analysis was performed. For instance, the patients on MTX at baseline may have been started on this treatment for indications, such as peripheral arthritis and elevated CRP that could be associated with a better treatment response. **Fig. 2** summarizes the frequency of antibodies against TNF blockers.

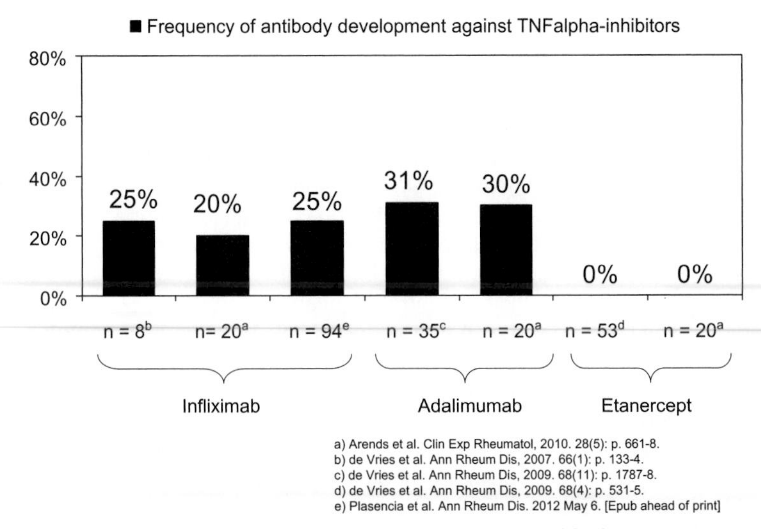

Fig. 2. Frequency of development of antibodies against TNF-α–blocking agents.

A second retrospective study from France evaluating 91 patients with SpA treated with IFX came to similar conclusions.[62] High concentrations of IFX during treatment initiation reduced the development of antibodies to IFX and the absence of such antibodies was associated with prolonged maintenance of IFX. Those who were treated concomitantly with MTX had a lower risk of developing anti-IFX antibodies than patients not taking MTX. Infusion reactions occurred in 52% of those with anti-IFX antibodies compared with only 1% without. It was unclear, however, whether treatment with MTX had any beneficial clinical effect.

In summary, several studies now show that patients with AS develop antibodies against ADA or IFX and the most recent data indicate that this is delayed compared with rheumatoid arthritis (RA) and that at least a year of follow-up is appropriate. The question is whether this is clinically relevant and whether antibody formation could be prevented by adding an immunosuppressant drug (such as MTX or azathioprine), which has been associated with a lower frequency of antidrug antibody expression in RA[63,64] and CD.[65]

This question arises because there are some studies with IFX in AS indicating that there is no difference whether or not IFX is combined with MTX in patients with AS,[66,67] including data from the Norwegian registry suggesting that drug survival in AS after 1 year is not different between patients who receive a combination of a TNF blocker plus MTX or TNF blocker alone,[68] which is different in PsA or RA registries.[68] Moreover, a recent extensive pharmacokinetic analysis has shown that combination of MTX and IFX does not increase the exposure to IFX over IFX alone in patients with AS and the 2 groups did not differ in disease activity or biomarkers of inflammation.[69]

To summarize, although evidence supporting a role for anti-IFX antibodies in reduced clinical response to IFX is compelling, there is insufficient evidence to warrant institution of MTX therapy as concomitant treatment for SpA, particularly because there are no controlled data that show that this agent has a beneficial effect in SpA. Because there is no proved intervention mitigating the development of anti-TNF blocker antibodies, the role of measuring these antibodies in routine clinical practice remains unclear.

CONTROVERSY 4: WHAT IS THE IMPLICATION OF RESIDUAL ACTIVE INFLAMMATION ON MRI IN PATIENTS TREATED WITH TNF BLOCKERS IN RELATION TO RADIOGRAPHIC PROGRESSION AND DOES MRI CONSTITUTE AN APPROPRIATE ENDPOINT FOR A TREAT-TO-TARGET THERAPEUTIC STRATEGY?

With the use of TNF blockers, a marked decrease of active inflammation on MRI can be observed of approximately 40% to 50% in the sacroiliac joints[70,71] and approximately 60% in the spine.[70–72] Nevertheless, this indicates that a significant amount of inflammatory burden remains and raises the question as to its impact on the course of disease. In particular, is there a relationship between inflammation and structural progression, and does the apparent lack of impact of TNF blocker therapies on structural progression reflect insufficient control of inflammation?

Several studies have now shown that vertebral inflammation as detected on short tau inversion recovery sequence (STIR) MRI predicts the development of new syndesmophytes.[73–78] But it has also been shown that the majority of syndesmophytes develop from vertebral corners, which appear normal on the STIR sequence. It has thus been argued that inflammation and ankylosis are uncoupled. It should be noted, however, that sample size calculations show that the TNF blocker trials of ETN, IFX, and ADA are only powered to detect treatment group differences of at least 80% in the modified Stokes Ankylosing Spondylitis Spinal*Score* and lesser degrees of reduction in that score with active therapy would not be captured.[79] The most recent study has confirmed the link between inflammation and new bone formation at vertebral corners but also shows that acute inflammatory lesions resolve completely without sequelae whereas more complex mature lesions, especially those where there is evidence of fat metaplasia as well as inflammation, resolve but are still associated with development of new syndesmophytes.[78] The majority of new syndesmophytes develop from vertebral corners with either inflammation on STIR images or fat metaplasia on T1-weighted sequence. Two reports have shown that inflammatory lesions undergo fat metaplasia.[80,81] The data, therefore, support a window of opportunity hypothesis for disease modification whereby early and effective intervention with anti-inflammatory therapy may prevent structural progression. The typical patients recruited to clinical trials of TNF blockers have a mix of acute and more complex inflammatory lesions and the overall development of new bone during TNF blocker therapy may, therefore, depend on the balance between the number of early and more mature inflammatory lesions. This hypothesis also predicts that with prolonged follow up it should be possible to demonstrate a beneficial effect of anti-TNF therapy on structural progression because continued treatment will prevent development of new inflammatory lesions.

Because recent data also suggest that NSAIDs may slow down radiographic progression[82–84] in AS patients with pre-existing syndesmophytes and elevated CRP levels, it is of special interest to know whether a combination of a TNF blocker and an NSAID is superior to TNF blocker monotherapy.

CONTROVERSY 5: IS SWITCHING BETWEEN TNF BLOCKERS EFFECTIVE? ARE THERE SPECIFIC SWITCHES THAT WORK BEST? CAN RESPONSE TO ANTI-TNF SWITCH BE PREDICTED?

Despite the good efficacy of TNF blockers, rheumatologists have to deal with the problem of nonresponders. The question is whether after failure of a first TNF blocker, a second or even third TNF blocker should be prescribed, and, if so, whether there are predictors for response to anti-TNF switch.

The first studies describing successful switching between TNF blockers included small numbers of patients and mostly reported switching from IFX to ETN (**Table 1**).[85–90]

A retrospective French study analyzed 222 SpA patients,[85] 93% of whom approximately fulfilled the new ASAS classification criteria for axial SpA.[91] The first TNF blocker treatment included ETN (52.7%), ADA (27.0%), or IFX (20.3%); 111 (50%) stopped the first TNF blocker treatment for different reasons. In 32%, a second TNF blocker was given, and approximately 50% of these patients also stopped the second TNF blocker. It was shown that switchers more frequently suffered from enthesitis and arthritis. Retention rates at 1 year were similar for the first and second TNF blocker (60%–65%). In this analysis, no predictor could be identified that predicted retention rates for the second TNF blocker.

Two-year data from real world practice are provided by the Norwegian registry of 514 TNF-naïve patients, of whom 15% (77/514) switched to a second TNF blocker.[92] Response rates after 3 months were higher for nonswitchers compared with switchers (ASAS 20 53% vs 40%, ASAS 40 38% vs 31%, and BASDAI 50 50% vs 28%). There was no difference regarding the efficacy for the second TNF blocker between switchers due to adverse events or due to nonresponse. Retention rates after 2 years were better for nonswitchers compared with switchers (65% vs 60%). Among patients on a second TNF blocker, patients who switched due to inadequate response had

Table 1
Overview of different studies in which TNF blockers were switched in AS

Study	Switch	Study Design	% of Switchers	Result	More Information
Delaunay et al,[86] 2005	IFX → ETN	Retrospective study, follow-up of 10 mo, France	(7 AS patients)	Clinical response achieved in 43% (3/7)	7 of 15 patients with AS (6 with former IR)
Cantini et al,[87] 2006	IFX → ETN	54-Wk prospective follow-up study, Italy	23 AS patients	At week 54 ASAS 20 = 74 and ASAS remission 74% and 22%	18/23 With former IR
Coates et al,[88] 2008	Not specified	Retrospective, >2-y follow-up, UK	13% (15 of 113)	93% of Switchers with good result	Similar outcomes regardless of drug used, disease duration, and HLA-B27 status
Conti et al,[89] 2007	IFX → ETN	Observational, prospective, Italy	6 AS patients of 165 with SpAs	83.3% Responders after 3 mo	Similar outcome regardless of switch due to AE or IR
Pradeep et al,[90] 2008	Not specified	Retrospective, UK; 33-mo follow-up, UK	15% (16/108)	65% Responders at 3 mo	Switching due to AE with slightly better response compared with IE
Rudwaleit et al,[91] 2010	IFX → ADA (n = 162) ETN → ADA (n = 85) IFX or ETN → ADA (79)	Open-label RCT, 12 wk, international RCT	26% of Patients in this RCT were TNF exposed (326/1250)	BASDAI 50 at wk = 41%, ASAS 40 = 38%	Odds of achieving BASDAI 50 response significantly greater for IFX→ ADA vs ETN→ ADA
Lie et al,[92] 2010	ETN→ IFX (n = 18) ETN → ADA (n = 14) IFX → ETA (n = 27) IFX → ADA (n = 14) ADA → ETN (n = 4)	Longitudinal study in Norway, 3-mo follow-up	15% (77/514)	At 3 mo: BASDAI 50 = 25% and ASAS 40 = 30% for first switchers	Similar outcome regardless of switch due to AE or IR
Dadoun et al,[85] 2011	Not specified	Retrospective study, 29-mo follow-up, SpA patients	32% (72/222)	50% Still on second TNF blocker at end of follow-up	No predictive factors identified for retention of the second TNF blocker

Abbreviations: AE, adverse event; ASAS 20/ASAS 40/ASAS remission, response of the ASAS criteria for 20% composite response (ASAS 20), ASA S40, and ASAS criteria for partial remission; IR, inadequate response.

slightly better retention rates compared with patients who had switched due to adverse events. Inadequate response, however, was not further defined, so it could mean primary nonresponse, partial response, and also secondary nonresponse (loss of response). In this study, there was not enough statistical power to compare the effectiveness of switches between TNF blockers with different mechanisms of action.

In the open-label phase 3 clinical trial of ADA in AS (RHAPSODY), the response to ADA was compared in TNF blocker–naïve AS patients (n = 924) versus TNF blocker–exposed AS patients (ETN or IFX) (n = 326).[93] Patients who had been treated with TNF blockers before had received IFX before the study (n = 162), ETN (n = 85), or both IFX and ETN (n = 79). Although the response was better in the TNF-naïve group, there was also a significant response in the TNF-exposed group (BASDAI 50 63% vs 41% and ASAS 40 59% vs 38%). The probability of reaching a BASDAI 50 response was significantly higher for patients who had received only IFX compared with only ETN before the study (BASDAI 50 48% vs 33%). The number of patients who only received ETN as a first TNF blocker, however, was small. It was also shown that response rates on ADA treatment after 12 weeks were higher in patients who had discontinued the prior TNF blocker (ETN or IFX) because of secondary failure/intolerance compared with primary failure (BASDAI 50 42%/46% vs 26%; ASAS 40 43%/39% vs 26%). So, in this study patients who initially showed a response to a first TNF blocker were more likely to also show a response to a second TNF blocker, especially when the type of agent was similar (monocloncal antibody).[93]

Glintborg and colleagues[94] recently presented data on 1436 AS patients from the Danish DANBIO registry with a follow-up of 2.6 years; 30% of these patients switched to a second TNF blocker and 10% to a third TNF blocker. IFX was the first TNF blocker in 45% of patients, ADA in 37%, and ETN in 16%. Switchers compared with non-switchers were more often female, had higher BASDAI and BASFI levels values, exhibited a low CRP, and were of older age. Although the number needed to treat to achieve a good response at 6 months increased with each TNF blocker (number needed to treat 1.7, 2.4 and 3.0 for first, second, and third TNF blocker, respectively), patients who switched still showed a significant response. Two years after starting the TNF blocker treatment, 52% of switchers had a good clinical response. Drug survival rates were 3.1, 1.6, and 1.8 years for the first, second, and third TNF blockers, respectively. Predictors that were identified for longer adherence to the second TNF blocker included male gender and a low baseline functional index.

In summary, there are observational data supporting the current practice of switching between TNF -blockers. Because treatment options for TNF blocker failures are limited in AS,[95] these data may be biased and controlled studies are necessary. Among the switch options, there is only evidence from the RHAPSODY trial that switching from IFX to ADA might work better than switching from ETN to ADA. These data are limited, however, and more data are needed from controlled studies.

CONTROVERSY 6: IS THE BASDAI CUTOFF GREATER THAN OR EQUAL TO 4 AN APPROPRIATE CUTOFF TO RECOMMEND INITIATION OF TNF BLOCKER THERAPY AND SHOULD OBJECTIVE EVIDENCE OF ACTIVE DISEASE, EITHER ELEVATED CRP OR EVIDENCE OF BONE MARROW EDEMA ON MRI, BE USED TO SELECT PATIENTS FOR TNF BLOCKER THERAPY?

There is some consensus that predictors for a major clinical response include shorter disease duration, young age, elevated CRP, and higher degree of inflammatory burden on MRI.[49,93,96,97] This is particularly evident in patients with early SpA.[49,98]

The BASDAI does not seem, however, to be a consistent predictor. The BASDAI cutoff of 4 was arbitrarily proposed a decade ago and has since been adopted without any validation.[99] The cutoff seems to reflect a patient's self-reported experience with respect to level of impairment and quality of life[100] and other reports have shown that it discriminates between patients reporting satisfactory symptom state and inadequate symptom control.[101,102] A recent report has shown, however, that there is no significant difference in objective measures of inflammation as recorded by the CRP and MRI between patients with BASDAI greater than or equal to 4 and those less than 4.[103] Moreover, there is evidence that patients with BASDAI less than 4 respond to TNF blocker therapy.[104,105]

The treatment of patient symptoms is paramount but if it could be shown that objective features of disease activity, such as CRP and MRI inflammation, are associated with radiographic progression, there could be a strong argument to treat patients even if the BASDAI is less than 4. This remains an open question, so it is unclear whether and to what degree the decision to treat should be influenced by expert opinion based on objective measures of inflammation. Although previous treatment recommendations have suggested the incorporation of objective measures of inflammation into the decision-making process, the Canadian Rheumatology Association/SPARCC treatment recommendations[106] explicitly call for the use of TNF blockers if there is evidence of active disease as defined by at least 2 of the following:

- BASDAI $\geq$4
- Elevated CRP and/or erythrocyte sedimentation rate
- Inflammatory lesions in the sacroiliac joints and/or spine on MRI

There are concerns regarding access to MRI, lack of familiarity with interpretation of MRI features of AS on the part of both rheumatologists and radiologists, and insufficient data on its predictive validity as regards radiographic progression. Although there is increasing evidence that the presence of objective features of inflammation plus short disease duration are predictive of clinical response to TNF blocker therapy, there are insufficient data as to the percentage of patients without elevated CRP or active MRI inflammation but BASDAI greater than 4 who still achieve a major clinical response to TNF blocker therapy. This is likely to vary according to age, disease duration, and Bath Ankylosing Spondylitis Functional Index (BASFI). Nevertheless, the key question remains—does the absence of any objective measure of active disease constitute justifiable grounds, clinical and pharmacoeconomic, for long-term therapy with TNF blockers?

CONTROVERSY 7: BIOSIMILARS—DO THEY OFFER ADVANTAGES FOR PATIENTS WITH AS?

TNF blockers are potent anti-inflammatory drugs. They are also, however, expensive. With more and more biosimilars in the pipeline, treating rheumatologists at some time will be faced with the question of whether they should or would prescribe biosimilars for their patients if they are approved.[107]

In the field of AS, recent data from an international, multicenter, phase I randomized controlled trial (RCT) were presented using an IFX biosimilar.[108] AS patients (N = 250) were randomized to receive the IFX biosimilar, CT-P13 (n = 125), or IFX (5 mg/kg) (n = 125) at weeks 0, 2, and 6 (dose-loading phase) and at weeks 14, 22, and 30 (maintenance phase). The primary outcome was a comparison of ratios of geometric means of primary pharmacokinetic parameters (AUC_τ and Cmax ss) between weeks 22 and 30 and these were comparable between treatment arms. Secondary parameters at week 30 were also comparable, including safety aspects and ASAS 20 and ASAS 40 response rates (70.5% for CT-P13 vs 72.4% for IFX and 51.8% vs 47.4%, respectively).

Examples of safety issues include cases of red cell aplasia in renal dialysis patients receiving erythropoietin alfa[109–111]; however, other biosimilars—erythropoietin alfa, somatropin, and filgrastim—have been used in Europe for at least 4 to 5 years and there have been no reports of serious adverse events submitted to the EMA. It remains to be seen whether biologics for the treatment of rheumatic diseases, such as RA, PsA, and AS, will be approved in Europe and the United States and how they will perform regarding efficacy and especially safety.

CONTROVERSY 8: IS MALIGNANCY A CONCERN IN AS PATIENTS ON ANTI-TNF AGENTS? WHAT SHOULD PATIENTS BE TOLD?

Data about the occurrence of solid malignant tumors or lymphoma are mainly derived from patients with RA. A recent review by Keystone[112] summarizes and discusses the risk for serious infections and cancer in patients with RA.

Regarding the risk for malignant diseases, data from RCTs and from observational studies are conflicting. In the meta-analysis by Bongartz and colleagues,[113] including ADA and IFX RCT data, a significantly increased risk for malignant diseases was found for the TNF blockers, but this could not be reproduced in subsequent meta-analyses.[114,115] An increased malignancy risk was also not found in observational studies, such as from the US National Data Bank for Rheumatic Diseases, where users of biologics were compared with nonusers,[116] except for an increased risk of basal cell cancer (odds ratio [OR] 1.5; 95% CI, 1.2–1.8) and possibly melanoma (OR 2.3; 95% CI, 0.9–5.4).

Further reassuring data come from 2 observational studies, which showed no significant risk of incident or recurrent malignant diseases in TNF blocker–treated RA compared with disease-modifying antirheumatic drug–treated RA patients with prior malignancies in the British Society for Rheumatology Biologics Register registry and the German biologics registry.[117,118]

Regarding lymphoma, earlier reports from the Swedish Biologics Register showed an increased lymphoma risk during TNF blocker treatment in RA patients.[119] The subsequent studies could not confirm, however, an increased lymphoma risk over the elevated lymphoma risk in RA patients in general.[120] In particular, the incidence and relative risk for cancers overall did not increase over time or with cumulative duration of TNF blocker treatment.[121] Unlike RA, AS has not been associated with an increased risk for lymphoma.[122]

A French registry, RATIO, analyzed lymphoma cases that occurred during TNF blocker treatment by performing a case-control-study.[123] It found 38 patients with lymphoma, including 31 patients with non-Hodgkin lymphoma, 5 with Hodgkin lymphoma, and 2 described as Hodgkin-like lymphoma. Among the patients were 27 with RA and 7 with SpA (3 PsA and 4 AS). Patients receiving ADA or IFX had a higher risk compared with those treated with ETN; the respective standardized incidence ratios were 4.1 (2.3–7.1) and 3.6 (2.3–5.6) versus 0.9 (0.4–1.8). The exposure to ADA or IFX versus ETN was found an independent risk factor for lymphoma in the case-control study with ORs of 4.7 (1.3–17.7) and 4.1 (1.4–12.5), respectively. For RA and SpA, the standardized incidence ratio (SIR) was 2.3 (1.6–3.3; $P<.0001$) and 1.9 (0.9–4.0; $P = .09$), respectively. Because of the small number of cases, no definitive conclusion may be drawn from these data in SpA patients.

A recent meta-analysis requested by the European Medicines Agency assessed the short-term risk by analyzing 74 RCTs (28 ETN, 23 ADA, and 23 IFX), including a total of more than 20,000 patients.[124] Trial durations were between 4 weeks and less than 6 months, and the RCTs included patients with RA, psoriasis, PsA, AS, and CD; 0.84% of patients (130 of 15.418) randomized to the TNF blockers ADA, ETN, or IFX were diagnosed with cancer compared with 0.64% (48 of 7486) in the comparator group. The relative risk with all TNF blockers was not elevated with 0.99 (95% CI, 0.61–1.68) for cancers (excluding nonmelanoma skin cancers) in contrast to an elevated risk of 2.02 (95% CI, 1.11–3.95) for nonmelanoma skin cancers. For AS no conclusive data were provided.

To summarize, TNF blockers seem to have an acceptable safety profile. The treating doctors should be aware of an increased risk for nonmelanoma skin cancer. As for lymphoproliferative diseases, including lymphoma, no definitive conclusions can be drawn and larger data sets need to be analyzed.

REFERENCES

1. van der Heijde D, Sieper J, Maksymowych W, et al. 2010 Update of the international ASAS recommendations for the use of anti-TNF agents in patients with axial spondyloarthritis. Ann Rheum Dis 2011;70(6):905–8.
2. van der Heijde D, Dijkmans B, Geusens P, et al. Efficacy and safety of infliximab in patients with ankylosing spondylitis: results of a randomized, placebo-controlled trial (ASSERT). Arthritis Rheum 2005;52(2):582–91.
3. van der Heijde D, Kivitz A, Schiff MH, et al. Efficacy and safety of adalimumab in patients with ankylosing spondylitis: results of a multicenter, randomized, double-blind, placebo-controlled trial. Arthritis Rheum 2006;54(7):2136–46.
4. Davis JC Jr, Van Der Heijde D, Braun J, et al. Recombinant human tumor necrosis factor receptor (etanercept) for treating ankylosing spondylitis: a randomized, controlled trial. Arthritis Rheum 2003;48(11):3230–6.
5. Inman RD, Davis JC Jr, Heijde D, et al. Efficacy and safety of golimumab in patients with ankylosing spondylitis: results of a randomized, double-blind, placebo-controlled, phase III trial. Arthritis Rheum 2008;58(11):3402–12.
6. Lee JH, Jun JB, Jung S, et al. Higher prevalence of peripheral arthritis among ankylosing spondylitis patients. J Korean Med Sci 2002;17(5):669–73.
7. Khan MA. Update on spondyloarthropathies. Ann Intern Med 2002;136(12): 896–907.
8. Elewaut D, Matucci-Cerinic M. Treatment of ankylosing spondylitis and extra-articular manifestations in everyday rheumatology practice. Rheumatology (Oxford) 2009;48(9):1029–35.
9. Vander Cruyssen B, Ribbens C, Boonen A, et al. The epidemiology of ankylosing spondylitis and the commencement of anti-TNF therapy in daily rheumatology practice. Ann Rheum Dis 2007;66(8):1072–7.
10. Rosenbaum JT. Effect of etanercept on iritis in patients with ankylosing spondylitis. Arthritis Rheum 2004;50(11):3736–7.
11. Smith JR, Levinson RD, Holland GN, et al. Differential efficacy of tumor necrosis factor inhibition in the management of inflammatory eye disease and associated rheumatic disease. Arthritis Rheum 2001;45(3):252–7.
12. Monnet D, Moachon L, Dougados M, et al. Severe uveitis in an HLA-B27-positive patient with ankylosing spondylitis. Nat Clin Pract Rheumatol 2006; 2(7):393–7.
13. Coates LC, McGonagle DG, Bennett AN, et al. Uveitis and tumour necrosis factor blockade in ankylosing spondylitis. Ann Rheum Dis 2008;67(5):729–30.

14. Wendling D, Paccou J, Berthelot JM, et al. New onset of uveitis during anti-tumor necrosis factor treatment for rheumatic diseases. Semin Arthritis Rheum 2011; 41(3):503–10.
15. Guignard S, Gossec L, Salliot C, et al. Efficacy of tumour necrosis factor blockers in reducing uveitis flares in patients with spondylarthropathy: a retrospective study. Ann Rheum Dis 2006;65(12):1631–4.
16. Cobo-Ibanez T, del Carmen Ordonez M, Munoz-Fernandez S, et al. Do TNF-blockers reduce or induce uveitis? Rheumatology (Oxford) 2008;47(5):731–2.
17. Lim LL, Fraunfelder FW, Rosenbaum JT. Do tumor necrosis factor inhibitors cause uveitis? A registry-based study. Arthritis Rheum 2007;56(10):3248–52.
18. Rudwaleit M, Rodevand E, Holck P, et al. Adalimumab effectively reduces the rate of anterior uveitis flares in patients with active ankylosing spondylitis: results of a prospective open-label study. Ann Rheum Dis 2009;68(5):696–701.
19. Braun J, Baraliakos X, Listing J, et al. Decreased incidence of anterior uveitis in patients with ankylosing spondylitis treated with the anti-tumor necrosis factor agents infliximab and etanercept. Arthritis Rheum 2005;52(8):2447–51.
20. Sieper J, Koenig A, Baumgartner S, et al. Analysis of uveitis rates across all etanercept ankylosing spondylitis clinical trials. Ann Rheum Dis 2010;69(1): 226–9.
21. Van den Bosch F, Kruithof E, De Vos M, et al. Crohn's disease associated with spondyloarthropathy: effect of TNF-alpha blockade with infliximab on articular symptoms. Lancet 2000;356(9244):1821–2.
22. Generini S, Giacomelli R, Fedi R, et al. Infliximab in spondyloarthropathy associated with Crohn's disease: an open study on the efficacy of inducing and maintaining remission of musculoskeletal and gut manifestations. Ann Rheum Dis 2004;63(12):1664–9.
23. Humira® (Adalimumab) Summary of Product Characteristics (SPC). February 2008.
24. Marzo-Ortega H, McGonagle D, O'Connor P, et al. Efficacy of etanercept for treatment of Crohn's related spondyloarthritis but not colitis. Ann Rheum Dis 2003;62(1):74–6.
25. Enbrel® (Etanercept) Summary of Product Characteristics (SPC). July 2008.
26. Sandborn WJ, Hanauer SB, Katz S, et al. Etanercept for active Crohn's disease: a randomized, double-blind, placebo-controlled trial. Gastroenterology 2001; 121(5):1088–94.
27. Song IH, Appel H, Haibel H, et al. New onset of Crohn's disease during treatment of active ankylosing spondylitis with etanercept. J Rheumatol 2008; 35(3):532–6.
28. Remicade® (Infliximab) Summary of Product Characteristics (SPC). August 2008.
29. van der Heijde D, Calin A, Dougados M, et al. Selection of instruments in the core set for DC-ART, SMARD, physical therapy, and clinical record keeping in ankylosing spondylitis. Progress report of the ASAS Working Group. Assessments in Ankylosing Spondylitis. J Rheumatol 1999;26(4):951–4.
30. Rudwaleit M, Landewe R, van der Heijde D, et al. The development of Assessment of SpondyloArthritis international Society classification criteria for axial spondyloarthritis (part I): classification of paper patients by expert opinion including uncertainty appraisal. Ann Rheum Dis 2009;68(6):770–6.
31. Dougados M, van der Linden S, Juhlin R, et al. The European Spondylarthropathy Study Group preliminary criteria for the classification of spondylarthropathy. Arthritis Rheum 1991;34(10):1218–27.

32. Rudwaleit M, Haibel H, Baraliakos X, et al. The early disease stage in axial spondylarthritis: results from the German Spondyloarthritis Inception Cohort. Arthritis Rheum 2009;60(3):717–27.
33. Mander M, Simpson JM, McLellan A, et al. Studies with an enthesis index as a method of clinical assessment in ankylosing spondylitis. Ann Rheum Dis 1987;46(3):197–202.
34. Dawes PT. Stoke ankylosing spondylitis spine score. J Rheumatol 1999;26(4): 993–6.
35. Gorman JD, Sack KE, Davis JC Jr. Treatment of ankylosing spondylitis by inhibition of tumor necrosis factor alpha. N Engl J Med 2002;346(18):1349–56.
36. Heuft-Dorenbosch L, Spoorenberg A, van Tubergen A, et al. Assessment of enthesitis in ankylosing spondylitis. Ann Rheum Dis 2003;62(2):127–32.
37. Brandt J, Khariouzov A, Listing J, et al. Six-month results of a double-blind, placebo-controlled trial of etanercept treatment in patients with active ankylosing spondylitis. Arthritis Rheum 2003;48(6):1667–75.
38. Maksymowych WP, Mallon C, Morrow S, et al. Development and validation of the Spondyloarthritis Research Consortium of Canada (SPARCC) Enthesitis Index. Ann Rheum Dis 2009;68(6):948–53.
39. Sieper J, Van der Heijde D, Dougados M, et al. Efficacy and safety of adalimumab in patients with non-radiographic axial spondyloarthritis: results of a randomised, placebo-controlled trial (ABILITY-1). Ann Rheum Dis 2012. [Epub ahead of print].
40. Dougados M, Combe B, Braun J, et al. A randomised, multicentre, double-blind, placebo-controlled trial of etanercept in adults with refractory heel enthesitis in spondyloarthritis: the HEEL trial. Ann Rheum Dis 2010;69(8):1430–5.
41. Song IH, Hermann K, Haibel H, et al. Effects of etanercept versus sulfasalazine in early axial spondyloarthritis on active inflammatory lesions as detected by whole-body MRI (ESTHER): a 48-week randomised controlled trial. Ann Rheum Dis 2011;70(4):590–6.
42. Weber U, Lambert RG, Rufibach K, et al. Anterior chest wall inflammation by whole-body magnetic resonance imaging in patients with spondyloarthritis: lack of association between clinical and imaging findings in a cross-sectional study. Arthritis Res Ther 2012;14(1):R3.
43. Navarro-Compan V, Moreira V, Ariza-Ariza R, et al. Low doses of etanercept can be effective in ankylosing spondylitis patients who achieve remission of the disease. Clin Rheumatol 2011;30(7):993–6.
44. Lee J, Noh JW, Hwang JW, et al. Extended dosing of etanercept 25 mg can be effective in patients with ankylosing spondylitis: a retrospective analysis. Clin Rheumatol 2010;29(10):1149–54.
45. Lee SH, Lee YA, Hong SJ, et al. Etanercept 25 mg/week is effective enough to maintain remission for ankylosing spondylitis among Korean patients. Clin Rheumatol 2008;27(2):179–81.
46. Paccou J, Bacle-Boutry MA, Solau-Gervais E, et al. Dosage adjustment of anti-tumor necrosis factor-alpha inhibitor in ankylosing spondylitis is effective in maintaining remission in clinical practice. J Rheumatol 2012;39(7):1418–23.
47. Baraliakos X, Listing J, Rudwaleit M, et al. Safety and efficacy of readministration of infliximab after longterm continuous therapy and withdrawal in patients with ankylosing spondylitis. J Rheumatol 2007;34(3):510–5.
48. Brandt J, Listing J, Haibel H, et al. Long-term efficacy and safety of etanercept after readministration in patients with active ankylosing spondylitis. Rheumatology (Oxford) 2005;44(3):342–8.

49. Haibel H, Rudwaleit M, Listing J, et al. Efficacy of adalimumab in the treatment of axial spondylarthritis without radiographically defined sacroiliitis: results of a twelve-week randomized, double-blind, placebo-controlled trial followed by an open-label extension up to week fifty-two. Arthritis Rheum 2008;58(7):1981–91.
50. Ash R, Barkham N, McGonagle DG, et al. Long term results of a remission induction approach to early axial spondyloarthritis: still looking for the window of opportunity. Arthritis Rheum 2011;63(Suppl 10):S503.
51. Song IH, Althoff CE, Haibel H, et al. Frequency and duration of drug-free remission after 1 year of treatment with etanercept versus sulfasalazine in early axial spondyloarthritis: 2 year data of the ESTHER trial. Ann Rheum Dis 2012;71(7): 1212–5.
52. Anderson JJ, Baron G, van der Heijde D, et al. Ankylosing spondylitis assessment group preliminary definition of short-term improvement in ankylosing spondylitis. Arthritis Rheum 2001;44(8):1876–86.
53. Machado P, Landewe R, Lie E, et al. Ankylosing Spondylitis Disease Activity Score (ASDAS): defining cut-off values for disease activity states and improvement scores. Ann Rheum Dis 2011;70(1):47–53.
54. Navarro-Sarabia F, Fernandez-Sueiro JL, Torre-Alonso JC, et al. High-dose etanercept in ankylosing spondylitis: results of a 12-week randomized, double blind, controlled multicentre study (LOADET study). Rheumatology (Oxford) 2011;50(10):1828–37.
55. Bartelds GM, Krieckaert CL, Nurmohamed MT, et al. Development of antidrug antibodies against adalimumab and association with disease activity and treatment failure during long-term follow-up. JAMA 2011;305(14):1460–8.
56. Arends S, Lebbink HR, Spoorenberg A, et al. The formation of autoantibodies and antibodies to TNF-alpha blocking agents in relation to clinical response in patients with ankylosing spondylitis. Clin Exp Rheumatol 2010;28(5):661–8.
57. de Vries MK, Wolbink GJ, Stapel SO, et al. Inefficacy of infliximab in ankylosing spondylitis is correlated with antibody formation. Ann Rheum Dis 2007;66(1):133–4.
58. de Vries MK, Brouwer E, van der Horst-Bruinsma IE, et al. Decreased clinical response to adalimumab in ankylosing spondylitis is associated with antibody formation. Ann Rheum Dis 2009;68(11):1787–8.
59. de Vries MK, van der Horst-Bruinsma IE, Nurmohamed MT, et al. Immunogenicity does not influence treatment with etanercept in patients with ankylosing spondylitis. Ann Rheum Dis 2009;68(4):531–5.
60. Emi Aikawa N, de Carvalho JF, Artur Almeida Silva C, et al. Immunogenicity of Anti-TNF-alpha agents in autoimmune diseases. Clin Rev Allergy Immunol 2010;38(2–3):82–9.
61. Plasencia C, Pascual-Salcedo D, Nuno L, et al. Influence of immunogenicity on the efficacy of long-term treatment of spondyloarthritis with infliximab. Ann Rheum Dis 2012.
62. Ducourau E, Mulleman D, Paintaud G, et al. Antibodies toward infliximab are associated with low infliximab concentration at treatment initiation and poor infliximab maintenance in rheumatic diseases. Arthritis Res Ther 2011;13(3):R105.
63. Bartelds GM, Wijbrandts CA, Nurmohamed MT, et al. Clinical response to adalimumab: relationship to anti-adalimumab antibodies and serum adalimumab concentrations in rheumatoid arthritis. Ann Rheum Dis 2007;66(7):921–6.
64. Maini RN, Breedveld FC, Kalden JR, et al. Therapeutic efficacy of multiple intravenous infusions of anti-tumor necrosis factor alpha monoclonal antibody combined with low-dose weekly methotrexate in rheumatoid arthritis. Arthritis Rheum 1998;41(9):1552–63.

65. Colombel JF, Sandborn WJ, Reinisch W, et al. Infliximab, azathioprine, or combination therapy for Crohn's disease. N Engl J Med 2010;362(15):1383–95.
66. Li EK, Griffith JF, Lee VW, et al. Short-term efficacy of combination methotrexate and infliximab in patients with ankylosing spondylitis: a clinical and magnetic resonance imaging correlation. Rheumatology (Oxford) 2008;47(9):1358–63.
67. Breban M, Ravaud P, Claudepierre P, et al. Maintenance of infliximab treatment in ankylosing spondylitis: results of a one-year randomized controlled trial comparing systematic versus on-demand treatment. Arthritis Rheum 2008; 58(1):88–97.
68. Heiberg MS, Koldingsnes W, Mikkelsen K, et al. The comparative one-year performance of anti-tumor necrosis factor alpha drugs in patients with rheumatoid arthritis, psoriatic arthritis, and ankylosing spondylitis: results from a longitudinal, observational, multicenter study. Arthritis Rheum 2008;59(2):234–40.
69. Mulleman D, Lauferon F, Wendling D, et al. Infliximab in ankylosing spondylitis: alone or in combination with methotrexate? A pharmacokinetic comparative study. Arthritis Res Ther 2011;13(3):R82.
70. Rudwaleit M, Baraliakos X, Listing J, et al. Magnetic resonance imaging of the spine and the sacroiliac joints in ankylosing spondylitis and undifferentiated spondyloarthritis during treatment with etanercept. Ann Rheum Dis 2005; 64(9):1305–10.
71. Lambert RG, Salonen D, Rahman P, et al. Adalimumab significantly reduces both spinal and sacroiliac joint inflammation in patients with ankylosing spondylitis: a multicenter, randomized, double-blind, placebo-controlled study. Arthritis Rheum 2007;56(12):4005–14.
72. Maksymowych WP, Salonen D, Inman RD, et al. Low-dose infliximab (3 mg/kg) significantly reduces spinal inflammation on magnetic resonance imaging in patients with ankylosing spondylitis: a randomized placebo-controlled study. J Rheumatol 2010;37(8):1728–34.
73. Baraliakos X, Listing J, Rudwaleit M, et al. The relationship between inflammation and new bone formation in patients with ankylosing spondylitis. Arthritis Res Ther 2008;10(5):R104.
74. van der Heijde D, Machado P, Braun J, et al. MRI inflammation at the vertebral unit only marginally predicts new syndesmophyte formation: a multilevel analysis in patients with ankylosing spondylitis. Ann Rheum Dis 2012;71(3):369–73.
75. Maksymowych WP, Chiowchanwisawakit P, Clare T, et al. Inflammatory lesions of the spine on magnetic resonance imaging predict the development of new syndesmophytes in ankylosing spondylitis: evidence of a relationship between inflammation and new bone formation. Arthritis Rheum 2009;60(1):93–102.
76. Chiowchanwisawakit P, Lambert RG, Conner-Spady B, et al. Focal fat lesions at vertebral corners on magnetic resonance imaging predict the development of new syndesmophytes in ankylosing spondylitis. Arthritis Rheum 2011;63(8): 2215–25.
77. Pedersen SJ, Chiowchanwisawakit P, Lambert RG, et al. Resolution of inflammation following treatment of ankylosing spondylitis is associated with new bone formation. J Rheumatol 2011;38(7):1349–54.
78. Maksymowych WP, Morency N, Conner-Spady B, et al. Suppression of inflammation and effects on new bone formation in ankylosing spondylitis: evidence for a window of opportunity in disease modification. Ann Rheum Dis 2012 [Epub ahead of print].
79. Maksymowych WP. Disease modification in ankylosing spondylitis. Nat Rev Rheumatol 2010;6(2):75–81.

80. Chiowchanwisawakit P, Lambert RG, Maksymowych W. What is the association between inflammation and focal fat infiltration in AS and does treatment matter? Ann Rheum Dis 2010;69(Suppl 3):262.
81. Song IH, Hermann KG, Haibel H, et al. Relationship between active inflammatory lesions in the spine and sacroiliac joints and new development of chronic lesions on whole-body MRI in early axial spondyloarthritis: results of the ESTHER trial at week 48. Ann Rheum Dis 2011;70(7):1257–63.
82. Wanders A, Heijde D, Landewe R, et al. Nonsteroidal antiinflammatory drugs reduce radiographic progression in patients with ankylosing spondylitis: a randomized clinical trial. Arthritis Rheum 2005;52(6):1756–65.
83. Poddubnyy D, Rudwaleit M, Haibel H, et al. Effect of non-steroidal anti-inflammatory drugs on radiographic spinal progression in patients with axial spondyloarthritis: results from the German Spondyloarthritis Inception Cohort. Ann Rheum Dis 2012. [Epub ahead of print].
84. Kroon F, Landewé R, Dougados M, van der Heijde D. Continuous NSAID use reverts the effects of inflammation on radiographic progression in patients with ankylosing spondylitis. Annals Rheum Dis 2012. [Epub ahead of print].
85. Dadoun S, Geri G, Paternotte S, et al. Switching between tumour necrosis factor blockers in spondyloarthritis: a retrospective monocentre study of 222 patients. Clin Exp Rheumatol 2011;29(6):1010–3.
86. Delaunay C, Farrenq V, Marini-Portugal A, et al. Infliximab to etanercept switch in patients with spondyloarthropathies and psoriatic arthritis: preliminary data. J Rheumatol 2005;32(11):2183–5.
87. Cantini F, Niccoli L, Benucci M, et al. Switching from infliximab to once-weekly administration of 50 mg etanercept in resistant or intolerant patients with ankylosing spondylitis: results of a fifty-four-week study. Arthritis Rheum 2006;55(5): 812–6.
88. Coates LC, Cawkwell LS, Ng NW, et al. Real life experience confirms sustained response to long-term biologics and switching in ankylosing spondylitis. Rheumatology (Oxford) 2008;47(6):897–900.
89. Conti F, Ceccarelli F, Marocchi E, et al. Switching tumour necrosis factor alpha antagonists in patients with ankylosing spondylitis and psoriatic arthritis: an observational study over a 5-year period. Ann Rheum Dis 2007;66(10):1393–7.
90. Pradeep DJ, Keat AC, Gaffney K, et al. Switching anti-TNF therapy in ankylosing spondylitis. Rheumatology (Oxford) 2008;47(11):1726–7.
91. Rudwaleit M, Van den Bosch F, Kron M, et al. Effectiveness and safety of adalimumab in patients with ankylosing spondylitis or psoriatic arthritis and history of anti-tumor necrosis factor therapy. Arthritis Res Ther 2010;12(3):R117.
92. Lie E, van der Heijde D, Uhlig T, et al. Effectiveness of switching between TNF inhibitors in ankylosing spondylitis: data from the NOR-DMARD register. Ann Rheum Dis 2011;70(1):157–63.
93. Rudwaleit M, van der Heijde D, Landewe R, et al. The development of Assessment of SpondyloArthritis international Society classification criteria for axial spondyloarthritis (part II): validation and final selection. Ann Rheum Dis 2009; 68(6):777–83.
94. Glintborg B, Ostergaard M, Krogh N, et al. Clinical response, drug survival and predictors thereof in 432 patients with ankylosing spondylitis switching anti tumor necrosis factor α therapy: results form the Danish nationwide DANBIO registry. Ann Rheum Dis 2012;71(Suppl 3):111.
95. Song IH, Poddubnyy D. New treatment targets in ankylosing spondylitis and other spondyloarthritides. Curr Opin Rheumatol 2011;23(4):346–51.

96. Rudwaleit M, Listing J, Brandt J, et al. Prediction of a major clinical response (BASDAI 50) to tumour necrosis factor alpha blockers in ankylosing spondylitis. Ann Rheum Dis 2004;63(6):665–70.
97. Rudwaleit M, Claudepierre P, Wordsworth P, et al. Effectiveness, safety, and predictors of good clinical response in 1250 patients treated with adalimumab for active ankylosing spondylitis. J Rheumatol 2009;36(4):801–8.
98. Barkham N, Keen HI, Coates LC, et al. Clinical and imaging efficacy of infliximab in HLA-B27-Positive patients with magnetic resonance imaging-determined early sacroiliitis. Arthritis Rheum 2009;60(4):946–54.
99. Brandt J, Haibel H, Cornely D, et al. Successful treatment of active ankylosing spondylitis with the anti-tumor necrosis factor alpha monoclonal antibody infliximab. Arthritis Rheum 2000;43(6):1346–52.
100. Barkham N, Kong KO, Tennant A, et al. The unmet need for anti-tumour necrosis factor (anti-TNF) therapy in ankylosing spondylitis. Rheumatology (Oxford) 2005;44(10):1277–81.
101. Cohen JD, Cunin P, Farrenq V, et al. Estimation of the Bath Ankylosing Spondylitis Disease Activity Index cutoff for perceived symptom relief in patients with spondyloarthropathies. J Rheumatol 2006;33(1):79–81.
102. Maksymowych WP, Richardson R, Mallon C, et al. Evaluation and validation of the patient acceptable symptom state (PASS) in patients with ankylosing spondylitis. Arthritis Rheum 2007;57(1):133–9.
103. Kiltz U, Baraliakos X, Karakostas P, et al. How much inflammation do patients with axial spondyloarthritis have who report low levels of disease activity? A prospective cohort study. Ann Rheum Dis 2011;70(Suppl 3):521.
104. Breban M, Vignon E, Claudepierre P, et al. Efficacy of infliximab in refractory ankylosing spondylitis: results of a six-month open-label study. Rheumatology (Oxford) 2002;41(11):1280–5.
105. Heiberg MS, Lie E, Van der Heijde D, et al. A substantial proportioin of AS patients respond to TNF inhibitors despite not fulfilling the criteria for initiating anti-TNF therapy according to the ASAS/EULAR recommendations. Ann Rheum Dis 2009;68(Suppl 3):631.
106. Maksymowych WP, Gladman D, Rahman P, et al. The Canadian Rheumatology Association/ Spondyloarthritis Research Consortium of Canada treatment recommendations for the management of spondyloarthritis: a national multidisciplinary stakeholder project. J Rheumatol 2007;34(11):2273–84.
107. Colbert RA, Cronstein BN. Biosimilars: the debate continues. Arthritis Rheum 2011;63(10):2848–50.
108. Park W, Hrycaj P, Kovalenko V, et al. Randomized, double-blind, phase 1 study demonstrates equivalence in pharmacokinetics, safety, and efficacy of CT-P13 and infliximab in patients with ankylosing spondylitis. Ann Rheum Dis 2012; 71(Suppl3):111.
109. Dranitsaris G, Amir E, Dorward K. Biosimilars of biological drug therapies: regulatory, clinical and commercial considerations. Drugs 2011;71(12): 1527–36.
110. Mellstedt H, Niederwieser D, Ludwig H. The challenge of biosimilars. Ann Oncol 2008;19(3):411–9.
111. Roger SD. Biosimilars: current status and future directions. Expert Opin Biol Ther 2010;10(7):1011–8.
112. Keystone EC. Does anti-tumor necrosis factor-alpha therapy affect risk of serious infection and cancer in patients with rheumatoid arthritis?: a review of longterm data. J Rheumatol 2011;38(8):1552–62.

113. Bongartz T, Sutton AJ, Sweeting MJ, et al. Anti-TNF antibody therapy in rheumatoid arthritis and the risk of serious infections and malignancies: systematic review and meta-analysis of rare harmful effects in randomized controlled trials. JAMA 2006;295(19):2275–85.
114. Alonso-Ruiz A, Pijoan JI, Ansuategui E, et al. Tumor necrosis factor alpha drugs in rheumatoid arthritis: systematic review and metaanalysis of efficacy and safety. BMC Musculoskelet Disord 2008;9:52.
115. Leombruno JP, Einarson TR, Keystone EC. The safety of anti-tumour necrosis factor treatments in rheumatoid arthritis: meta and exposure-adjusted pooled analyses of serious adverse events. Ann Rheum Dis 2009;68(7):1136–45.
116. Wolfe F, Michaud K. Biologic treatment of rheumatoid arthritis and the risk of malignancy: analyses from a large US observational study. Arthritis Rheum 2007;56(9):2886–95.
117. Dixon WG, Watson KD, Lunt M, et al. Influence of anti-tumor necrosis factor therapy on cancer incidence in patients with rheumatoid arthritis who have had a prior malignancy: results from the British Society for Rheumatology Biologics Register. Arthritis Care Res (Hoboken) 2010;62(6):755–63.
118. Strangfeld A, Hierse F, Rau R, et al. Risk of incident or recurrent malignancies among patients with rheumatoid arthritis exposed to biologic therapy in the German biologics register RABBIT. Arthritis Res Ther 2010;12(1):R5.
119. Geborek P, Bladstrom A, Turesson C, et al. Tumour necrosis factor blockers do not increase overall tumour risk in patients with rheumatoid arthritis, but may be associated with an increased risk of lymphomas. Ann Rheum Dis 2005;64(5): 699–703.
120. Askling J, Baecklund E, Granath F, et al. Anti-tumour necrosis factor therapy in rheumatoid arthritis and risk of malignant lymphomas: relative risks and time trends in the Swedish Biologics Register. Ann Rheum Dis 2009;68(5):648–53.
121. Askling J, van Vollenhoven RF, Granath F, et al. Cancer risk in patients with rheumatoid arthritis treated with anti-tumor necrosis factor alpha therapies: does the risk change with the time since start of treatment? Arthritis Rheum 2009;60(11): 3180–9.
122. Askling J, Klareskog L, Blomqvist P, et al. Risk for malignant lymphoma in ankylosing spondylitis: a nationwide Swedish case-control study. Ann Rheum Dis 2006;65(9):1184–7.
123. Mariette X, Tubach F, Bagheri H, et al. Lymphoma in patients treated with anti-TNF: results of the 3-year prospective French RATIO registry. Ann Rheum Dis 2010;69(2):400–8.
124. Askling J, Fahrbach K, Nordstrom B, et al. Cancer risk with tumor necrosis factor alpha (TNF) inhibitors: meta-analysis of randomized controlled trials of adalimumab, etanercept, and infliximab using patient level data. Pharmacoepidemiol Drug Saf 2011;20(2):119–30.

How Important is Early Therapy in Axial Spondyloarthritis?

Joachim Sieper, MD[a,*], Jürgen Braun, MD[b]

KEYWORDS

- Axial spondyloarthritis • TNF blockers • NSAIDs

KEY POINTS

- Patients with axial spondyloarthritis respond best to TNF-blocker therapy if treated early in the course of their disease. Patients seem also to respond better to NSAiDs if treated early.
- There is currently no clear evidence that early therapeutic intervention is mandatory in axial SpA to,prevent structural damage. More research is needed in this area. NSAIDs seem to prevent sturctural damage in established ankylosing spondylitis.

INTRODUCTION

Currently there are mainly 2 groups of drugs that have been shown effective in the treatment of patients with axSpA, NSAIDs and TNF-α blockers, which have been approved for those patients who do not adequately respond to NSAID treatment.[1] Conventional disease-modifying antirheumatic drugs and some other biologics, such as anakinra[2] and abatacept,[3] have not been shown so far to be clinically efficacious in this disease.

Most of the early treatment trials in axSpA have been performed in patients with ankylosing spondylitis (AS) classified according to the modified New York criteria—implying that patients already had structural changes in the SI joints (radiographic sacroiliitis). The mean symptom duration of patients included in treatment trials both with NSAIDs and TNF blockers has been between 10 and 14 years. Although short symptom duration and young age have been identified as parameters predictive of good response rates,[4] there were, until recently, no data available addressing the question of whether axSpA patients respond better when treated earlier. The development of the ASAS classification criteria for axSpA[5] was a big step forward in that regard because they allow including patients in treatment trials at an early phase of their disease before the occurrence of radiographic changes in the SI joints. This

[a] Section of Rheumatology, Campus Benjamin Franklin, Charité University, Hindenburgdamm 30, Berlin 12200, Germany; [b] Rheumazentrum Ruhrgebiet, Herne and Ruhr Universität Bochum, Germany
* Corresponding author.
E-mail address: Joachim.sieper@charite.de

Rheum Dis Clin N Am 38 (2012) 635–642
http://dx.doi.org/10.1016/j.rdc.2012.08.001 **rheumatic.theclinics.com**
0889-857X/12/$ – see front matter

group has recently be termed as nonradiographic axSpA (nr-axSpA). The ASAS classification criteria for the whole group of axSpA are fulfilled if patients have chronic back pain greater than 3 months, if symptoms start at an age younger than 45 years, and if they have either active inflammation in the SI joints on MRI plus 1 additional clinical or laboratory feature typical of SpA, or if they are positive for HLA-B27 plus 2 additional other SpA features.

This overview discusses the available data on whether early treatment strategies in patients with axSpA have an effect on (1) the percentage of patients reaching clinical remission, (2) achieving drug-free remission, and (3) the progress of radiographic progression in the spine as a parameter for structural damage.

THE EFFECT OF ANTI-TNF THERAPY ON CLINICAL PARAMETERS DEPENDS ON SYMPTOM DURATION

This article focuses on clinical remission rates according to the ASAS definition[6] but also reports on Bath Ankylosing Spondylitis Disease Activity Index (BASDAI) 50% and/or ASAS 40% response rates[6] if data on remission are not available. These data are summarized in **Table 1**. Clinical remission was reached in TNF blocker trials in approximately 25% of patients with established AS,[7–9] but AS patients with a symptom duration of less than 10 years showed a better response rate than patients with a symptom duration of between 10 and 20 or more years.[4] In another analysis of an open-label AS trial, remission was reached in 50% of patients younger than 30 years in contrast to only 19% of patients between the age of 40 and 49 years, whereas young age as predictor of a good response was largely overlapping with short symptom duration.[10]

The first TNF blocker trial in patients with nr-axSpA was performed with adalimumab in the usual dosage (40 mg subcutaneous every 2 weeks).[11] Although these patients did not yet fulfill the modified New York criteria for radiographic sacroiliitis, the mean symptom duration was still 7 to 8 years. Remission was reached in 22.7% (in comparison to 0% in the placebo group)—a percentage similar to the 22.1% of patients in the AS treatment trial with adalimumab.[8] The remission rate went up to 50%, however, when concentrating on the patients with symptom duration less than 3 years—which was considerably higher than the 16% in those with symptom duration greater than 3 years.[11] A larger, phase III trial with 185 nr-axSpA patients treated with adalimumab (using the same dosing) or placebo for 12 weeks followed.[12] Again, the mean symptom duration at inclusion was approximately 10 years. An ASAS 40 response rate was achieved in 36.3% of the adalimumab-treated patients versus 14.9% in the placebo group. The difference between the 2 groups, however, was larger in the subgroup of patients with less than 5 years symptom duration: 49% versus 6%, compared with 31% versus 20%, in patients with symptom duration greater than 5 years, respectively. In another study performed in the United Kingdom with infliximab (5 mg/kg 4 times intravenously until week 12), axSpA patients were included if the symptom duration was less than 3 years, if they had active inflammation in the SI joints detected by MRI, and if they complained about inflammatory back pain and were HLA-B27 positive.[13] Only approximately 12% of these patients already had radiographic sacroiliitis. The remission rate at week 16 in these patients with short symptom duration and a positive MRI was as high as 55.6% versus 12.5% in the placebo group. In another nonblinded but prospective randomized head-to-head trial performed within axSpA patients who had a symptom duration less than 5 years and a positive MRI at inclusion, the remission rate was 50% after 1 year of treatment with etanercept (50mg per week s.c) versus 19% in the group treated with sulfasazine.[14]

Table 1
Clinical response rates in axSpA, including nr-axSpA and AS, in relation to symptom duration

Name of Study	Treatment[a]	Subgroup	No. of Patients	Symptom Duration	Clinical Remission (%)[a,b]	BASDAI 50 or ASAS 40 (%)[b]	Ref.
ASSERT	Infliximab	AS	201	7.7	22.4		7
ATLAS	Adalimumab	AS	208	11.3	22.1		8
International etanercept study	Etanercept	AS	138	10.1	17		9
Pooled AS data	Infliximab Etanercept	AS	99	14.8		56	4
<10 y						73	
10–20 y						58	
>20 y						31	
German nr-axSpA study	Adalimumab	nr-axSpr	22	7	22.7	54.5	11
≤3 y					50		
>3 y					16		
ESTHER	Etanercept	axSpA[c]	40	<5 y	50		14
Leeds axSpA study	Infliximab	axSpA[c]	20	<3 y	55.6		13
ABILITY-1	Adalimumab	nr-axSpA	91	10.1	16	36	12
≤5 y						48	
>5 y						31	
INFAST	Infliximab	axSpA[c]	105	<3 y	61.9		12

[a] Patients were treated between 12 and 52 weeks.
[b] According to the ASAS definition.[6]
[c] axSpA includes both patients with nr-axSpA and AS.

Half of these patients did not have radiographic sacroiliitis and could thus be labeled as having nr-axSpA, whereas the other half already had structural changes. The symptom duration and the baseline disease activity were similar in both groups. The observation that the response rate was similar in these 2 groups indicates that presence or absence of radiographic sacroiliitis does not matter regarding the response rate if the other parameters are similar.[15]

In a recent treatment trial (Infliximab as First line Therapy in Patients with Early Active Spondyloarthritis Trial [INFAST]), axSpA patients with a symptom duration of less than 3 years, who were not allowed to be included when they had already been refractory to NSAIDs, were treated blindly for 28 weeks either with infliximab (5 mg/kg in the usual sequence of dosing) plus naproxen (1000 mg/d) or just with naproxen plus placebo.[16] In this study the, until now, highest remission rate was achieved in the group treated with both compounds: 62% versus 35% in the group treated with naproxen only.

THE EFFECT OF NSAID THERAPY ON CLINICAL PARAMETERS ALSO DEPENDS ON SYMPTOM DURATION

The vast majority of NSAID trials have been performed in patients with established AS, and remission rates between 11% and 15% are reported.[6,17,18] As discussed previously, in the only early study performed in patients with axSpA (symptom duration <3 years), a remission rate of 33% was found.[16] These results indicate that an early and consequent treatment with NSAIDs (patients in this study were treated with naproxen 1000 mg/d for 28 weeks) in active axSpA patients seems effective and that good response rates can be expected when therapy starts early. There was even a constant increase in the remission rate over time up to week 28. This may indicate that patients need to be treated continuously for longer periods of time and/or that the natural course of the disease may be more favorable in some patients. Alternatively, the response rate has been augmented artificially by excluding patients who were already known not to respond to NSAIDs sufficiently, but this also was the case in all previous NSAID trials of AS.

POTENTIAL EFFECT OF EARLY TREATMENT ON REACHING DRUG-FREE REMISSION

In all TNF blocker trials performed in patients with axSpA so far, the relapse rates after drug withdrawal were high, indicating a chronic inflammatory disease and that TNF blocker therapies are not curative. Nonetheless, although there were only minor differences in the relapse rates reported in these trials, a shorter symptom duration may have some effect on these rates: in patients with a symptom duration greater than 10 years,[19] 7 to 8 years,[20] 2.9 years,[21] or 15 months,[22] a clinical relapse was found in 95% to 100%, 84%, 77%, and 60% of patients, respectively. In the INFAST trial, in which active patients were treated who were either NSAID-naïve or were not yet treated with a full doses of NSAIDs, the remission rate after follow-up of half a year without TNF blockers was the highest, with 40% to 50% of patients remaining in remission.[23] Thus, the question about the potential of very early treatment to reach drug-free remission is open and justifies, in the authors' opinion, further investigations.

Half of the patients who had reached remission at week 28 with either of the 2 treatment strategies compared in the INFAST trial were randomized to continue on naproxen (1000 mg/d) for another 6 months whereas the other half of the patients were completely taken off drugs. The remission rates were 46% and 41%, respectively, a difference that was not significant.[23] Thus, continuation of NSAID treatment in axSpA in remission does not seem to have a major influence on clinical remission rates. This may be different in longer-term follow-up studies, however, and it may be different for other outcome parameters, such as structural progression.

POTENTIAL EFFECT OF EARLY TREATMENT ON STOPPING OR RETARDING STRUCTURAL PROGRESSION

Structural progression has been quantified in nearly all axSpA studies by measuring structural damage in the spine, most often by applying the Modified Stroke Ankylosing Spondylitis Spinal Score (mSASSS),[24] which is predominantly but not exclusively a score for new bone formation. Although NSAIDs seem to have a retarding effect on radiographic progression in AS patients[25–27] (discussed in more detail by Poddubnyy and colleagues elsewhere in this issue), this seems not to be the case in patients with nr-axSpA. This may be explained, however, by methodologic and anatomic issues. Little is known about radiographic progression in the spine (as compared with the SI joints) in early stages of the disease, but a major progression in the spine in early disease in patients with nr-axSpA seems unlikely and has not been found in the German Spondyloarthritis Inception Cohort.[26] Therefore, using mSASSS, any interventional effect is difficult to measure. More sensitive techniques may become available in the future (for example, low-dose CT), which have a higher sensitivity to change for the detection of small structural changes—potentially including the thoracic spine where most of the spinal changes are known to occur.[28,29] Nonetheless, currently there are no data to support an indication for early treatment of axSpA with NSAIDs to prevent structural damage. TNF blockers, in contrast to NSAIDs, have not been shown to inhibit progression of structural changes in patients with established AS.[30] It remains to be seen, however, whether this might be different in cases of early intervention.[31] A question in this regard is whether fatty changes as detected by MRI[31] are the main predecessors of bone formation and how they may be influenced by therapeutic interventions.

WHAT IS THE OPTIMAL STRATEGY IN THE MANAGEMENT OF PATIENTS WITH AXSPA?

There are at least 2 areas of discussion. The first question is, Which is more important—identifying patients with axSpA at any disease stage, concentrating on inflammation regardless of symptom duration and treating whenever there is evidence of that, or trying to detect patients with axSpA as early as possible to suppress inflammation as early as possible? These strategies are not exclusive, and the former is clinical routine in most rheumatologic settings around the world. In an analogy to rheumatoid arthritis, however, the potential of inhibition of structural damage, which is mainly new bone formation in AS, requires additional investigations in the future. The 2 main points in the context of early therapeutic intervention are, Can structural changes in the SI joints be prevented? and Can progression in the spine be prevented by early intervention? There are not sufficient data available to answer these questions at the moment.

Another question relates to the argument of comparing improvement rates and how to deal with recent concepts of predicting response to therapy.[32–34] What is the cutoff for an acceptable response rate, if any, and what does this mean for the treatment of individual patients? Related to these questions, it was recently shown that the BASDAI cutoff of 4 may not be the best tool to identify patients in need of anti-TNF therapy.[35] Using the Ankylosing Spondylitis Disease Activity Score seems an alternative,[36] but the BASDAI is easier to handle and all approvals[37] relate to that partly arbitrary cutoff.

Thus, there are several open questions that cannot be answered with a simple yes or no at present. More research in this area is needed.

SUMMARY

There is growing evidence that patients with axSpA respond better to TNF blocker therapy if started early. This is not only the case for patients with AS but also for those with nr-axSpA. Which part of the complaints in the subgroup of axSpA patients with longstanding disease, with low grade of structural damage and with low grade of inflammation as detected by CRP and MRI can be explained by fibromyalgia has yet to be investigated. Treatment with NSAIDs seems to result in superior improvement rates of measures of clinical disease activity if treatment of patients with axSpA starts in early disease stages. Recent data have suggested that early treatment with TNF blockers may induce drug-free remission in a higher percentage of patients treated early compared with those with later treatment. These rates are still low, however, and the majority of patients seem to need continuous anti-inflammatory therapy. There are currently no data available to show that early therapeutic intervention is able to retard progression of structural damage in patients with axSpA. As it stands now, the recommendation remains that patients with persistent active disease should be treated with an optimal dose of NSAIDs continuously and that anti-TNF therapy should be started if that does not lead to an acceptable symptom state and suppression of inflammation. Further research in this important area of management of patients with axSpA is necessary.

REFERENCES

1. Braun J, van den Berg R, Baraliakos X, et al. 2010 Update of the ASAS/EULAR recommendations for the management of ankylosing spondylitis. Ann Rheum Dis 2011;70(6):896–904.
2. Haibel H, Rudwaleit M, Listing J, et al. Open label trial of anakinra in active ankylosing spondylitis over 24 weeks. Ann Rheum Dis 2005;64(2):296–8.
3. Song IH, Heldmann F, Rudwaleit M, et al. Treatment of active ankylosing spondylitis with abatacept: an open-label, 24-week pilot study. Ann Rheum Dis 2011; 70(6):1108–10.
4. Rudwaleit M, Listing J, Brandt J, et al. Prediction of a major clinical response (BASDAI 50) to tumour necrosis factor alpha blockers in ankylosing spondylitis. Ann Rheum Dis 2004;63(6):665–70.
5. Rudwaleit M, van der Heijde D, Landewe R, et al. The development of assessment of SpondyloArthritis International Society classification criteria for axial spondyloarthritis (part II): validation and final selection. Ann Rheum Dis 2009; 68(6):777–83.
6. Anderson JJ, Baron G, van der Heijde D, et al. Ankylosing spondylitis assessment group preliminary definition of short-term improvement in ankylosing spondylitis. Arthritis Rheum 2001;44(8):1876–86.
7. van der Heijde D, Dijkmans B, Geusens P, et al. Efficacy and safety of infliximab in patients with ankylosing spondylitis: results of a randomized, placebo-controlled trial (ASSERT). Arthritis Rheum 2005;52(2):582–91.
8. van der Heijde D, Kivitz A, Schiff MH, et al. Efficacy and safety of adalimumab in patients with ankylosing spondylitis: results of a multicenter, randomized, double-blind, placebo-controlled trial. Arthritis Rheum 2006;54(7):2136–46.
9. Davis JC Jr, Van Der Heijde D, Braun J, et al. Recombinant human tumor necrosis factor receptor (etanercept) for treating ankylosing spondylitis: a randomized, controlled trial. Arthritis Rheum 2003;48(11):3230–6.
10. Rudwaleit M, Claudepierre P, Wordsworth P, et al. Effectiveness, safety, and predictors of good clinical response in 1250 patients treated with adalimumab for active ankylosing spondylitis. J Rheumatol 2009;36(4):801–8.

11. Haibel H, Rudwaleit M, Listing J, et al. Efficacy of adalimumab in the treatment of axial spondylarthritis without radiographically defined sacroiliitis: results of a twelve-week randomized, double-blind, placebo-controlled trial followed by an open-label extension up to week fifty-two. Arthritis Rheum 2008;58(7):1981–91.
12. Sieper J, van der Heijde D, Dougados M, et al. Efficacy and safety of adalimumab in patients with non-radiographic axial spondyloarthritis: results of a randomised placebo-controlled trial (ABILITY-1). Ann Rheum Dis 2012. [Epub ahead of print].
13. Barkham N, Keen HI, Coates LC, et al. Clinical and imaging efficacy of infliximab in HLA-B27-Positive patients with magnetic resonance imaging-determined early sacroiliitis. Arthritis Rheum 2009;60(4):946–54.
14. Song IH, Hermann K, Haibel H, et al. Effects of etanercept versus sulfasalazine in early axial spondyloarthritis on active inflammatory lesions as detected by whole-body MRI (ESTHER): a 48-week randomised controlled trial. Ann Rheum Dis 2011;70(4):590–6.
15. Song IH, Hermann KG, Haibel H, et al. Similar response rates in patients with ankylosing spondylitis and non-radiographic axial spondyloarthritis after one year of treatment with etanercept—results from the ESTHER trial. Ann Rheum Dis 2012;71(Suppl 3):247.
16. Sieper J, Lenaerts J, Wollenhaupt J, et al. Double-blind, placebo-controlled, 28-week trial of efficacy and safety of infliximab plus naproxen vs naproxen alone in patients with early active spondyloarthritis treated with a submaximal dose of NSAIDs: preliminary results of INFAST part I. Ann Rheum Dis 2012;71(Suppl 3):247.
17. van der Heijde D, Baraf HS, Ramos-Remus C, et al. Evaluation of the efficacy of etoricoxib in ankylosing spondylitis: results of a fifty-two-week, randomized, controlled study. Arthritis Rheum 2005;52(4):1205–15.
18. Sieper J, Klopsch T, Richter M, et al. Comparison of two different dosages of celecoxib with diclofenac for the treatment of active ankylosing spondylitis: results of a 12-week randomised, double-blind, controlled study. Ann Rheum Dis 2008; 67(3):323–9.
19. Baraliakos X, Listing J, Brandt J, et al. Clinical response to discontinuation of anti-TNF therapy in patients with ankylosing spondylitis after 3 years of continuous treatment with infliximab. Arthritis Res Ther 2005;7(3):R439–44.
20. Haibel H, Heldmann F, Rudwaleit M, et al. Long-term efficacy of adalimumab for patients with active, non-radiographic, axial spondyloarthritis who relapsed following adalimumab withdrawal. Ann Rheum Dis 2010;69:59.
21. Song IH, Althoff CE, Haibel H, et al. Frequency and duration of drug-free remission after 1 year of treatment with etanercept versus sulfasalazine in early axial spondyloarthritis: 2 year data of the ESTHER trial. Ann Rheum Dis 2012;71(7):1212–5.
22. Barkham N, Keen HI, Coates LC, et al. Clinical response and time to active disease following infliximab therapy in patients with HLA-B27 positive very early ankylosing spondylitis. Ann Rheum Dis 2009;68(Suppl 3):72.
23. Sieper J, Lenaerts J, Wollenhaupt J, et al. Double-blind, placebo-controlled, 28-week trial of efficacy and safety of infliximab plus naproxen vs naproxen alone in patients with early active spondyloarthritis treated with a submaximal dose of NSAIDs: preliminary results of INFAST part II. Ann Rheum Dis 2012;71(Suppl 3):247.
24. Creemers MC, Franssen MJ, van't Hof MA, et al. Assessment of outcome in ankylosing spondylitis: an extended radiographic scoring system. Ann Rheum Dis 2005;64(1):127–9.
25. Wanders A, Heijde D, Landewe R, et al. Nonsteroidal antiinflammatory drugs reduce radiographic progression in patients with ankylosing spondylitis: a randomized clinical trial. Arthritis Rheum 2005;52(6):1756–65.

26. Poddubnyy D, Rudwaleit M, Haibel H, et al. Effect of non-steroidal anti-inflammatory drugs on radiographic spinal progression in patients with axial spondyloarthritis: results from the German Spondyloarthritis Inception Cohort. Ann Rheum Dis 2012. [Epub ahead of print].
27. Kroon F, Landewe R, Dougados M, et al. Continuous NSAID use reverts the effects of inflammation on radiographic progression in patients with ankylosing spondylitis. Ann Rheum Dis 2012. [Epub ahead of print].
28. Baraliakos X, Landewe R, Hermann KG, et al. Inflammation in ankylosing spondylitis: a systematic description of the extent and frequency of acute spinal changes using magnetic resonance imaging. Ann Rheum Dis 2005;64(5):730–4.
29. Althoff CE, Sieper J, Song IH, et al. Active inflammation and structural change in early active axial spondyloarthritis as detected by whole-body MRI. Ann Rheum Dis 2012. [Epub ahead of print].
30. van der Heijde D, Landewe R, Baraliakos X, et al. Radiographic findings following two years of infliximab therapy in patients with ankylosing spondylitis. Arthritis Rheum 2008;58(10):3063–70.
31. Song IH, Hermann KG, Haibel H, et al. Relationship between active inflammatory lesions in the spine and sacroiliac joints and new development of chronic lesions on whole-body MRI in early axial spondyloarthritis: results of the ESTHER trial at week 48. Ann Rheum Dis 2011;70(7):1257–63.
32. Vastesaeger N, van der Heijde D, Inman RD, et al. Predicting the outcome of ankylosing spondylitis therapy. Ann Rheum Dis 2011;70(6):973–81.
33. Rudwaleit M, Schwarzlose S, Hilgert ES, et al. MRI in predicting a major clinical response to anti-tumour necrosis factor treatment in ankylosing spondylitis. Ann Rheum Dis 2008;67(9):1276–81.
34. Sieper J, van der Heijde D, Dougados M, et al. Early response to adalimumab predicts long-term remission through 5 years of treatment in patients with ankylosing spondylitis. Ann Rheum Dis 2012;71(5):700–6.
35. Kiltz U, Baraliakos X, Karakostas P, et al. The degree of spinal inflammation is similar in patients with axial spondyloarthritis who report high or low levels of disease activity: a cohort study. Ann Rheum Dis 2012;71(7):1207–11.
36. van der Heijde D, Lie E, Kvien TK, et al. ASDAS, a highly discriminatory ASAS-endorsed disease activity score in patients with ankylosing spondylitis. Ann Rheum Dis 2009;68(12):1811–8.
37. van der Heijde D, Sieper J, Maksymowych WP, et al. 2010 update of the international ASAS recommendations for the use of anti-TNF agents in patients with axial spondyloarthritis. Ann Rheum Dis 2011;70(6):905–8.

Index

Note: Page numbers of article titles are in **boldface** type.

Rheum Dis Clin N Am 38 (2012) 643–652
http://dx.doi.org/10.1016/S0889-857X(12)00105-6 rheumatic.theclinics.com
0889-857X/12/$ – see front matter

I

O

P

R

U

V

W

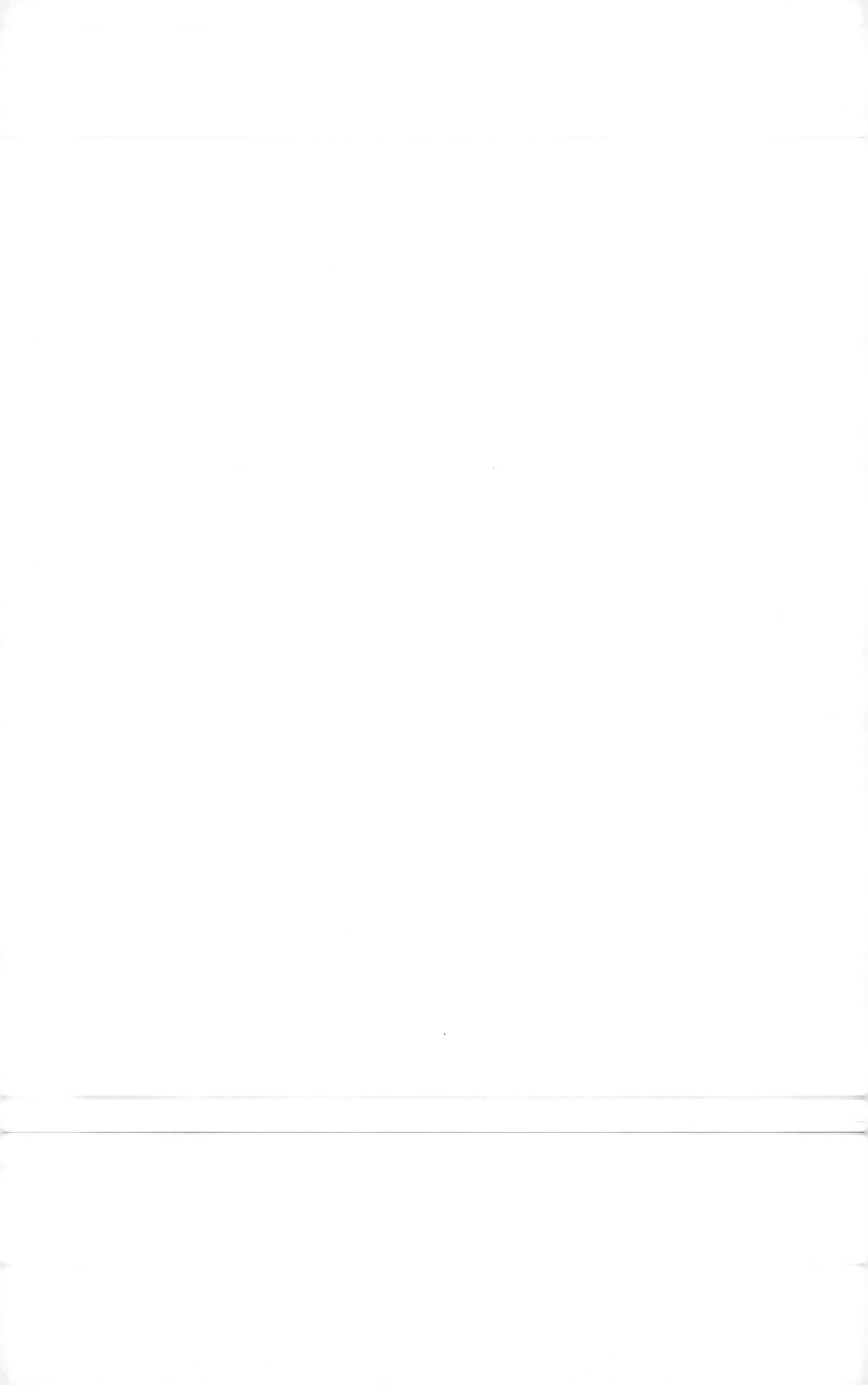

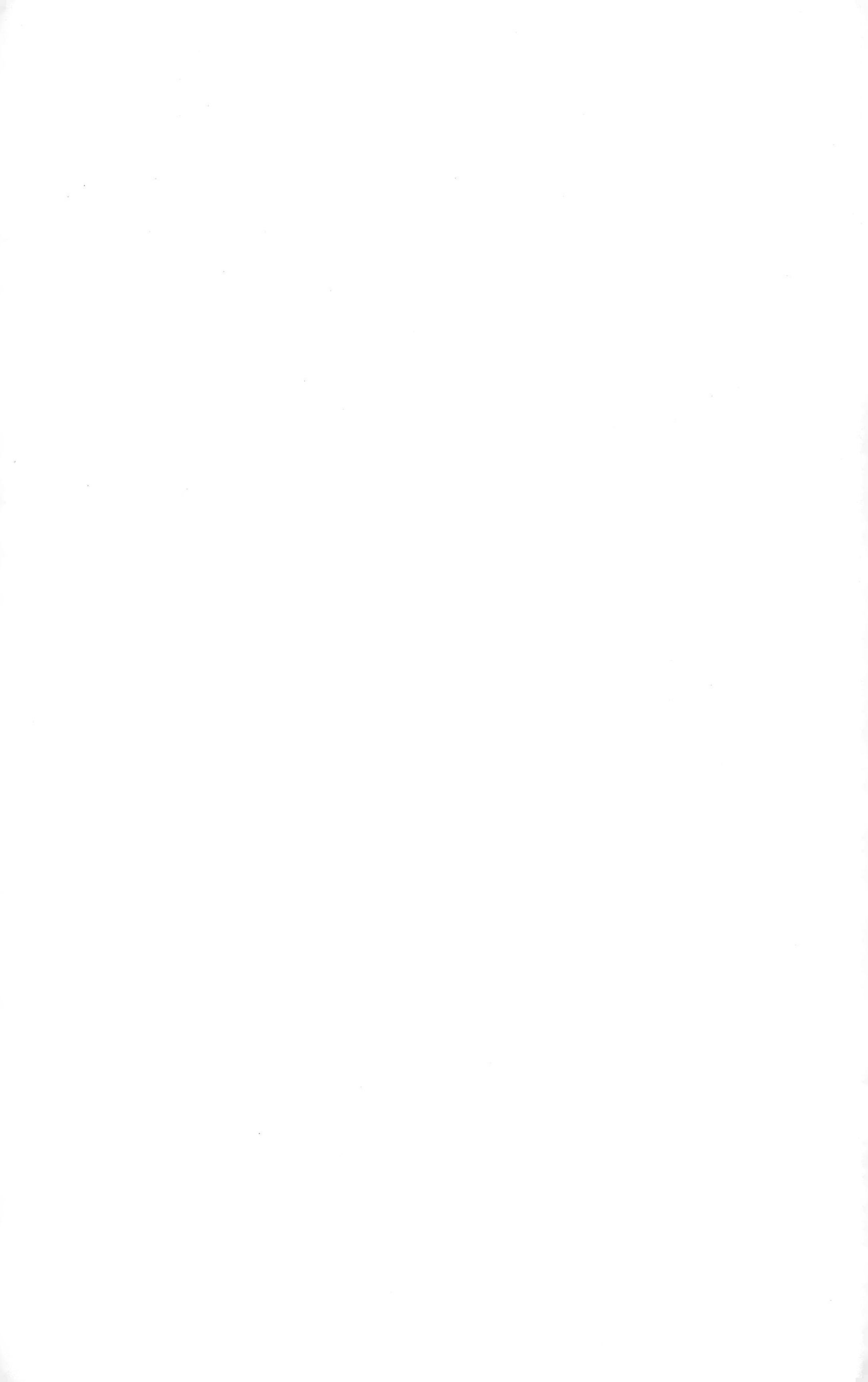